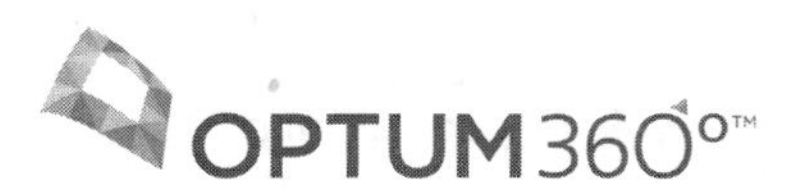

2017

Clinical Documentation Improvement Desk Reference for ICD-10-CM and Procedure Coding

The Clinician's Checklist for ICD-10-CM
Your copy of this manual includes *The Clinician's Checklist for ICD-10-CM*, a trifold card with documentation tips for the most important chronic and acute medical conditions. Use this card to help clinicians understand the documentation needed for accurate ICD-10-CM coding.

Optum360 Notice

Clinical Documentation Improvement Desk Reference for ICD-10-CM and Procedure Coding is designed to be an accurate and authoritative source regarding coding and every reasonable effort has been made to ensure accuracy and completeness of the content. However, Optum360 makes no guarantee, warranty, or representation that this publication is accurate, complete, or without errors. It is understood that Optum360 is not rendering any legal or other professional services or advice in this publication and that Optum360 bears no liability for any results or consequences which may arise from the use of this book.

Optum360
2525 Lake Park Blvd
Salt Lake City, UT 84120

Our Commitment to Accuracy

Optum360 is committed to producing accurate and reliable materials.

To report corrections, please visit www.optum360coding.com/accuracy or email accuracy@optum.com. You can also reach customer service by calling 1.800.464.3649.

American Medical Association Notice

Copyright

Made in the USA
ISBN 978-1-62254-269-7

Acknowledgments

Michael Grambo, *Product Manager*
Karen Schmidt, BSN, *Technical Director*
Stacy Perry, *Manager, Desktop Publishing*
Lisa Singley, *Project Manager*
Deborah C. Hall, *Clinical/Technical Editor*
Leanne Patterson, CPC, *Clinical/Technical Editor*
Tom Darr, *MD*
Tracy Betzler, *Senior Desktop Publishing Specialist*
Hope M. Dunn, *Senior Desktop Publishing Specialist*
Katie Russell, *Desktop Publishing Specialist*
Jean Parkinson, *Editor*

About the Technical Editors

Deborah C. Hall

Ms. Hall is a new product subject matter expert for Optum360. She has more than 35 years of experience in the health care field. Ms. Hall's experience includes 10 years as practice administrator for large multi-specialty medical practices. She has written several multi-specialty newsletters and coding and reimbursement manuals, and served as a health care consultant. She has taught seminars on CPT/HCPCS and ICD-9-CM coding and physician fee schedules.

Leanne Patterson, CPC

Ms. Patterson has more than 10 years of experience in the health care profession. She has an extensive background in professional component coding, with expertise in E/M coding and auditing, and HIPAA compliance. Her experience includes general surgery coding, serving as Director of Compliance, and conducting chart-to-claim audits and physician education. She has been responsible for coding and denial management in large multi-specialty physician practices and most recently served as a practice manager where she supervised implementation of a new EHR system. Ms. Patterson is credentialed by the American Academy of Professional Coders (AAPC) as a Certified Professional Coder (CPC).

Tom Darr, MD

Tom Darr, MD, is the VP of Clinical Solutions for Optum360. Through his clinical expertise and 20 years of business experience related to the revenue cycle, Dr. Darr brings a patient focus to Optum360's technology solutions and services, designed to simplify and improve the patient experience so patients and health care providers can focus their attention on treatment, healing, and care. He is certified by the American Board of Emergency Medicine and is a practicing emergency medicine physician with more than 30 years' experience.

Contents

Section 1: Introduction

Medical record documentation, whether paper or electronic, is one of the cornerstones of our health system today. Only accurate, consistent, and complete documentation can translate into the data and information necessary to ensure clinical quality, substantiate medical necessity, and determine the most appropriate reimbursement. No matter the setting, the health record documentation, as designated by the physician provider, remains the foundation upon which many decisions are based. As a result, efforts to improve the quality of that documentation have been on-going for many years.

Origins of Clinical Documentation Improvement (CDI) Efforts

Providers' focus on clinical documentation has its beginnings in the administration of President Ronald W. Reagan in the early 1980s. Ironically, President Reagan's initial opposition to government intervention in private industry gave way to the heavily regulated payment systems that characterize Medicare today. Following the creation of the Medicare program in the 1960s, Medicare costs increased rapidly. By the late 1970s, it was a "runaway" program that had thwarted all voluntary efforts by hospitals to slow costs.

However, as voluntary restraints proved to be ineffective at controlling the costs of the Medicare program, President Reagan and Congress pragmatically turned to prospective payment. The resulting diagnosis related group (DRG) system pays hospitals on the basis of a patient's medical condition and other factors, including procedures provided. Clinical documentation is a fundamental element in securing appropriate provider payment under the DRG payment system. Under DRGs, poor documentation results in lower payments.

Since its inception, Medicare's DRG payment system has saved the government hundreds of billions of dollars. Due to its success, the Centers for Medicare and Medicaid Services (CMS) has expanded its use of prospective payment systems (PPS) and introduced other payment methodologies to control Medicare program costs. In each instance, provider reimbursement hinges on documentation. CMS's intent to move to "value-based payments" is the latest example. Demonstrating value means showing how a patient's medical condition has improved or has been addressed by specific care, as found in the physician quality reporting system. Communicating a patient's improved condition relies upon clinical documentation.

The Clinician's View of CDI

There has been a long battle between administrative staff and clinicians over clinical documentation. Too often, clinical detail is lacking in clinical documentation, which makes it difficult to code claims and answer auditor's questions. There are two issues that contribute to a misalignment of physician and facility interests:

- Physicians have traditionally been paid based on procedures performed, with the patient diagnosis considered secondary. The procedure was either performed, or not performed. It is a simple matter in the mind of the physician and does not require detailed documentation. Today, however, diagnosis documentation has become more important in order to confirm medical necessity for procedures and to accurately identify the patient's medical condition. Additionally, the lack of detail of the service or procedure performed often leads to a less complex procedure or service being reported on the claim and, therefore, reimbursement is at a lower rate.
- Clinical detail required for billing is not usually an independent clinician's first concern. Extra work or effort from clinicians to help billing does not reward physicians.

Several factors, however, are now working to enhance clinician motivation toward improving documentation, including audits of professional claims by payers, such as Medicare's recovery audit contractors (RAC), and concerted efforts by billing personnel and auditors to gain clinician cooperation with documentation through CDI programs. Both internal and payer auditors find that lack of documentation is the most common reason for claim denials. But in a broader way, clinicians are now more aware of documentation issues as a result of the change from ICD-9 to ICD-10 coding systems and CMS's intention to shift payments in a way that requires more clinical detail for demonstrating value-based care.

Gain Share is Encouraging Documentation Improvement

The health plans participating in CMS's Medicare Advantage program now have nearly a third of all Medicare beneficiaries enrolled, with a significant number of the nation's physicians serving these beneficiaries. Payments to the health plans are made on a capitated, per-member, per-month basis, with rates adjusted by the patient's medical condition. Medicare Advantage plans are allowed to keep the portion of premiums not spent for care, and increasingly, physicians serving these beneficiaries are invited to participate in gain sharing. In these arrangements, physicians receive some part of the health plan revenues. Physicians contribute to health plan revenue largely by providing complete and accurate clinical documentation that earns higher capitated payments for individual patients. Involvement with gain sharing arrangements has elevated some physicians' attention to clinical documentation improvement.

In the physician office/clinic setting, reimbursement has been tied directly to diagnosis codes by substantiating the medical necessity of the service or procedure performed. Additionally, for Medicare Advantage or Part C claims, diagnosis coding can affect reimbursement under the Medicare Hierarchical Condition Category (HCC) regulations. The latest regulatory initiative that increased these efforts was the move from the ICD-9-CM coding system to ICD-10-CM for diagnoses.

Because of the increased number of codes available and their corresponding level of detail, the documentation driving that code assignment must be just as detailed and provide the additional information. Additional regulatory efforts to prevent health care fraud and abuse also require concise, complete, and accurate medical record documentation that supports the procedures or services reported.

Optum360's *Guide to Clinical Validation, Documentation and Coding* is a suggested companion to this desk reference. Visit www.Optum360Coding.com for more details.

Reasons to Implement Clinical Documentation Improvement

Clinical documentation improvement provides a number of benefits and the reasons to implement are far reaching. Some of the reasons to implement a CDI program are the following:

- To identify and clarify any confusing, incomplete, conflicting, or missing information in the physician-documented portion of the health record that is related to diagnoses or procedures
- To foster and enhance communication between members of the CDI team (such as CDI staff and coders) and the medical staff
- To provide education to medical staff members on the increased granularity inherent in ICD-10-CM and how it necessitates more detailed documentation in the medical record
- To provide continuity of care for the patient, between members of the health care team that rely on documentation in the health record for determining ongoing treatment decisions
- To provide a more robust and accurate depiction of patient severity
- To provide education to coding staff members to increase their clinical knowledge, particularly as it relates to the increased specificity in conditions, diseases, procedures, and services
- To support clinical quality initiatives, including those related to outcome scores and pay-for-performance programs
- To provide more robust clinical data to the clinical community to assist in data-driven decisions
- To decrease the provider's compliance risk as it relates to medical necessity and coverage, coding and billing, and other issues related to regulatory compliance
- To provide a defense for regulatory compliance reviews, such as those by RACs, zone program integrity contractors (ZPIC) and Medicaid integrity contractors programs
- To decrease the number of delayed or denied claims due to insufficient documentation

- To promote the goal of the hospital medical record being as complete as possible during an acute care admission
- To ensure appropriate reimbursement for the medically necessary services provided, regardless of the reimbursement mechanism

CDI and ICD-10-CM

It is generally understood that ICD-10-CM has seemingly exponentially more codes than its predecessor, ICD-9-CM. But there are many other attributes of ICD-10-CM that help drive its specificity and ability to "tell the patient's story" in a much more robust way. Examples of these differences appear in the table below:

ICD-9-CM Diagnosis Codes	ICD-10-CM Diagnosis Codes
3–5 characters per code	3–7 characters per code
All codes begin with a number (except V & E codes); remainder of code is numeric	Most begin with alpha character and two numeric, with some exceptions
17 chapters and two supplemental chapters (V codes and E codes)	21 chapters, all considered part of the core classification
Not specific; considerable use of "unspecified" and "other specified" options	Very specific; "unspecified" and "other specified" options available, but in a much more specific framework
Some codes contain only a word or two; the user must refer to the subcategory or category level for the complete code title	All code descriptions are complete and stand alone
No laterality included	Includes laterality
Limited combination codes	Many combination codes for conditions and their associated symptoms and manifestations
Does not support international disease tracking and other initiatives due to no other country using ICD-9	Supports international disease tracking and other initiatives due to other countries' use of ICD-10
No distinction of episode of care or encounter	Episode of care/encounter represented in 7th character (e.g., initial encounter, subsequent encounter, etc.)
Limited or no space for new conditions	Due to alpha-numeric structure, much more room in the classification system

Supporting Documentation for Reporting Procedures and Services

Medical record documentation is also essential for determining the most appropriate CPT® code. The CPT code book contains many code for procedures which, while very similar, have distinct components that differentiate them. This could be something as easily identifiable as the morphology of a lesion, or something more difficult, such as specific instrumentation. The difficulty lies in educating clinicians on the exact information needed for documentation as well as the coder or CDI experts understanding the key terms that identify these components.

Failing to adequately document medical services and procedures can lead to inaccurately reported services, claim delays, claim denials or even, after postpayment review by an insurer, recoupment of payments, or allegations of fraud and abuse.

How to Use This Book

The Optum360 *Clinical Documentation Improvement Desk Reference for ICD-10-CM and Procedure Coding* is designed for use by providers and all others who are involved in the documentation and coding processes in any setting. It is organized in an easy-to-use alphabetic format, focusing on those diagnoses, services, and procedures with significant differences in the type and specificity required for accurate code assignment. This allows greater ease in providing very specific and focused information for physicians in certain specialties who provide documentation.

For example, a pulmonologist may want to review the differences in documentation requirements between ICD-9-CM and ICD-10-CM codes for a condition such as asthma. The chapter related to Diseases of the Respiratory System contains a section for asthma, and at first glance, it is apparent that the code axes, or the major way in which the codes are arranged and classified, have changed. Instead of the "extrinsic" and "intrinsic" categories in ICD-9-CM, the asthma codes in ICD-10-CM fall into the following major categories:

- Mild intermittent asthma
- Mild persistent asthma
- Moderate persistent asthma
- Severe persistent asthma
- Other and unspecified asthma

The second code axis is related to presentation of disease: Is the patient suffering from an acute exacerbation, is status asthmaticus present, or is this a chronic and uncomplicated case? The answers to these questions relate to the fifth-digit subclassification under each of the major categories listed above.

The Clinical Documentation Improvement Desk Reference for ICD-10-CM and Procedure Coding manual provides definitions for each of the major types of asthma, so that the pulmonologist may share the information with the office staff, residents, interns, and any others that may be reviewing the healthrecord documentation. These differentiating factors (mild versus moderate, intermittent versus persistent) should be clearly documented, according to the definitions provided. Obviously, the severity level determination is affected by whether any of the secondary axis items (acute exacerbation, status asthmaticus) are also documented.

In addition to conditions, *The Clinical Documentation Improvement Desk Reference for ICD-10-CM and Procedure Coding* also provides key documentation requirements that differentiate between select procedures. For example, the topic Abortion illustrates the differences between the treatment of different types of abortions and the differences in the documentation requirements for each.

A new feature for the 2017 edition is the Clinician Documentation Checklist. For most entries, diagnosis or procedure, this manual provides a listing of clinical issues that need to be addressed in clinical documentation in order to help coders assign appropriate codes and distinguish a medical condition from similar but different conditions. In the example below for Ulcerative Colitis, the clinician is prompted to identify evidence of the medical condition, and distinguish the manifestation from among the alternatives. Finally, the checklist asks about associated conditions.

Clinician Documentation Checklist

Clinician documentation should indicate the following:

- Identify manifestation such as pyoderma gangrenosum
- Type
  - ulcerative (chronic) pancolitis
    - backwash ileitis
  - ulcerative (chronic) proctitis
  - ulcerative (chronic) rectosigmoiditis
  - inflammatory polyps of colon
  - left sided colitis
    - left hemicolitis
    - other ulcerative colitis
  - unspecified ulcerative colitis
- Associated
  - without complication
  - with complication
    - rectal bleeding
    - intestinal obstruction
    - fistula
    - abscess
    - other complication
    - unspecified complications

Another helpful tool incorporated into *The Clinical Documentation Improvement Desk Reference for ICD-10-CM and Procedure Coding* manual is

"Key Terms." Under each section or condition, alternate terminology is provided that may be found in the medical record documentation. These alternative clinical descriptions ensure that all involved in the documentation and coding processes are clear concerning which conditions or services may have the same meaning and be classified together, and which conditions or services may be slightly different and should be classified elsewhere.

For example, a medical record may be documented with "idiosyncratic asthma," which is found on the list of conditions in the "Key Terms" section related to asthma. This means that the terminology is one of the inclusion conditions found under the J45 Asthma section of ICD-10-CM. Conversely, if "wood asthma" is documented, it is not on this list of conditions. While the list itself is not all-inclusive, the condition should be reviewed more closely; the ICD-10-CM index indicates that the condition wood asthma should be classified to another code under category J67.

The Clinical Documentation Improvement Desk Reference for ICD-10-CM and Procedure Coding manual also provides, where appropriate, clinical tips. For example, the topic Nerve Blocks contains a clinical tip that identifies the components of the somatic nerves and the required documentation elements that should be included when performing nerve blocks on one of these nerves.

Clinical Tip

Somatic nerves are a part of the peripheral nervous system and are associated with the voluntary control of body movements through the skeletal muscles.

Documentation should also include the reason for the nerve block and the response of prior treatment if any.

Although this manual is not considered a coding instructional manual, coding instructional notes that affect documentation are also included. For instance, under the main category for asthma (J45), an instructional note appears:

Use additional code to identify:

exposure to environmental tobacco smoke (Z77.22)
exposure to tobacco smoke in the perinatal period (P96.81)
history of nicotine dependence (Z87.891)
occupational exposure to environmental tobacco smoke (Z57.31)
nicotine dependence (F17.-)
tobacco use (Z72.Ø)

Because clinical researchers have identified links between use or exposure to tobacco smoke and asthma, the instructional note indicates that these conditions should be coded in addition to the code for asthma. References within the Clinical Documentation Improvement Desk Reference for ICD-10-CM and Procedure Coding manual prompt the physician to provide documentation for related conditions such as these, that provide detail and a more complete clinical picture.

The Clinical Documentation Improvement Desk Reference for ICD-10-CM and Procedure Coding manual also provides, in appendix 1, templates and instructions for accurately and compliantly developing physician query documents. The physician query, particularly those that seek to clarify certain conflicting or missing information, is one of the most commonly used tools to improve physician documentation. These queries must be constructed in a correct and nonleading manner in order to be compliant.

Appendix 2 contains the 2017 *ICD-10-CM Official Guidelines for Coding and Reporting*. These guidelines provide useful information regarding the documentation required, as well as reporting guidelines for the ICD-10-CM classification system.

Appendix 3 contains mapping tables for the conditions discussed in this manual. These tables allow the user to determine the ICD-9-CM code that was previously used to report the condition.

The process of clinical documentation improvement should be a collaborative one, involving those who provide the documentation and those who interpret it and translate the verbiage to the most appropriate numeric code. Being proactive in assisting the physician provider with the detailed information that will be necessary under the ICD-10-CM coding system can only enhance that collaboration.

Section 2: Clinical Documentation Improvement Processes—Best Practices

As mentioned earlier, the clinical documentation improvement process should be a collaborative one in order to be successful. The health care setting and whether the clinical conditions treated involve only a few, such as in a specialty clinic, or encompass the entire spectrum of diseases and disorders, such as in a full-service acute care hospital, will determine the scope and breadth of the program. However, there are many attributes that are commonly seen in successful programs of any size. Many physicians have found that participating in a CDI program at their local hospital also improves documentation in the office setting as well.

There are three main components to a successful clinical documentation improvement program: assessment, implementation, and sustainability.

Assessment

The first step in any CDI program must be an assessment. The assessment will identify those areas that are compliant as well as areas where improvement is needed.

There are several steps involved in performing the CDI assessment:

- Develop a CDI team
- Develop a review process
- Identify areas of risk
- Identify the root cause

Staffing

Before an assessment can take place, a clinical documentation improvement team must be established. This team should include members from all groups involved (e.g., clinicians, coders, information technology, etc.). Each team member can provide particular insight into what is needed for his or her particular responsibilities.

Staff members who will work on the CDI program can come from a variety of different backgrounds. Typically they include health information management (HIM) coding professionals, compliance officers, physicians, nursing staff, and other professionals with either a coding or clinical background. Some programs involve a variety of the above-mentioned individuals and job titles are not as important as specific attributes and skills, such as: clinical knowledge of the the individual code sets and the reporting guidelines associated with that code set; understanding health care compliance as it relates to documentation, coding, and billing; and strong written and verbal communication skills. The importance of strong verbal skills cannot be overemphasized; these staff members will be communicating with physicians on a daily basis and must convey

professionalism and significant clinical and coding knowledge. Many successful programs have one or more physician "champions," who act both as advisors to the other staff members in the program and are liaisons with the medical staff providing the documentation.

Physician Advisor or Liaison

Many CDI professionals believe that a major component of a successful program is a strong physician advisor. This major role is to act as a liaison between the CDI staff members, HIM coding, and the medical staff and to facilitate accurate coding and representation of acuity and severity. As a result, the corresponding reimbursement should also be enhanced, regardless of the setting.

Just as importantly, the physician advisor is responsible for communicating with and educating the medical staff in both the general concepts of severity and acuity as they relate to documentation and coding, and in encouraging and recommending specific documentation enhancements. To accomplish these goals, the physician advisor should have knowledge related to physician performance profiling, physician E/M payment and pay for performance, and appropriate documentation for hospital reimbursement and profiling (if working in that setting). Publicly available data tools are available that can be incorporated in the CDI strategy, including the Surgical Care Improvement Project (SCIP) outcomes, risk of mortality (ROM), and severity-of-illness (SOI) data instruments. Helping other physicians become more aware of outcomes data and the documentation and coding effect on them is a very successful way of reaching those most responsible for providing the documentation upon which these data instruments are based.

Physician advisors can also emphasize the continuity of care approach to other physicians on the medical staff. This approach reinforces the fact that what is documented accurately represents not only the patient conditions, but what was done for the patient. Other physicians participating in the care of the patient need to ensure that what they review in the medical record is accurate and complete to provide additional input and/or services. Continuity of care is an essential goal of any CDI program and should be the number one reason that conflicting information in the medical record is addressed quickly and thoroughly via the CDI process.

In addition, the physician advisor should meet on a regular basis with the CDI professionals to review selected medical records, particularly those involving traditionally confusing conditions or those with a somewhat varied set of clinical definitions. Examples of these conditions include those with respiratory failure, acute blood loss anemia, renal insufficiency versus chronic kidney disease, acute kidney injury, and urosepsis. In some cases, internal definitions of these conditions can be formulated through a collaborative process. Taking a proactive stance in handling these cases that can cause confusion on the part of both CDI/coding and the medical staff can alleviate future problems and can significantly decrease the number of physician queries required.

When physician queries are necessary, the physician advisor can provide assistance in several ways. First, the physician advisor can determine whether a query is necessary based on the initial documentation in the medical record. Secondly, he or she can help formulate physician queries that are not leading in nature, but that provide enough clinical information to make the query relevant and compliant. If queries on a particular condition become repetitive over time, the physician advisor can assist in the development of a query template, which makes further questions on the topic easier to initiate and can develop and facilitate provider education.

Another important aspect of the physician advisor role involves providing feedback to medical staff physicians on the effect of their documentation on some of the patient severity and acuity data instruments mentioned above. Providing this last link between the documentation and the resulting movement in acuity or other scores is extremely valuable, can add legitimacy, and reinforce the importance of accurate and complete documentation.

Review Process

After the team has been established, a review process should be developed. The process should be customizable depending on the particular type of review being performed. For example, a review may be to determine the completeness of the clinicians' documentation of conditions, procedures, or services or a review may be performed to determine if other clinicians can determine the patient's medical status based on the documentation in the medical record.

When developing the process, it should also be determined if the process will take place concurrently (while the patient is being treated) or retrospectively (after the patient has received treatment). In most instances, in a physician practice, concurrent review occurs prior to the submission of the claim. It may also occur at the time care is being provided. A clinician reviewer (e.g., another physician or a medical assistant trained to recognize the necessary data points) can review the medical record before the patient leaves the office.

Retrospective review usually occurs once the claim has been processed. Both types of review have benefits and it may be that each would be performed depending on the type of documentation that will be reviewed.

Regardless of the type of review selected, both can result in more detailed, accurate, and complete documentation that improves code assignment and reduces liability risk.

Implementation

Policies and procedures must be implemented for each CDI program, depending upon the size of the program, whether records consist of paper or are electronic, and staffing. The example below is a procedure for a hospital program that uses paper records:

1. After midnight, generate and obtain a hospital census report, which includes admissions. The report should, at a minimum, include the following information:
   - Patient name

- Admission date
- Insurance information
- Attending physician name
- Admitting diagnosis

2. Each CDI staff member reviews each admission to his or her assigned floor or location in the facility. The frequency of reviews depends upon program guidelines and policies, but is typically every one to two days. Some facilities target high potential cases according to admitting diagnosis.
3. CDI staff produces an initial new admission worksheet for all new cases and the worksheet is placed in the specified location in the patient's medical record on the hospital floor. The worksheet should, at a minimum, include the following information:
   - Patient name
   - Medical record or encounter number
   - Admission date
   - Attending physician
   - Principal diagnosis
   - Secondary diagnoses
   - Principal procedure (if applicable)
   - Secondary procedures (if applicable)
4. If no query opportunity is identified, the CDI staff member reviews the case records periodically, according to facility policies. If a query opportunity is identified, the CDI staff member initiates it according to the most appropriate method (i.e., verbal, written, or electronic), detailing its existence, reason, and date on the CDI worksheet.
5. CDI physician queries are followed concurrently. If there is no response to the query within a predetermined amount of time, the physician advisor is contacted to review the current documentation and query. If appropriate, the physician advisor contacts the physician responsible for the missing or conflicting documentation.
6. After patient discharge, the coder assigns codes based on the final documentation in the medical record and any answered queries. Cases with no discrepancies are final billed. Cases with discrepancies are routed to the CDI staff member for an additional review and a physician query may be initiated after this review.
7. All cases are tracked and trended, particularly those with physician queries. The facility has a policy on the retention of queries, whether in the medical record itself or elsewhere.
8. CDI staff members meet monthly (or at other designated intervals) with the physician advisor to discuss trends in the program and any issue related to queries or documentation.
9. Quarterly meetings are scheduled between the CDI team and physician leadership and administration. Metrics and benchmarks for measuring success are reviewed, along with discussions of recently identified successes or potential problems.

Generally speaking, many of the same procedures listed above can be used in a physician practice.

1. The practice runs reports at the beginning of a month to determine possible areas where clinical documentation improvement may be needed. For example, a report may be run to determine the number of "unspecified" or "other specified" codes where assigned or the practice may wish to run a report indicating those claims that were denied because of medical necessity issues.
2. A CDI staff member reviews the reports to determine if there are patterns. For example, a report indicates that 86 percent of Dr. Smith's claims for patients with complete blood counts are performed for unspecified anemia or 62 percent of all flexible sigmoidoscopy claims are unpaid because of medical necessity issues.
3. CDI staff produces an initial CDI review worksheet for all new cases and the worksheet is placed in the specified location in the patient's medical record. The worksheet should, at a minimum, include the following information:
   - Patient name
   - Medical record or encounter number
   - Admission date
   - Attending physician
   - Principal diagnosis
   - Secondary diagnoses
   - Principal procedure (if applicable)
   - Secondary procedures (if applicable)
   - Claim denial codes (if applicable)
4. The medical record is reviewed to determine if further clinical documentation could have resulted in a better understanding of what was performed during the encounter and the reason for the service. If a query opportunity is identified, the CDI staff member initiates it according to the most appropriate method (i.e., verbal, written, or electronic), detailing its existence, reason, and date on the CDI worksheet.
5. CDI physician queries are followed concurrently. If there is no response to the query within a predetermined amount of time, the physician advisor is contacted to review the current documentation and query. If appropriate, the physician advisor contacts the physician responsible for the missing or conflicting documentation.
6. After including any additional information to the medical record that may potentially affect code assignment, the CDI staff member updates the CDI worksheet. **Note:** Care is taken that any additions/addenda to the medical record are made in accordance with standard clinical documentation guidelines.
7. The case is circulated back to the coder who assigns codes based on the final documentation and submits or resubmits the claim as necessary. When a claim is resubmitted, payer guidelines are carefully followed.
8. All cases are tracked and trended, particularly those with physician queries. The practice has a policy on the retention of queries, whether in the medical record itself, or elsewhere.
9. CDI staff members meet monthly (or at other designated intervals) with the physician advisor to discuss trends in the program and any issue related to queries or documentation. It is determined during these

meetings if formal education is necessary and if the education is to be provided to a specific clinician or to the entire clinical staff.

10. Quarterly meetings are scheduled between the CDI team and physician leadership and administration. Metrics and benchmarks for measuring success are reviewed along with discussions of recently identified successes or potential problems.

The Query Process

Because the physician query process is a major component of a CDI program, each facility or practice should have a policy related to query development, format, and management. The policy should specify when to query, how to format the query appropriately, and the retention policy of the query. Some programs rely heavily on one type of query, such as the written query, while others use a combination of approaches, including verbal and electronic methods. Queries may be used to request further specificity or to clarify the severity of a documented condition, to clarify a cause-and-effect relationship, or to present clinical indicators of an undocumented condition.

Appendix 1, "Physician Query Samples" in this manual, provides numerous examples of physician queries.

The following six criteria should be used when reviewing documentation and in determining whether a query is necessary:

Legibility: Poor penmanship, improper use of photocopies, poor document scans, "cut-and-paste" errors, use of templates, or improperly correcting an error in a medical record can cause problems with legibility, omissions, or additions in text that can result in errors of documentation and code assignment: does a condition warrant reporting that is a result of "cut and paste" documentation from a previous encounter problem list which was not addressed on the current encounter?

Consistency: Documentation that is conflicting, inadequate, incomplete, ambiguous, or inconsistent: is the condition exacerbated or is it stable; was the suspected condition ruled out; what is the clinical significance of the abnormal test results; or, does the provider confirm the consultant's diagnosis?

Relationships: Clinical indicators noted without a stated related diagnosis, diagnostic work-up without stated reason, treatment without identified indication or manifestations not linked to an underlying cause: does the notation ↑ Na represent a clinically significant diagnosis; what is the reason for the need of continuous O2; what was the indication and final conclusion for the performance of a glucose test; is the ulcer due to a complication of the underlying diabetes?

Specificity: Clinical results, including pathology reports, response to treatment, and/or the patient's clinical condition suggest a more specific diagnosis or level of severity than is documented: based on culture and sensitivity and patient response to treatment, can the condition be further specified as to a causative organism; can the post-op/final diagnosis be further specified due to the pathology report findings; based on the pathology report findings, which additional sites of metastasis are clinically significant?

Clinical validation: When there is a lack of clinical data or insufficient indicator(s)needed to determine a diagnosis or the necessary level of specificity necessary for reporting the most appropriate ICD-10-CM code, the decision to query a clinician may be required. For example, the PACU note stating "post-op respiratory failure" during the routine post-op intubation period without correlating clinical indicators represent a complication due to surgery, other condition, or an expected outcome immediately postsurgery; is the diagnosis of acute exacerbation supported by clinical findings, adjustment of regimen/treatment or clinical manifestation?

Other issues related to queries include the following:

When not to query: In some instances, physicians must make clinical diagnostic decisions that may not appear to agree with test results or other findings. Queries should not be formulated that question a provider's clinical judgment, but only to clarify documentation when it fails to meet one of the six criteria listed above. To help avoid clinical validation issues, the physician should indicate why a critical clinical indicator is not met for the patient when stating his or her diagnostic statement; for example, pneumonia ruled in based on clinical scenario with negative chest x-ray due to severe dehydration. Also, queries are not necessary for every unaddressed issue or discrepancy in the medical record. Insignificant or irrelevant findings typically do not warrant a query.

Clinical validation escalation policy: All entities and physician practices should have a written policy and procedure that identifies what constitutes the need for a clinical validation query, those who are part of the escalation team, and that outlines their role and the chain of responsibility.

How to notify the physician that a query has been placed in the medical record: Because a variety of members of the health care team has access to and may frequently be reviewing the medical record, it may be a challenge to ensure that the appropriate physician sees the query. Some organizations handle the issue by electronically notifying the physician when a query is placed in the record.

Ensuring that the resulting answer to a query is documented appropriately in the medical record: This issue relates to query retention. Many organizations do not consider the query form itself a part of the medical record. In that case, the physician must document the answer to the query elsewhere in the medical record, typically in the progress notes or discharge summary. The other issue related to the timing of unanswered queries involves how to track the unanswered queries. Each organization should have a policy regarding this process, including how to address a lack of response, and strategies for record completion.

Query timing for resolved conditions: Some physicians may be reluctant to document a condition, particularly an acute condition, if it has resolved by the time of the query. In this instance, it is helpful to provide information regarding patient severity. Regardless of the timing of the treatment, if the patient was treated for the condition, it should be documented and coded for appropriate acuity.

Queries for conditions not documented in the record: Queries must be based on physician documentation within the medical record and the link between the data and the condition must be made in order to support the query. For example, the routine lab test performed after a minor surgery shows slightly below normal H/H levels and the provider simply notes the lab results in a progress note; the patient's pre-op baseline is unknown and there is no mention of a condition in the progress notes nor is there any documentation of the need for monitoring or treatment of a condition. This scenario would not warrant a query: the labs were routine and not specifically ordered to monitor or evaluate for a condition and although the provider noted the results, there was no mention of their clinical significance and in fact there is no indication they were significant as there is no documentation the patient was symptomatic or required treatment.

Verbal queries: This is more commonplace when used in concurrent programs and CDI staff members are interacting with physicians on a real-time basis. These must follow the same format as written queries but in condensed form including the question and its clinical support. Each program should have a policy regarding documentation of verbal queries.

Query documentation: The use of queries on easily removable and discardable notes (such as sticky notes or scratch paper) is disallowed regardless of whether or not the query form becomes a part of the final medical record. Preferred documentation includes the CDI program-approved query template or general query form, secure email electronic form, or approved form on an IT messaging system.

Leading queries: Queries should include clinical indications and information and should ask the physician to make a clinical interpretation of these facts based on professional judgment. Queries that clearly ask the physician to document a specific condition or that illicit a specific response are inappropriate and could lead to allegations of upcoding. Queries should also never indicate that any particular response would impact reimbursement or any other measurable instrument (such as a quality reporting system).

Query formats:

Narrative: Clinical scenario is succinctly noted, followed by clinical data citing document and date, summary of clinical judgment, diagnostic statement, note of decision making including treatment plan, and patient response to therapy. The query must include relevant points and identify the need for further clarification (etiology, specificity, link, severity, clinical validation, etc.). The question must not be worded for a yes or no answer nor should it indicate a specified diagnosis or procedure. Anticipate possible answers and word the query in such a way to include them; this may prompt the need for an additional or follow-up question for an anticipated answer.

Query templates should not be titled with a diagnosis that has not already been documented in the record, as this may be considered leading. If a diagnosis of pneumonia is not already documented in the record then the written query should not be titled "pneumonia." However, if a diagnosis of pneumonia is already documented and the query is to further specify the pneumonia, then the query may be titled "pneumonia" and request further specificity/type.

Multiple choice: Clinical scenario is succinctly noted, followed by clinical data citing document and date, summary of clinical judgment, diagnostic statement, note of decision making including treatment plan and patient response to therapy. The query must include relevant points and identify the need for further clarification (etiology, specificity, link, severity, etc.). The question must not be worded for a yes or no answer. Clinically possible diagnostic choices are presented in a bulleted list along with choices of "other," "undetermined," "clinically insignificant," "integral" or "unspecified." This format allows a new diagnosis as an option, as long as it meets the clinical scenario and data from the record.

Yes/no/other choice: Clinical scenario is succinctly noted, followed by clinical data citing document and date, summary of clinical judgment, diagnostic statement, and, as appropriate, note of decision making including treatment plan and patient response to therapy. The query must include relevant points and identify the need for further clarification after review of pathology, consult, or other report findings. This format involves confirmation of an existing diagnosis from the report either as an additional or a more specified diagnosis or to resolve conflicting documentation. The list of answer choices are yes, no, other, clinically undetermined, integral, or clinically insignificant.

Multiple query questions: Multiple questions may be formulated on one physician query as long as they are distinct and none are leading. For example, in a patient with diabetes mellitus and chronic kidney failure, one query question may involve the type of diabetes (type 1, 2, drug-induced, etc.), one may involve the relationship between the diabetes and the kidney failure, and one may involve the specific renal manifestation.

Post-bill queries: Most queries of this type are a result of an internal or external audit and refer to the fact that the claim has been submitted or the remittance advice or EOB indicates the claim was paid. Most organizations have policies to help determine whether to generate physician queries at this point in time. Issues to consider include payer-specific rebilling time frames and determining the reliability of the query response given the time frame.

Query Program Sustainability

Each CDI program management should establish an auditing and monitoring program related to physician queries. Not only will this policy make queries more consistent across the organization, but it will also identify areas that require additional education and training. Three major questions should be answered after review of any query:

- Was the query necessary?
- Was the language in the query leading or in any way inappropriate?
- Did the query introduce any new diagnostic information that was not previously in the medical record?

Based on the findings from that audit, educational activities can be scheduled to ensure accurate and appropriate queries are formulated in the future.

Additional auditing activities related to queries can take the following forms:

Sampling: At regular intervals, random or targeted sampling should be done for each staff member that is formulating queries. The review should include not only the content of the query but the format as well. This auditing activity will also target areas for further education.

Tracking query response results: The response to a query can have varying effects on code assignments. A tracking form should categorize the various types of results in order to identify query effectiveness. The topic (e.g., sepsis, acute respiratory failure, excisional debridement, etc.) should also be noted to identify and quantify which issues are queried and the frequency.

Individual physician provider tracking: The total number of queries per provider should decrease over time, indicating an improvement in documentation patterns. This is also a success metric for the clinical documentation improvement program. The response time for a physician should also be tracked to identify those who fail to respond or who habitually respond beyond the specified period resulting in billing delays.

High risk, historically problematic, or confusing conditions: It is especially instructive to measure queries for problematic diagnoses before and after educational sessions, to determine educational program success.

CDI Success Metrics

One of the most important aspects of a clinical documentation improvement program is the establishment and performance of a success metrics system. Some of the data elements to consider tracking include the following:

- Risk of mortality (ROM) and severity of illness (SOI)
- Total volume of queries formulated and released per month
- Diagnoses with high volume of queries
- Physicians most often queried
- Proportion of successful versus unsuccessful queries
- Clinical or patient care area which originates highest volume of queries
- Trended elements, including query, condition, physician, CDI staff member, case-mix-index (CMI) data (if hospital-based program)
- Case-mix-index (CMI) movement as a result of the CDI program (for hospital-based programs)
- Documentation habit changes as a result of the CDI program

Most organizations have an internal average measurement of coded data that is tracked over time. In the physician office/clinic setting it may track the hierarchical condition category (HCC) conditions; in the hospital setting it typically involves the case-mix index, which can be tracked in several different ways (e.g., by coder, by physician, by clinical service area, etc.). Any unexpected change in one of these metrics may represent a potential problem with clinical documentation. It is important to be able to isolate the factor causing the metric movement in order to address it appropriately.

Using Technology for Clinical Documentation Improvement

There are a number of electronic solutions that are currently in use in the health care arena today that can and will affect clinical documentation improvement. Although the reasons for a CDI program and the benefits of a program will not change, the use of some of these automated tools can alter the day-to-day activities, scope, roles, and duties for many of the staff members in a CDI program. Several of these tools and their resulting effects and benefits are listed below.

Electronic Health Record

A significant proportion of hospitals and physician practices have transitioned to electronic health records (EHR) and, even if not in a completely paper-free environment, they use a hybrid medical record with a sizable amount of information collected and stored electronically. While this can eliminate issues related to legibility and entirely missing documentation, it may also potentially produce other problems such as overwhelming staff with the sheer amount of required documentation or the tendency to "overcode." Written policies should be in place that address the copy, paste, and clone functions in the EHR. Specific documentation should be provided for each and every patient, and each should consist of "stand-alone" information that does not rely on data from other sources that may not be present at the time of a CDI process or coding.

The EHR can be a useful tool in providing feedback and prompts to physicians for more specific documentation, if structured in a thoughtful and consistent way. The goal is not to overwhelm the providers with too many prompts and requests for further information, but to provide very specific pointers, some in template fashion that will remind the physician that more specificity is required. This will be particularly crucial after the transition to ICD-10-CM. For example, in a pulmonology practice, the EHR template should prompt the physician for more information when "asthma" is documented. In ICD-10-CM there are 18 different codes in category J45 that represent asthma. Code subcategories related to "mild intermittent," "mild persistent," "moderate persistent," and "severe persistent" are available, along with combination code components related to the presence of status asthmaticus or an acute exacerbation. Similarly, a diagnostic statement of "acute respiratory failure" is no longer sufficient. An additional piece of information related to whether coexisting hypoxia or hypercapnia is present is also required. Any CDI program must be integrated with the facility or practice EHR in order to be most efficient and effective.

Computer-assisted Coding

Computer-assisted coding (CAC) is a method of providing coded information for a variety of purposes. Its use has grown exponentially during the last several years as facilities and physicians are asked to do more with less, coupled with a need for increased coding productivity and consistency. CAC uses natural language processing (NLP) technology, which generates structured data from unstructured text. As the health care community implements ICD-10-CM and CPT coding with its greater need for specificity, the CAC tool provides a method for positively affecting both coder productivity and documentation specificity. Some CAC programs are run concurrently, along with the CDI process, in order to address documentation deficiencies immediately, at the point of care.

Most CAC systems are able to "read" input documentation and generate a list of "initial" or working ICD-10-CM, CPT, or HCPCS codes. The coding professional is then required to review the list of codes and determine whether the codes are accurate and complete and ready to be billed. The process changes the role of the coder from one that reads documentation and assigns codes to that of an auditor, which in most cases does not require as much time, thus improving productivity. However, this does require a change in the "thought" process and, therefore, additional instruction and training should be provided to the coder to ensure accuracy and efficiencies. In addition, some CAC systems can review patient documentation in real time and target cases that require CDI review and intervention. In this way, a higher proportion of the total patient population is evaluated, leading to overall consistency throughout the facility or practice.

As technology progresses, it appears that many of the electronic solutions will be integrated and provide more than one function. For example, an EHR and a computer-assisted CDI program, perhaps with CAC, may be integrated and provide several solutions concurrently. While it may be only one automated system, a need will still exist for staffing related to a coding professional, a clinical documentation specialist, a case manager, and a physician liaison; each role is distinct.

CDI Brings Many Improvements

CDI programs have become more essential under ICD-10-CM, as the increased specificity and granularity require a correspondingly higher specificity in the clinical documentation provided in the health record.

The overriding goal of clinical documentation improvement should be to ethically improve the accuracy, completeness, and specificity of clinical documentation through assessment, education, review, communication, clarification, querying, and analysis of clinical documentation patterns. Additionally, all of this must be accomplished without overburdening the clinician, confusing the clinician regarding what does or does not need to be documented as well as avoiding the tendency to "overcode" because of the additional documentation that was previously unclear or unavailable. If successful, improvements will be seen in programs related to care coordination, quality and severity of illness reporting, meaningful use initiatives, pay-for-performance programs, bundled payments of various types, RAC and other fraud and abuse auditing, and code-based reimbursement.

Section 3: Documentation Issues

This section is organized in an easy-to-use alphabetic format according to the condition or procedure addressed.

For ICD-10-CM codes the, focus is on those diagnoses with significant differences in the type and specificity required for accurate code assignment. The code axes are listed, which may include the component subcategories or each code in the section to be discussed. Information related to the entire section of codes appears next, whether related to the ICD-10-CM classification itself or to the CDI process.

The procedures included are those that have documentation issues as well as those for which multiple coding options are available.

Each topic includes clinical definitions that indicate differentiating factors that can affect code assignment. Clinical data such as physical examination findings, laboratory tests commonly ordered, and/or abnormal laboratory findings, ancillary testing results, therapeutic procedures performed, and other significant information that may support reporting the condition are also included. A Clinician Documentation Checklist that displays the clinical factors that the clinician should document is also provided.

In addition to the elements listed above, within each of the topics covered the following components may also appear:

Clinical Tip: Provides the clinical definitions and information that must be documented in order to classify the condition, service, or procedure to this particular code or ICD-10-CM subcategory.

Documentation Tip: Provides information regarding specific elements that are needed in the documentation to differentiate the condition or procedure from other similar conditions or procedures.

CPT Alert: Identifies information that may be found in the documentation that could possibly affect procedure code assignment.

CDI Alert: Contains helpful tips for the CDI professional or other staff member who may be reviewing the physician documentation. Suggestions for ensuring the most appropriate and complete documentation appear here.

I-10 Alert: Provides information that, when found in the clinical documentation, could affect ICD-10-CM code assignment.

Key Terms: Lists synonyms or other clinical terms that may be documented in the medical record that are also classified to the code.

Clinician Note: Shares tips related to documentation for the physician practice setting, which may impact professional component reimbursement and quality initiatives.

CDI ALERT

Contains helpful tips for the CDI professional or other staff member who may be reviewing the physician documentation. Suggestions for ensuring the most appropriate and complete documentation appear here.

⇨ **I-10 ALERT**

Alerts the user to classification concepts unique to this code subcategory or code section along with assignment tips and/or differentiating factors. Instructions for additional coding requirements may also appear here.

Abnormal Auditory Perceptions and Acoustic (Auditory) Nerve Disorders

Code Axes

Other abnormal auditory perceptions	**H93.2**
Auditory recruitment	**H93.21**
Diplacusis	**H93.22**
Hyperacusis	**H93.23**
Temporary auditory threshold shift	**H93.24**
Central auditory processing disorder	**H93.25**
Other abnormal auditory perceptions	**H93.29**
Disorders of acoustic nerve	**H93.3X**

Description of Condition

Abnormal auditory perceptions and acoustic (auditory) nerve disorders

Clinical Tip
In auditory perception disorders, the patient is unable to process auditory sounds or objects, but the function of the auditory nerve is intact. The origin of dysfunction is postulated to occur in the central nervous system, not the ear or auditory nerve, and is not associated with peripheral hearing loss.

In auditory nerve disorder, there is a malfunction or compromise of the acoustic (eighth cranial) nerve which may be associated with or caused by congenital anomaly, tumor, infection or other etiology.

Auditory perception disorder is an umbrella term that encompasses a wide range of disorders, which affect the processing (or translation) of auditory information.

Auditory processing disorder may be acquired by neurological problems including tumor, injury, stroke, neurological disorders, infection, or oxygen deficiency.

Temporary auditory threshold shift is a temporary hearing loss when the sensory structures of the cochlea (inner ear) have been overstimulated or fatigued; often due to exposure to loud noise. The threshold of hearing shifts in which the lowest (softest) decibel level is higher than usual.

Diplacusis is a cochlear dysfunction causing the patient to hear single auditory stimulus as two sounds (e.g., echo), whereas hyperacusis is an acute, though usually nonpainful, hearing sensitivity.

Key Terms

Key terms found in the documentation for auditory processing disorder may include:

Central auditory processing disorder (CAPD)

Congenital auditory imperception

Word deafness

Key terms found in the documentation may include:

Acoustic neuritis

Auditory neuropathy

Auditory or acoustic neuralgia

Eighth cranial nerve disorder

Documentation Tip

Ensure that all related conditions are coded appropriately, particularly if the condition is related to other underlying diseases or disorders (e.g., vascular disease, metabolic disturbances, congenital anomalies, infection, history of trauma).

⇨ I-10 ALERT

ICD-10-CM classifies disorders of the acoustic (auditory) nerve (H93.3X) separately from disorders of auditory perception (H93.2). In auditory perception disorders, the patient is unable to process auditory sounds or objects, but the function of the auditory nerve is intact. In auditory nerve disorder, there is a malfunction or compromise of the auditory (eighth cranial) nerve.

Auditory perception disorder is an umbrella term that encompasses a wide range of disorders, which affect the processing (or translation) of auditory information.

Note: Conditions classified to chapter 8 include laterality (right, left, bilateral) within the code structure. All conditions should specify the affected ear(s).

Disorders of acoustic nerve (H93.3X)

The acoustic nerve or sometimes documented as the eighth cranial nerve or vestibulocochlear nerve controls balance. Documentation will indicate that the patient complains of dizziness or feeling that he, she, or the environment, or both are spinning. Acoustic nerve disorders may also result in facial or head pain as well as tinnitus and hearing loss. Cranial nerve disorders can also cause various kinds of facial or head pain or a feeling of fullness in the ear.

CDI ALERT

When documentation indicates an acoustic neuroma or benign neoplasm of the acoustic nerve, ICD-10-CM code D33.3 is assigned.

Key Terms

Key terms found in the documentation may include:

Acoustic nerve compression

Cochleovestibular nerve compression syndrome

Microvascular compression syndrome

Clinical Findings

Physical Examination

History and review of systems may include:

- Visualization of the inner ear (otoscope)
- Basic hearing test
  - Weber's test
  - Rinne's test
  - free field test (whispering test)

Diagnostic Procedures and Services

- Laboratory
  - complete blood count
  - chemistry blood profile
- Imaging
  - MRI
  - CT
- Other
  - auditory brainstem response testing (ABR)
  - audiometry (hearing test)
  - tilt table test

Therapeutic Procedures and Services

- Microvascular decompression (MVD), if failure of medical (nonsurgical) therapy

Clinician Note

Documentation should list all symptoms including any circumstances that exacerbate the condition. Results of the physical examination, including normal findings should be recorded. Testing results should be included and any final diagnosis, including other conditions such as an acoustic neuroma, Meniere's disease or labyrinthitis, which are coded to other ICD-10-CM codes, should be identified.

Clinician Documentation Checklist

Clinician documentation should indicate the following:

- Symptoms
- Hearing loss
  - conversational hearing
  - percentage hearing loss
  - unilateral or bilateral
- Paroxysmal positional vertigo, if present
  - vestibulo-ocular reflex (Dix-Hallpike test)
- Procedures performed
  - MRI
  - CT
  - laboratory studies
  - auditory brainstem response testing (ABR)
  - audiometry (hearing test)
  - tilt table test
- Treatment
  - Medical intervention including medications prescribed
  - Neurology consult

Clinician Note

Specify the type of abnormal auditory perception. Differentiate between auditory recruitment, diplacusis, hyperacusis, auditory threshold shift, and auditory processing disorders.

Document whether these conditions exist in combination with other systemic disease or auditory disorder. Specify any contributory history of trauma, infection or other related condition or status (e.g., congenital anomaly, family history).

Document the laterality of the affected site (i.e., left, right, bilateral).

CDI ALERT

Documentation must include the type of abnormal auditory perception to avoid reporting nonspecific diagnoses. The provider should qualify the disorder as:

- Auditory recruitment
- Diplacusis
- Hyperacusis
- Temporary auditory threshold shift
- Central auditory processing disorder
- Other (specify)

Documentation of laterality (right, left, bilateral) of affected ear or nerve should be thorough and specific to avoid reporting unspecified codes.

Abortion

Code Axes

Procedure	Codes
Surgical treatment of incomplete abortion	**59812**
Surgical treatment of missed abortion	**59820–59821**
Surgical treatment of septic abortion	**59830**
Induced abortion	**59840–59857**

Description of Procedure

An abortion is the expulsion or extraction of the products of conception. Carefully review the medical record documentation to determine if the abortion is spontaneous, induced, complete, incomplete or induced as well as what type of surgical intervention was required.

Treatment of incomplete abortion, any trimester, completed surgically (59812)

An incomplete abortion occurs when some but not all of the products of conception are expelled. This code is most commonly used when reporting the surgical treatment after a woman spontaneously aborts part of the products of conception. Usually, the treatment requires dilation and curettage but, depending upon the gestation age, it may be necessary to perform dilation and vacuum extraction.

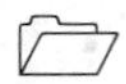

CPT ALERT

This code should not be reported when documentation indicates that the dilation and curettage or evacuation was performed to terminate a viable pregnancy. In these instances, see codes 59840–59841, 59851, 59856.

Key Terms

Key terms found in the documentation may include:

- Ab with retained products of conception with D&C
- D&C for retained products of conception
- Miscarriage with D&C
- Partial ab with D&C
- Partial ab with D&E

CDI ALERT

When documentation indicates that there was early fetal death, but the products of conception were retained, it is inappropriate to report 59812 for this procedure. In these instances, the service is considered the treatment of a missed abortion.

Clinician Note

Documentation should include the gestational age of the fetus as well as the specific type of surgical intervention required (dilation and curettage or dilation and evacuation) and any complicating factors such as infection or excessive bleeding.

Treatment of missed abortion, completed surgically, first trimester (59820)

Treatment of missed abortion, completed surgically, second trimester (59821)

A missed abortion is the death of the fetus before the completion of 22 weeks; however, the products of conception are retained and must be surgically extracted. In missed abortion, the fetus remains in the uterus four to eight weeks following its death. Code 59820 describes the treatment of a missed abortion in the first trimester and is usually accomplished by suction curettage. Code 59821 is used to report the surgical treatment of a missed abortion during the second trimester and may include dilation and vacuum extraction. Documentation will indicate that the provider dilated the cervical canal and then inserted a cannula into the uterus after which time the uterine contents are evacuated by rotation of the cannula. After suction curettage, a sharp curette may be used to gently scrape the uterus to ensure that the uterus is empty.

Key Terms

Key terms found in the documentation may include:

D&C for missed ab

Treatment missed miscarriage

Treatment of missed ab

Clinician Note

Because appropriate code selection is dependent upon the gestation age of the fetus, it is imperative that the gestation age be recorded.

Clinical Tip

Ultrasonography may be needed to determine the size of the fetus to determine the type of procedures required prior to the procedure and is reported separately.

CDI ALERT

Gestational age is often recorded by the number of weeks gestation completed. The chart below can be used to convert the gestation age to the trimester.

Weeks Completed	Trimester
1–13	First
14–27	Second
28–42	Third

Treatment of septic abortion, completed surgically (59830)

A septic abortion is one complicated by generalized fever and infection. Documentation will also indicate inflammation and infection of the endometrium and in the cellular tissue around the uterus. The infection is treated with intravenous antibiotics and blood transfusions as necessary and, when treated surgically, will indicate that the provider performed a dilation and curettage or vacuum extraction of the products of conception.

Key Terms

Key terms found in the documentation may include:

D&C for septic abortion

Septic abortion treated surgically

Clinician Note

When known, the specific infectious agent should be recorded in the medical record documentation.

Induced abortion, by dilation and curettage (59840)

Induced abortion, by dilation and evacuation (59841)

Induced abortion, by 1 or more intra-amniotic injections (59850–59852)

Induced abortion, by 1 or more vaginal suppositories (59855–59857)

Code 59840 is used to report the termination by dilation and curettage (D&C). Code 59841 describes the termination by dilation and evacuation (D&E). Because D&E requires wider cervical dilation than curettage, the physician may dilate the cervix with a laminaria several hours to several days before the procedure. For pregnancies through 16 weeks, the cannula will usually evacuate the pregnancy. For later pregnancies, the cannula is used to drain amniotic fluid and to draw tissue into the lower uterus for extraction by forceps. In either case, a sharp curette may be used to gently scrape the uterus to ensure that it is empty. These types of induced abortions are commonly performed for the legal termination of the pregnancy.

Examination of the documentation may also indicate that the termination of a pregnancy was performed by inducing labor with amniocentesis and intra-amniotic injections (59850–59852). This method is usually used after the first trimester (13 weeks or more). Documentation will indicate that the physician inserts an amniocentesis needle into the abdomen to obtain a free flow of clear amniotic fluid. A hypertonic solution is then administered by gravity drip. The hypertonic solution results in fetal death and labor usually results. Code 59851 is used when this method fails to expel all products of conception, and documentation supporting the assignment of this code includes indications that a dilation and curettage and/or evacuation were used to remove the remaining tissue. Code 59852 is used when documentation indicates that an incision in the abdominal wall and uterus was made in order to remove the remaining tissue.

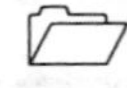

CPT Alert

When medical record documentation indicates that the abortive service was performed to reduce the number of fetuses, otherwise known as multifetal pregnancy reduction or MPR, see CPT code 59866.

Termination can also be by means of vaginal suppositories. In this method labor is induced with vaginal suppositories. Before using the suppositories, documentation may indicate that a laminaria, which is an applicator made of kelp or synthetic material, was inserted in the cervix to soften and expand the cervical canal. Once the cervix is ready, the physician inserts the vaginal suppositories and labor usually results. The fetus and placenta are delivered through the vagina (59855). Code 59856 is used when this method fails to expel all products of conception, and a dilation and curettage and/or evacuation is used to remove the remaining tissue. Code 59857 is used when this method fails to expel all products of conception, and a hysterotomy, through an incision in the abdominal wall and uterus, is used to remove the remaining tissue.

Key Terms

Key terms found in the documentation may include:

Induced abortion

Legal abortion

Termination of pregnancy

Clinical Findings

Physical Examination

History and review of systems may include:

- Review of GU and GI symptoms including vaginal bleeding and urinary tract infection.
- Determine if vaginal bleeding is present for an inevitable, incomplete, or complete abortion.
- Determine if dilation is present in cervical os. Cervical os may be closed in spontaneous, threatened, inevitable, incomplete, or missed abortion.
- Determine if fever, chills, constant abdominal or pelvic pain and/or purulent vaginal discharge is present in septic abortion. Cervical os is opened in septic abortion.
- Palpate abdomen for tenderness, rebound, rigidity, and guarding.
- Perform fetal Doppler for fetal heart sounds.

Diagnostic Procedures and Services

- Laboratory studies
  - β-hCG

Gestation weeks	Whole HCG units
<1	5–50
2	50–500
3	100–10,000
4	1,000–30,000
5	3,500–115,000
6–8	12,000–270,000
12	15,000–270,000

Note: HCG units may indicate a dropping level when the pregnancy is no longer viable.

  - CBC
  - blood type with Rh typing
- Imaging
  - ultrasound for fetal viability in cases of suspected inevitable, incomplete, or complete abortion

Therapeutic Procedures and Services

- Surgical intervention including dilation and curettage, dilation and evacuation or intra-amniotic injections

Clinician Documentation Checklist

Clinician documentation should indicate the following:

- Type of abortion
  - spontaneous
  - induced
  - complete
  - incomplete
- Surgical intervention
  - D&C
  - D&E
- Gestation age of fetus (weeks)
- Septic abortion

Acute Myocardial Infarction (AMI)

Code Axes

ST elevation (STEMI) myocardial infarction of anterior wall	**I21.Ø1, I21.Ø2, I21.Ø9**
ST elevation (STEMI) myocardial infarction of inferior wall	**I21.11, I21.19**
ST elevation (STEMI) myocardial infarction of other and unspecified sites	**I21.21, I21.29, I21.3**
Non-ST elevation (NSTEMI) myocardial infarction	**I21.4**
Subsequent ST elevation (STEMI) myocardial infarction of anterior/inferior walls	**I22.Ø, I22.1**
Subsequent non-ST elevation (NSTEMI) myocardial infarction	**I22.2**
Subsequent ST elevation (STEMI) myocardial infarction of other/unspecified site	**I22.8, I22.9**
Old myocardial infarction	**I25.2**
Intraoperative acute myocardial infarction, during cardiac surgery	**I97.79Ø**
Intraoperative acute myocardial infarction, during other surgery	**I97.791**
Postprocedural acute myocardial infarction, following cardiac surgery	**I97.19Ø**
Postprocedural acute myocardial infarction, following other surgery	**I97.191**

Description of Condition

ST elevation (STEMI) myocardial infarction (I21.Ø-, I21.1-, I21.2-, I21.3)

An ST elevation myocardial infarction (STEMI) involves electrocardiogram (ECG) evidence of the ST-segment elevation, meaning that there is active and ongoing transmural myocardial damage due to the coronary artery being totally blocked. Patients with STEMI can develop Q-waves, which indicate an area of dead myocardium and irreversible damage. STEMI AMIs reflect a higher severity level than non-STEMI AMIs.

Clinical Tip

AMIs may affect the anterior wall, which includes the following:

- Left main coronary artery
- Left anterior descending coronary artery
- Diagonal coronary artery

⇨ I-10 ALERT

The ICD-10-CM definition of initial acute myocardial infarction (category I21) is that with a stated duration of four weeks (28 days) or less from onset. A subsequent AMI is defined as one occurring within four weeks (28 days) of a previous AMI. If a patient is still receiving treatment for the myocardial infarction after the four week time frame, an appropriate aftercare code should be reported.

- Anteroapical, anterolateral, or anteroseptal AMIs

The inferior wall AMIs include the following:

- Right coronary artery
- Inferolateral AMI

Other areas where AMIs may occur include:

- Left circumflex coronary artery
- Apical-lateral, basal-lateral, high lateral, posterobasal, posterolateral, posteroseptal

Key Terms
Key terms found in the documentation may include:

AMI with ST elevation
Coronary artery embolism, occlusion, rupture, or thrombosis
Infarction of heart, myocardium, or ventricle
ST AMI
Transmural Q-wave infarction

Clinician Note
Clinician documentation should also include information indicating tPA status and tobacco exposure, use, or dependence since these should be coded additionally. Similarly, when the body mass index (BMI) is documented, the appropriate code should be reported additionally.

CDI ALERT

If a STEMI AMI converts to an NSTEMI due to thrombolytic therapy, it is still classified as a STEMI, due to the higher severity level of the STEMI and the fact that the patient was treated for the condition. If an NSTEMI evolves into a STEMI, then it is classified as a STEMI AMI. Review documentation carefully if both STEMI and NSTEMI appear in the medical record.

Non-ST elevation (NSTEMI) myocardial infarction (I21.4)

A non-STEMI acute myocardial infarction results from a partially blocked coronary artery and is diagnosed on ECG, which indicates no ST-elevation. In a non-STEMI AMI there is less permanent damage to the myocardium. The non-STEMI is also known as a non-transmural AMI because the damage does not involve the entire thickness of the ventricular wall.

Key Terms
Key terms found in the documentation may include:

Acute subendocardial myocardial infarction
Coronary artery embolism, occlusion, rupture, or thrombosis
Non-Q wave myocardial infarction
Nontransmural myocardial infarction

CDI ALERT

Review documentation carefully for AMI cases, particularly as it involves timeframes and patients who have been readmitted. An acute MI is defined in ICD-10-CM terms as that occurring within the last 28 days. The definition of "subsequent" has changed between ICD-9-CM and ICD-10-CM, making clear and accurate documentation much more important. In ICD-10-CM terms, a "subsequent" AMI is defined as an additional AMI that has occurred within 28 days of another previous AMI. Documentation should also be reviewed carefully to ensure that there is no confusion between a non-STEMI AMI and acute coronary syndrome, with symptoms of unstable angina. If an acute MI is more than 28 days old, it should be classified as an old myocardial infarction (I25.2).

Subsequent ST elevation (STEMI) and non-ST elevation myocardial infarction (I22.Ø–I22.9)

The definitions related to STEMI versus NSTEMI and locations of AMI for subsequent AMIs are the same as those for initial AMIs. The differentiating factor involves the timing of the AMI, and whether multiple AMIs have occurred.

Documentation Tip

Heart auscultation for timing and ST heart sound and second heart sound: documentation indicates a click or snap for valve murmurs and gallops or rubs.

Documentation indicating possible myocardial infarction include tachycardia, bradycardia, tachypnea, hypotension, shortness of breath, asymmetric breath sounds or pulses, new heart murmurs and pulses paradoxus.

Clinical Findings

Physical Examination

History and review of systems may include:

- Other cardiac conditions
  - myocardial ischemia
  - unstable angina
  - myocardial infarctions
  - coronary artery bypass graft
- Past medical conditions
  - hypertension
  - diabetes
  - risk of bleed
  - other
- Patient's complaints
  - chest discomfort
  - other associated symptoms
- Heart rate and blood pressure
- A brief, focused and limited neurological examination to determine cognitive deficits
- An inspection of the neck for venous distention and hepatojugular reflux
- An examination of lungs for presence of symmetry of breath sounds and signs of congestion such as dry or wet rales, pleural friction rubs or decreased breath sounds
- Examination of lower extremity to determine presence or absence of edema and arterial pulses.

Diagnostic Procedures and Services

- Laboratory
  - CBC

    - cardiac biomarkers/enzymes
    - myoglobin levels
    - chemistry panel
    - creatinine kinase MB
    - cardiac troponins (cTnI, cTnT, troponin C, troponin I troponin T)

Note: Increased cardiac enzymes support myocardial infarction.

- Imaging
    - cardiac MRI
    - echocardiography
- Other
    - EKG/ECG
        - findings that support a STEMI diagnosis:
            - new ST elevation at the J point in two contiguous leads of >0.1 mV in all leads other than leads V2–V3
            - for leads V2–V3, the following cut points apply: ≥0.2 mV in men ≥40 years, ≥0.25 mV in men <40 years, or ≥0.15 mV in women
            - the presence of reciprocal ST depression helps confirm the diagnosis
            - no Q-wave EKG findings support a non-STEMI diagnosis

Clinician Note

When ischemic dilated cardiomyopathy (IDCM) is documented prior to the MI, the medical necessity of an implantable cardioverter-defibrillator is supported.

Intraoperative acute myocardial infarction, during cardiac or other surgery (I97.79Ø, I97.791)

Postprocedural acute myocardial infarction, following cardiac or other surgery (I97.19Ø, I97.191)

Patients at increased risk of intraoperative or postprocedural acute myocardial infarction include those with a diagnosis of decompensated congestive heart failure, severe cardiac valvular diseases, significant arrhythmias, and unstable or severe angina. The vast majority of these cases develops by postoperative day two and can significantly affect clinical progress.

Clinician Note

If the cause-and-effect relationship between the medical intervention and the acute MI is not clearly documented in the medical record, however the relationship is suspected, the Clinician should be queried for additional information clarifying the relationship if present.

Other ischemic heart diseases: angina pectoris (I2Ø.-)

Some patients may experience acute ischemic cardiac conditions without progression to acute myocardial infarction. Documentation should be reviewed in order to appropriately classify these patients and ensure consistency. Documentation for angina must be specific; there are four ICD-10-CM codes for the condition, ranging from unstable angina to angina pectoris with documented spasm, to other and unspecified forms of the disease.

> ⇨ **I-10 ALERT**
>
> Work-up is the same as for myocardial infarction; however, EKG findings are negative and chest discomfort subsides with rest and medications.

Documentation Tip

Documentation for the cardiac work-up is the same as for myocardial infarction; however, EKG findings are negative and chest discomfort subsides with rest and medications.

Key Terms

Key terms found in the documentation for angina may include:

Accelerated or crescendo angina
Angina equivalent
Angiospastic or Prinzmetal angina
Cardiac angina
Coronary slow flow syndrome
De novo effort angina
Intermediate coronary syndrome
Ischemic chest pain
Preinfarction syndrome
Spasm-induced or variant angina

> ⇨ **I-10 ALERT**
>
> For codes in the angina category, only two codes (I2Ø.Ø and I2Ø.1), representing unstable angina and angina pectoris with documented spasm, are designated as CC (complication/comorbidity) conditions. Ensure that documentation is clear to support these codes.

Clinician Note

Documentation should include information regarding use, exposure to, history of, or dependence to tobacco products. Additionally, documentation should be reviewed to determine if the coronary atherosclerosis is due to lipid rich plaque. Look for terms such as fibrous atherosclerosis or coronary plaque.

Other acute ischemic heart diseases (I24.-)

Patients may experience acute ischemic conditions that do not progress to acute myocardial infarction; it is essential that documentation be clear and accurate, particularly in cases in which the patient had a coronary embolism, occlusion, or thromboembolism not related to AMI.

Dressler's syndrome, or postmyocardial infarction syndrome, involves a persistent low-grade fever, pleuritic chest pain, a pericardial friction rub, and/or a pericardial effusion. Most patients develop the condition three to six weeks following an acute MI. It is usually a self-limiting condition and is thought to be due to an autoimmune response.

Key Terms

Key terms found in the documentation for Dressler's syndrome may include:

Postcardiac injury syndrome

Postmyocardial infarction syndrome

Postpericardiotomy syndrome

Clinician Note

When documentation contains terms such as acute coronary embolism, occlusion, or thromboembolism but does not mention myocardial infarction, a code from category I24 may be supported.

Clinician Documentation Checklist

Clinician documentation should indicate the following:

- Episode of care
  - initial: initial infarction
  - subsequent: the second MI within the acute phase
- Time frame for acute phase of myocardial infarction (MI) is four weeks (a change from the eight weeks in ICD-9-CM)
- Document the site of the myocardial infarction
  - anterolateral
  - posterior
  - anterior wall
  - inferior wall
- Document the type of MI
  - non-STEMI
  - STEMI
- Document the involved vessel
  - left anterior descending
  - left main
  - right coronary artery
  - left circumflex
  - other coronary artery
    - if non-STEMI evolves into a STEMI, document STEMI only
    - if STEMI converts to non-STEMI due to thrombolytic therapy, document STEMI
- Sequencing of initial and subsequent MI
  - Depends on the circumstances of admission
  - If patient is admitted for AMI and has subsequent AMI during hospitalization, the first MI is sequenced first with the subsequent MI sequenced second
  - If patient is discharged following treatment for an initial AMI, then has subsequent AMI that requires readmission within the four-week acute phase of the initial AMI, the subsequent AMI is sequenced first followed by the initial AMI

- Types of subsequent MI
  - transmural MI of anterior wall
  - transmural (Q wave) MI of anterior wall NOS
  - anteroapical transmural (Q wave)
  - anterolateral transmural (Q wave)
  - anteroseptal transmural (Q wave)
  - transmural infarction (Q wave) diaphragmatic wall
  - transmural infarction (Q wave) inferior wall
  - inferolateral transmural (Q wave)
  - inferoposterior transmural (Q wave)
  - subendocardial MI
  - non-Q wave
  - nontransmural
  - apical-lateral transmural
  - basal-lateral transmural
  - high lateral transmural
  - transmural lateral wall NOS
  - posterior true transmural
  - posterobasal transmural
  - posterolateral transmural
  - posteroseptal transmural
  - septal NOS transmural
  - subsequent acute MI of unspecified site
  - subsequent MI (acute) NOS
- Complications of MI
  - hemopericardium
  - atrial septal defect
  - ventricular septal defect
  - rupture of cardiac wall
  - rupture of chordae tendineae
  - rupture of papillary muscle
  - thrombosis:
    - atrium
    - auricular appendage
    - ventricle
  - sequencing of myocardial infarction and complications is dependent on when the MI and complications occurred
- Old myocardial infarction should be documented, if applicable
- Use of TPA should be documented
  - previous facility
  - current facility

Alcohol Abuse

Code Axes

Alcohol abuse, uncomplicated	**F1Ø.1Ø**
Alcohol abuse with intoxication, uncomplicated	**F1Ø.12Ø**
Alcohol abuse with intoxication, delirium	**F1Ø.121**
Alcohol abuse with intoxication, unspecified	**F1Ø.129**
Alcohol abuse with alcohol-induced mood disorder	**F1Ø.14**
Alcohol abuse, with alcohol-induced psychotic disorder with delusions	**F1Ø.15Ø**
Alcohol abuse with alcohol-induced psychotic disorder with hallucinations	**F1Ø.151**
Alcohol abuse with alcohol-induced psychotic disorder, unspecified	**F1Ø.159**
Alcohol abuse with other alcohol-induced disorders, anxiety disorder	**F1Ø.18Ø**
Alcohol abuse with alcohol-induced sexual dysfunction	**F1Ø.181**
Alcohol abuse with alcohol-induced sleep disorder	**F1Ø.182**
Alcohol abuse with other alcohol-induced disorder To use this code, the other alcohol-related disorder must be specified and not found in any other subcategory.	**F1Ø.188**
Alcohol abuse with unspecified alcohol-induced disorder	**F1Ø.19**

⇨ I-10 ALERT

Report blood alcohol level (BAC), when available and clinically relevant.

Description of Condition

Alcohol abuse (F1Ø.1-)

Alcohol abuse is characterized by recurring misuse of alcohol in excess with identifiable harmful and dysfunctional behaviors and negative consequences for health, psychosocial state, and employment. It lacks the criteria of dependency. Time frame for consideration of abuse would be persisting for at least one month or has occurred repeatedly within a 12-month period.

Key Terms

Key terms found in the documentation may include:

Alcohol abuse

Dipsomania (without documentation of addiction)

ETHO abuse

Clinician Note

The provider must state the pattern of harmful usage (dependence, abuse or use) and its current clinical state (uncomplicated, intoxication, remission, etc.) and indicate the relationship to any identified mental, behavioral, or physical disorder or its relevance to the patient's status or encounter including its clinical significance.

First Listed Diagnosis Note

Admit for acute alcohol intoxication with alcohol abuse: The appropriate code from category F1Ø.1- will be the first listed diagnosis, followed by all reported alcohol-induced complications and comorbidities.

Admit for toxicity due to alcohol abuse and cocaine use with aspiration pneumonia: The appropriate code from the Table of Drugs and Chemicals for poisoning will be the first listed diagnosis (either alcohol (absolute, beverage) or cocaine), followed by all documented manifestations, complications, and comorbidities.

Admit for encephalopathy due to alcohol abuse: The appropriate code from the Table of Drugs and Chemicals for poisoning will be the first listed diagnosis (alcohol, absolute, beverage), followed by the code for alcohol abuse with other alcohol-related disorder, then toxic encephalopathy. Follow with all documented manifestations, complications, and comorbidities.

Clinical Findings

Physical Examination

Patient's history may indicate that there are findings of a failure to fulfill obligations, drinking in physically hazardous situations (such as driving or boating), legal issues arising from alcohol use or that there are social and/or interpersonal problems without the evidence of dependence.

Physical examination may indicate health issues such as:

- cardiac arrhythmia
- dyspepsia
- liver disease
- depression
- anxiety
- insomnia
- trauma related to alcohol use

The following screening questions may be asked when determining the level of alcohol-related problems:

- On any single occasion during the past three months have you had greater than five drinks containing alcohol?
- On a typical day when you drink, how many drinks do you have?
- What is the maximum number of drinks you had on any given day in the past month?

Clinician Documentation Checklist

Clinician documentation should indicate the following:

- Name of substance
  - alcohol
    - identify blood alcohol level
  - polysubstance
- Level of substance use
  - use
  - abuse
  - dependence
- Any additional description of use
  - intoxication
  - remission
  - withdrawal
- Associated psychoactive-induced disorders
  - anxiety
  - delirium
  - delusions
  - hallucinations
  - mood disorder
  - perception disturbance
  - persisting amnestic disorder
  - persisting dementia
  - psychotic disorder
  - sexual dysfunction
  - sleep disorder

Alcohol Dependence

Code Axes

Alcohol dependence, uncomplicated	**F1Ø.2Ø**
Alcohol dependence, in remission	**F1Ø.21**
Alcohol dependence with intoxication, uncomplicated	**F1Ø.22Ø**
Alcohol dependence with intoxication delirium	**F1Ø.221**
Alcohol dependence with intoxication, unspecified	**F1Ø.229**
Alcohol dependence with withdrawal, uncomplicated	**F1Ø.23Ø**
Alcohol dependence with withdrawal delirium	**F1Ø.231**
Alcohol dependence with withdrawal with perceptual disturbance	**F1Ø.232**
Alcohol dependence with withdrawal, unspecified	**F1Ø.239**
Alcohol dependence with alcohol-induced mood disorder	**F1Ø.24**
Alcohol dependence with alcohol-induced psychotic disorder with delusions	**F1Ø.25Ø**
Alcohol dependence with alcohol-induced psychotic disorder with hallucinations	**F1Ø.251**
Alcohol dependence with alcohol-induced psychotic disorder, unspecified	**F1Ø.259**
Alcohol dependence with alcohol-induced persisting amnestic disorder	**F1Ø.26**
Alcohol dependence with alcohol-induced persisting dementia	**F1Ø.27**
Alcohol dependence with other alcohol-induced disorders, anxiety	**F1Ø.28Ø**
Alcohol dependence with other alcohol-induced disorders, sexual dysfunction	**F1Ø.281**
Alcohol dependence with other alcohol-induced disorders, sleep disorder	**F1Ø.282**
Alcohol dependence with other alcohol-related disorder To use this code, the other alcohol-related disorder must be specified and not found in any other subcategory.	**F1Ø.288**
Alcohol dependence with unspecified alcohol-induced disorder	**F1Ø.29**

Description of Condition

Alcohol dependence (F1Ø.2-)

Alcohol dependence (i.e., alcoholism) is a chronic disorder characterized by large or frequent consumption of ethanol in which the individual becomes physically and mentally dependent upon to function. Long-term consequences are physical, psychological, and behavioral, some of which are liver disease, undernutrition with electrolyte disorders and vitamin deficiencies, coagulopathy, depression, dementia, psychosis, heart disease, and violent behavior. Criterion denoting dependence is increased tolerance and continued use despite impairment of health, social life, and job performance. Cessation results in withdrawal symptoms, including early seizures.

Key Terms

Key terms found in the documentation may include:

- Alcohol addiction
- Alcohol dependence
- Chronic alcoholism

Clinical Note

Beer potomania is severe hyponatremia accompanied by mental status changes occurring as a rare syndrome associated with binge beer ingestion and inadequate dietary intake.

Clinician Note

The provider must state the pattern of harmful usage (dependence, abuse, or use) and its current clinical state (uncomplicated, intoxication, remission, etc.) and indicate the relationship to any identified mental, behavioral, or physical disorder or its relevance to the patient's status or encounter including its clinical significance.

Documentation Tip

Detoxification treatment should be documented in orders and in the progress notes, including the drugs or substances used and their administration. Medication administration records completed by nursing staff should include date, start and end time, route, and substance.

First Listed Diagnosis Note

Admit for detoxification or rehab: The appropriate code from category F1Ø.2- will be the first listed diagnosis, followed by all reported alcohol-induced complications and comorbidities.

Admit for acute alcohol intoxication in alcoholism: The appropriate code from category F1Ø.2- will be the first listed diagnosis, followed by all reported alcohol-induced complications and comorbidities. Document and report any associated alcohol and drug dependence, abuse or use. Include the reason for the type of service-complexity (observation, outpatient, inpatient).

I-10 ALERT

Report the blood alcohol level (BAC), when available and clinically relevant.

I-10 ALERT

Delirium tremens (DTs) is reported in subcategories of F1Ø that identify "delirium."

CDI ALERT

Alcohol taken in conjunction with other drugs, prescribed or nonprescribed, that results in toxicity or other reaction as a consequence of the interaction between the alcohol and drug is classified as a poisoning. All manifestations (coma, seizure, respiratory failure, etc.) should be documented. If aspiration occurs, it should be specified as to the site of the aspiration (esophagus, trachea, bronchus, lung, etc.) and its clinical significance.

I-10 ALERT

Personal history of alcohol dependence is reported as alcohol dependence in remission.

Admit for toxicity due to alcohol and cocaine use with aspiration pneumonia: The appropriate code from the Table of Drugs and Chemicals for poisoning will be the first listed diagnosis (either alcohol (absolute, beverage) or cocaine), followed by all documented manifestations, complications, and comorbidities. Document and report any associated alcohol and drug dependence, abuse or use.

Admit for alcohol withdrawal with seizure: The code for alcohol dependence with withdrawal will be reported as the first listed diagnosis, followed by alcohol dependence with other alcohol-induced disorder, then seizure (other) code. Follow with all documented manifestations, complications and comorbidities.

CDI Alert

Documentation will indicate the consumption of large amounts of alcohol with ≥3 of the following:

- Tolerance
- Withdrawal symptoms
- Drinking larger amounts than intended
- Persistent decisions to reduce use without success
- Substantial time spent obtaining, drinking, or recovering from alcohol
- Sacrifice of other life events for drinking
- Continued use despite physical or psychological problems

Clinician Documentation Checklist

Clinician documentation should indicate the following:

- Name of substance
  - alcohol
    - identify blood alcohol level
  - polysubstance
- Level of substance use
  - use
  - abuse
  - dependence
- Any additional description of use
  - intoxication
  - remission
  - withdrawal
- Associated psychoactive-induced disorders
  - anxiety
  - delirium
  - delusions
  - hallucinations
  - mood disorder
  - perception disturbance
  - persisting amnestic disorder
  - persisting dementia
  - psychotic disorder
  - sexual dysfunction
  - sleep disorder

Alcohol Use

Code Axes

Alcohol use, unspecified with intoxication, uncomplicated	**F10.920**
Alcohol use, unspecified with intoxication, delirium	**F10.921**
Alcohol use, unspecified with intoxication, unspecified	**F10.929**
Alcohol use, unspecified with alcohol-induced mood disorder	**F10.94**
Alcohol use, unspecified with alcohol-induced psychotic disorder with delusions	**F10.950**
Alcohol use, unspecified with alcohol-induced psychotic disorder with hallucinations	**F10.951**
Alcohol use, unspecified with alcohol-induced psychotic disorder, unspecified	**F10.959**
Alcohol use, unspecified with alcohol-induced persisting amnesia disorder	**F10.96**
Alcohol use, unspecified with other alcohol-induced persisting dementia	**F10.97**
Alcohol use, unspecified with other alcohol-induced disorders, anxiety disorder	**F10.980**
Alcohol use, unspecified with alcohol-induced sexual dysfunction	**F10.981**
Alcohol use, unspecified with other alcohol-induced sleep disorder	**F10.982**
Alcohol use, unspecified with other alcohol-induced disorder	**F10.988**
Alcohol use, unspecified with unspecified alcohol-induced disorder	**F10.99**

Description of Condition

Alcohol use (F10.9-)

Harmful alcohol use is characterized by mental, behavioral and physical disorders due to alcohol use when dependency or abuse is not documented. Alcohol use without negative consequences documented, e.g., mere usage, is not reported with category F10. Provider documented BAC levels should be reported when the clinical significance is stated and has relevance to the encounter (Y90.-).

Key Terms

Key terms found in the documentation may include:

Alcohol intoxication

Alcohol intoxication, unknown usage

Alcohol use with clinical manifestation/state

Drunkenness

ETHO intoxication

Clinician Note

The provider must state the pattern of harmful usage (dependence, abuse or use) and its current clinical state (uncomplicated, intoxication, remission, etc.) and indicate the relationship to any identified mental, behavioral or physical disorder or its relevance to the patient's status or encounter including its clinical significance.

First Listed Diagnosis Note

Admission for acute alcohol poisoning with coma, teen with history of infrequent recreational use: The appropriate code from the Table of Drugs and Chemicals for poisoning will be the first listed diagnosis (alcohol, absolute, beverage), followed by the code for coma and alcohol use, unspecified with other alcohol-induced disorder.

Clinician Documentation Checklist

Clinician documentation should indicate the following:

- Name of substance
  - alcohol
    - identify blood alcohol level
  - polysubstance
- Level of substance use
  - use
  - abuse
  - dependence
- Any additional description of use
  - intoxication
  - remission
  - withdrawal
- Associated psychoactive-induced disorders
  - anxiety
  - delirium
  - delusions
  - hallucinations
  - mood disorder
  - perception disturbance
  - persisting amnestic disorder

- persisting dementia
- psychotic disorder
- sexual dysfunction
- sleep disorder

Anemia — Acquired Hemolytic

Code Axes

Drug-induced autoimmune hemolytic anemia	**D59.Ø**
Other autoimmune hemolytic anemias	**D59.1**
Drug-induced nonautoimmune hemolytic anemia	**D59.2**
Hemolytic-uremic syndrome	**D59.3**
Other nonautoimmune hemolytic anemias	**D59.4**
Paroxysmal nocturnal hemoglobinuria (Marchiafava-Micheli)	**D59.5**
Hemoglobinuria due to hemolysis from other external causes	**D59.6**
Other acquired hemolytic anemias	**D59.8**
Acquired hemolytic anemia, unspecified	**D59.9**

⇨ I-10 ALERT

The ICD-10-CM subcategories for acquired hemolytic anemia now include classifications for drug-induced conditions, whether autoimmune or nonautoimmune. When the condition is drug-induced, an additional adverse effect ICD-10-CM code should be assigned from categories T36 through T5Ø, with fifth or sixth character 5, indicating a therapeutic use adverse effect.

Description of Condition

Drug-induced autoimmune hemolytic anemia (D59.Ø)

Some therapeutic drugs may cause the patient's immune system to inappropriately target its own red blood cells for destruction through development of antibodies. These antibodies attach themselves to the red blood cells and cause early destruction. Cephalosporins are a class of antibiotics most commonly associated with the condition, but others are listed below:

- Cephalosporins
- Dapsone
- Levodopa
- Levofloxacin
- Methyldopa
- Nitrofurantoin
- Nonsteroidal anti-inflammatory drugs (NSAIDs)
- Penicillin and its derivatives
- Phenazopyridine (Pyridium)
- Quinidine

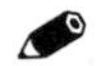 **CDI ALERT**

Ensure that the documentation specifies that the condition is determined to be drug-induced. Initial symptoms include dark urine, jaundice, tachycardia, shortness of breath, and weakness.

Key Terms

Key terms found in the documentation may include:

Acquired hemolytic anemia, chemical induced

Other autoimmune hemolytic anemias (D59.1)

There are two major types of disorders in this classification: cold antibody hemolytic anemia and warm antibody hemolytic anemia. In the cold antibody type, the autoantibodies become most active and attack red blood cells only at temperatures well below normal body temperature, whereas in the warm antibody type, the autoantibodies attach to and destroy red blood cells at temperatures equal to or higher than normal body temperature.

CDI ALERT

Diagnosis is typically made on the initial blood test, with an increase in the number of red blood cells that are immature (reticulocytes). Also, tests indicate increased amounts of certain antibodies, either attached to red blood cells (direct antiglobulin or direct Coombs' test) or in the liquid portion of the blood (indirect antiglobulin or indirect Coombs' test). Initial symptoms include dark urine, jaundice, tachycardia, shortness of breath, and weakness and may progress to splenomegaly.

Key Terms

Key terms found in the documentation may include:

- Autoimmune hemolytic disease
- Chronic cold hemagglutinin disease
- Cold agglutinin disease
- Cold agglutinin hemoglobinuria
- Immune complex hemolytic anemia
- Immunohemolytic anemia
- Secondary cold type hemolytic anemia
- Secondary warm type hemolytic anemia

Drug-induced nonautoimmune hemolytic anemia (D59.2)

This condition is similar to that listed above for code D59.Ø, except that the drug's adverse reaction is not associated with the body's autoimmune response. Instead, an oxidative mechanism occurs, where a component of the therapeutic drug binds to the red blood cells, resulting in oxygen deprivation and oxygen delivery to the tissues is impaired. This resulting condition is called methemoglobinemia.

CDI ALERT

Ensure that the documentation specifies that the condition is determined to be drug-induced. Initial symptoms include dark urine, jaundice, tachycardia, shortness of breath, and weakness.

Several of the drugs most commonly associated with the condition are listed below:

- Dapsone
- Phenazopyridine
- Primaquine
- Ribavirin

Key Terms

Key terms found in the documentation may include:

- Drug-induced enzyme deficiency anemia

I-10 ALERT

ICD-10-CM Instructional note: Use additional code for any associated: *E. coli* infection (B96.2-), pneumococcal pneumonia (J13), or *Shigella dysenteriae* (AØ3.9).

Hemolytic-uremic syndrome (D59.3)

Hemolytic-uremic syndrome (HUS) is a combination of three major components: hemolytic anemia (destruction of red blood cells), acute kidney failure, and a low platelet count (thrombocytopenia). The condition most commonly affects children and very often is preceded by an episode of infectious, sometimes bloody, diarrhea caused by *E. coli* O157:H7, which is acquired as a foodborne illness.

Key Terms

Key terms found in the documentation may include:

Drug-induced enzyme deficiency anemia

HUS

Clinical Tip

Acquired hemolytic anemias are uninherited disorders involving premature destruction of erythrocytes (red blood cells). Causes may include injury, infection, drugs, or blood transfusions (autoimmune). The condition is also classified as either intrinsic, where the cause is related to the red blood cell (RBC) itself, or extrinsic, where outside factors are believed to cause the disorder.

CDI ALERT

Review documentation carefully. Initially, HUS can be very hard to distinguish from thrombotic thrombocytopenic purpura, so documentation may appear in the medical record related to ruling out either condition.

Clinical Findings

Physical Examination

A complete physical examination with particular attention to pallor, abdominal distention, petechiae, and heart murmur. Hypoxia may also be indicated.

Diagnostic Procedures and Services

- Laboratory
  - CBC: Findings may indicate normochromic-monocystic, reticulocytosis or marrow erythroid hyperplasia
  - chemistry panel may indicate elevated serum bilirubin and LDH
  - stool guaiac: negative as anemia is not due to blood loss
  - ferritin
  - total iron binding capacity
  - serum iron
  - iron saturation

Note: Hemolytic anemia results usually note that a ferritin serum iron and iron saturation levels are normal and a TIBC are normal or low.

Therapeutic Procedures and Services

Type of treatment is dependent upon the severity and cause and may include the following:

- Blood transfusions
- Corticosteroid medications
- Treatment with intravenous immune globulin (to strengthen the immune system)
- Rituximab

Clinician Documentation Checklist

Clinician documentation should indicate the following:

- Type of acquired hemolytic anemia:
  - autoimmune or nonautoimmune
  - drug-induced autoimmune or nonautoimmune:
    - specify drug and any adverse effect
  - hemolytic-uremic syndrome
    - specify associated disorder
      - *Escherichia coli*
      - pneumococcal pneumonia
      - *Shigella dysenteriae*
  - paroxysmal nocturnal hemoglobinuria (Marchiafava-Micheli)
  - hemoglobinuria due to hemolysis from other external cause
    - Specify the external cause
      - from exertion
      - march hemoglobinuria
      - paroxysmal cold hemoglobinuria
- Other autoimmune types
  - autoimmune hemolytic disease (cold, warm)
  - chronic cold hemagglutinin disease
  - cold agglutinin disease
  - cold agglutinin hemoglobinuria
  - cold hemolytic anemia (secondary, symptomatic)
  - warm hemolytic anemia (secondary, symptomatic
- Other nonautoimmune types
  - mechanical hemolytic anemia
  - microangiopathic hemolytic anemia
  - toxic hemolytic anemia

Anemia — Iron-Deficiency

Code Axes

Iron deficiency anemia secondary to blood loss (chronic)	**D5Ø.Ø**
Other and unspecified iron deficiency anemias	**D5Ø.8, D5Ø.9**

CDI ALERT

Ensure that the anemia is specified as chronic (and not acute posthemorrhagic) to assign codes from this category.

Description of Condition

Iron deficiency anemia secondary to blood loss (chronic) (D5Ø.Ø)

Iron deficiency anemia due to chronic blood loss most commonly results from a recurrent bleeding lesion in the gastrointestinal tract, such as a gastric ulcer or diverticulitis. As with ICD-9-CM, acute posthemorrhagic anemia is excluded from this category. The two conditions are clinically very dissimilar and have different causes.

Key Terms

Key terms found in the documentation may include:

- Asiderotic anemia
- Chlorosis
- Chronic blood loss anemia
- Chronic posthemorrhagic anemia (D5Ø.Ø)
- Hypoferric anemia
- Hypochromic or microcytic anemia
- IDA due to inadequate nutrition
- Idiopathic hypochromic anemia

 **CDI ALERT**

Laboratory work-up typically reveals depleted iron stores and small, pale red blood cells (RBC), erythrocyte count less reduced than hemoglobin, serum ferritin below 12 ng/mL, low serum iron, and increased total iron-binding capacity. The physician must document the underlying cause of the anemia; no cause and effect may be assumed.

Other and unspecified iron deficiency anemias (D5Ø.8, D5Ø.9)

These classifications are available when the documentation indicates conditions that either have no specific code assignment, or there is no specific documentation for the condition. The previous ICD-9-CM code for iron deficiency anemia secondary to inadequate dietary iron intake is now indexed to code D5Ø.8.

Key Terms

Key terms found in the documentation may include:

- IDA due to inadequate nutrition
- Iron deficiency anemia due to inadequate dietary iron intake
- Refractory sideropenic anemia

Clinical Findings

Physical Examination

History and review of systems may include:

- Signs and symptoms
  - fatigue
  - loss of stamina
  - shortness of breath
  - weakness and pallor

Diagnostic Procedures and Services

- Laboratory
  - CBC: low hemoglobin and hematocrit are below normal levels (In early stages, the hemoglobin may be normal.)
  - serum iron
  - total iron binding
  - iron saturation
  - serum ferritin
  - bone marrow evaluation

Note: In uncomplicated iron deficiency anemia the ferritin and serum iron levels are below normal while the TIBC may be elevated. Iron saturation results are either normal or low.

Therapeutic Procedures and Services

In most instances iron supplements are provided either in the oral or intramuscular method.

Clinician Documentation Checklist

Clinician documentation should indicate the following:

- Type of iron deficient anemia
  - secondary to blood loss
  - due to inadequate dietary iron intake
  - due to inadequate nutrition
  - asiderotic
  - chlorosis
  - hypoferric
  - idiopathic hypochromic
  - refractory sideropenic

Anemia — Postoperative

Code Axes

Postoperative (postprocedural) anemia due to (acute) blood loss	**D62**
Postoperative (postprocedural) anemia, due to chronic blood loss	**D5Ø.Ø**
Postoperative (postprocedural) anemia, specified NEC	**D64.9**

Description of Condition

Postoperative (postprocedural) anemia due to (acute) blood loss (D62)

Anemia due to blood loss that is acute is the result of rapid, sudden loss of blood following trauma, a hemorrhagic condition, hemophilia, acute leukemia or loss during surgery. Postoperative anemia due to blood loss (posthemorrhagic) must be evidenced by clinically significant lab values that are indicative of the diagnosis. The diagnosis of anemia must be documented by the provider; the code cannot be reported based on lab values alone. The term 'acute' is not required to report postoperative blood loss anemia as D62, but the anemia *must* be described as "[due to] blood loss" *and* a stated link to the surgery/procedure would verify the cause/effect relationship with terms/phrases such as "postoperative," "due to," as "a result of" the surgery or procedure. It should be noted that this code is not a "complication" code but is identifying a condition that is occurring postoperatively or acutely due to bleeding/hemorrhage as "acute hemorrhagic anemia."

CDI ALERT

When the clinical scenario and clinical indicators are suggestive of anemia due to blood loss after a procedure or surgery, and only the diagnosis of anemia is made, a query would be appropriate to clarify the link and nature for specificity.

Key Terms

Key terms found in the documentation may include:

- Acute blood loss anemia
- Acute posthemorrhagic anemia
- Acute post-op anemia due to blood loss
- Acute post-op anemia due to blood loss as a result of surgery
- P/O blood loss anemia
- Post-op anemia due to blood loss
- Postprocedure blood loss anemia

CDI ALERT

Arrows: up and down arrows do not indicate a diagnosis. Query the provider as to the meaning of the symbols and request the information be fully stated including the clinical significance.

Clinical Note

If a diagnosis of anemia is specified in the absence of documentation of significant surgical blood loss, review operative records for documentation of administration of excessive fluids (e.g., colloids, crystalloids, plasma, etc.) intraoperatively which could result in iatrogenic dilutional anemia. An immediate drop in hemoglobin in the absence of significant blood loss during surgery may be indicative of a dilutional anemia rather than anemia due to acute blood loss. Any multiple choice clinician query for acute blood loss during surgery should also include the clinically reasonable choice of dilutional anemia along with any clinical indicators.

Documentation Tip

The baseline or preoperative H/H should be documented in order to qualify the type of anemia. Note that treatment is not required in order to report D62.

Arthroscopies

Code Axes

Arthroscopy, temporomandibular joint	**29800–29804**
Arthroscopy, shoulder	**29805–29828**
Arthroscopy, elbow	**29830–29838**
Arthroscopy, wrist	**29840–29848**
Arthroscopy, hip	**29860–29863, 29914–29916**
Arthroscopy, knee	**29866–29887**
Arthroscopy, ankle	**29891, 29894–29899**
Arthroscopy, metacarpophalangeal joint	**29900–29902**
Arthroscopy, subtalar joint	**29904–29907**

Description of Procedure

An arthroscopy is the visualization of a joint using a fiberoptic scope and may be performed as a diagnostic tool or as a surgical intervention. It requires two or more small surgical incisions and the scope and surgical instrumentation, often referred to as trocars, are inserted into the joint space. A number of surgical procedures may be performed through the scope, including but not limited to the removal of loose bodies (bone and/or cartilage), debridement, partial or complete synovectomy, or meniscus repairs.

When reviewing documentation to ascertain correct code selection, it is important to note the anatomical location (joint) but also additional terms such as medial, lateral, and the specific ligament being treated. The instrumentation used can also help to determine the exact type of surgical intervention being performed.

 **CDI ALERT**

The documentation should be carefully reviewed to determine what exact procedures were performed. There are times when the procedure performed and listed at the beginning of the operative report will not be the actual procedure described in the body of the report.

Key Terms

Key terms found in the documentation may include:

Arthroscopy with ______________

Debridement (debride): The smoothing of rough or torn cartilage as well as osteophytes and loose body removal that interfere with the motion of the joint Documentation may indicate the use of a shaver as well as other instruments such as rasps, curettes, spoons, and awls.

Meniscectomy (meni): The removal of the meniscus, a fibrocartilaginous structure that divides a joint space in half Meniscectomies are commonly performed knee arthroscopic procedures and physicians often use specialized instruments called meniscectomies when performing this service.

Synovectomy (syno): The partial removal of all or part of the synovium of a joint and documentation will often refer to motorized shaver.

Clinical Note

Documentation should clearly indicate any services or procedures performed at the time of arthroscopic examination and should clearly identify the location within the joint that the procedure is performed.

Clinician Documentation Checklist

Clinician documentation should indicate the following:

- Indicate the medical condition being treated
- Anatomical location
- Instrumentation
- Surgical procedures performed
  - removal of loose material
  - debridement
  - synovectomy
  - meniscus repair
  - other

Asthma

Code Axes

Note: All asthma codes (with the exception of subcategory J45.99) have fifth or sixth characters that represent the following three classification axes: uncomplicated, with (acute) exacerbation, with status asthmaticus: defined as an acute exacerbation of asthma that does not respond to standard treatments of bronchodilators and steroids.

Mild intermittent asthma	**J45.2**
Mild persistent asthma	**J45.3**
Moderate persistent asthma	**J45.4**
Severe persistent asthma	**J45.5**
Other and unspecified asthma	**J45.9**
Other asthma (exercise induced bronchospasm, cough variant asthma, other)	**J45.99**

I-10 ALERT

Classification axes for extrinsic and intrinsic asthma have been eliminated in ICD-10-CM. Instead, asthma severity levels, as have been defined by pulmonologists, have been introduced.

Description of Condition

Key Terms

Key terms found in the documentation may include:

Allergic asthma
Allergic bronchitis
Allergic rhinitis with asthma
Atopic asthma
Extrinsic allergic asthma
Hay fever with asthma
Idiosyncratic asthma
Intrinsic nonallergic asthma
Nonallergic asthma
Reactive airway disease

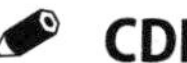

CDI ALERT

If there is an obstructive component to the patient's asthma, ensure that it is documented appropriately. These cases are coded and classified differently and require two codes, one from category J44 and one from category J45.

Clinical Tip

Respiratory insufficiency is integral to asthma. Hypoxemias are reported separately as it is not inherent.

Asthma Severity Levels

Mild intermittent asthma (J45.2-)

Mild intermittent asthma is the least severe of all types, involves a frequency of symptoms no more than two days a week, and nighttime symptoms no more than two times a month. This type of asthma typically does not interfere at all with daily activities.

Mild persistent asthma (J45.3-)

Patients with mild persistent asthma may have symptoms more than twice weekly, but not daily, and the condition can typically be controlled with one controller medication. A rescue inhaler may be used on a regular basis, but not daily. This type of asthma may interfere with daily activities in a minor way.

Moderate persistent asthma (J45.4-)

A classification of moderate persistent asthma requires that the patient have asthma symptoms daily that are controlled with two medications. A rescue inhaler may be used daily, and the patient may wake with asthma symptoms more than once a week, but not daily. The effect on daily activities is moderate.

Severe persistent asthma (J45.5-)

This is the most severe asthma classification and these patients have asthma symptoms daily. In some cases symptoms are experienced throughout the day, regardless of the use of two or more medications. The patient wakes from asthma symptoms nightly and must use a rescue inhaler multiple times a day. The effect on daily activities is extreme.

Exercise induced bronchospasm (J45.990)

This condition is defined as a reversible transient bronchoconstriction that affects patients both with and without a history of asthma. The symptoms of shortness of breath, wheezing, cough, or chest tightness occurs during strenuous exercise and may peak at five to ten minutes after exercising. Spirometry is commonly used to rule out underlying asthma.

Cough variant asthma (J45.991)

The major symptom of cough variant asthma is a dry non-productive cough that has persisted for six to eight weeks. There are no other more typical asthma symptoms, such as wheezing, or shortness of breath. The condition may be triggered by cold air or environmental allergens and is treated with a rescue inhaler.

Clinical Findings

Physical Examination

History and review of systems may indicate:

- Coughing
- Wheezing
- Chest tightness
- Shortness of breath

Diagnostic Procedures and Services

- Imaging
  - pulmonary function tests (PFT)
  - chest x-ray
  - electrocardiogram
  - allergy testing

Clinician Documentation Checklist

Clinician documentation should indicate the following:

- Identify any triggers
- Exposure to environmental tobacco smoke
- Exposure to tobacco smoke in the perinatal period
- History of tobacco use
- Occupational exposure to environmental tobacco smoke
- Tobacco dependence
- Tobacco use
- Include additional conditions
  - allergic (predominantly) asthma
  - allergic bronchitis
  - allergic rhinitis with asthma
  - atopic asthma
  - extrinsic allergic asthma
  - fever with asthma
  - idiosyncratic asthma
  - intrinsic nonallergic asthma
  - nonallergic asthma
- Type
  - mild intermittent
  - mild persistent
  - moderate persistent
  - severe persistent

- other
  - exercise-induced bronchospasm
  - cough variant asthma
- unspecified
  - asthmatic bronchitis
  - childhood asthma
  - late onset asthma
- document if any of the above type is:
  - uncomplicated
  - with (acute) exacerbation
  - with status asthmaticus

Atelectasis

Code Axes

Atelectasis	**J98.11**
Postprocedural atelectasis	**J95.89** **J98.11**

Description of Condition

Atelectasis (J98.11)

Atelectasis is an incomplete expansion of lung segments that may result in partial or complete lung collapse. It occurs to some degree in many patients undergoing upper abdominal or thoracic surgery. Prognosis depends on prompt removal of any airway obstruction, relief of hypoxia, and re-expansion of the collapsed lung. Prolonged immobility, anesthesia, mechanical ventilation, prolonged bed rest with few changes in position, underlying lung diseases, or any condition that inhibits full lung expansion or makes deep breathing painful, with shallow breathing are risk factors.

CDI Alert

When atelectasis is associated with significant findings, such as fever, or requires further diagnostic or therapeutic work up, such as chest x-ray (as part of work-up, not routinely/incidentally), urinalysis/blood culture, or respiratory therapy, or is linked to an extended hospital stay, then it is reportable.

Postprocedural atelectasis (J95.89, J98.11)

Atelectasis is an expected condition within the first 48 hours postoperatively when the patient has undergone a general anesthetic with moderately high oxygen concentrations. It is often an incidental x-ray/physical finding that is frequently self-limiting. It will usually resolve spontaneously without treatment. When it becomes symptomatic and requires work-up or additional monitoring or treatment, and it is documented as a complication of a procedure, it will be reported as a postprocedure complication.

Clinical Findings

Physical Examination

History and review of systems may include:

- Coarse lung sound and/or decreased lung sound
- Cough
- Dyspnea
- Shortness of breath
- Chest pain
- Transudate pleural effusion

Diagnostic Procedures and Services

- Imaging
  - chest x-ray
- Other
  - spirometry

Therapeutic Procedures and Services

- Nebulizer

Clinician Documentation Checklist

Clinician documentation should indicate the following:

- Recent procedures requiring general anesthesia
- Complications that occurred were
  - during procedure (intraoperative)
  - after procedure (postprocedural)
- Significant symptoms
  - shortness of breath
  - dyspnea
  - respiratory failure
  - decreased breath sounds
  - dullness to percussion
  - chest pain
  - transudate pleural effusion
  - fever
- Additional diagnostic or therapeutic workup
  - chest x-ray
  - blood culture
  - respiratory therapy
- Reason for an extended hospital stay

Body Mass Index

Code Axes

Body mass index (BMI) 25.Ø-29.9, adult	**Z68.25–Z68.29**
Body mass index (BMI) 3Ø.Ø-39.9, adult	**Z68.3Ø–Z68.39**
Body mass Index (BMI) ≥4Ø.Ø, adult	**Z68.41–Z68.45**

⇨ I-10 ALERT

Codes Z68.25–Z68.45 are unacceptable as principal diagnoses for facility billing.

Description of Condition

Overweight = Body Mass Index (BMI) 25.Ø–29.9, adult (Z68.25–Z68.29)

Key Terms

Key terms found in the documentation may include:

Dietary counseling

Overweight

Obesity = Body Mass Index (BMI) 3Ø.Ø–39.9, adult (Z68.3Ø–Z68.39)

Morbid Obesity = Body Mass Index (BMI) ≥4Ø.Ø, adult (Z68.41–Z68.45)

This disorder is defined as excess body weight. Causes are typically multifactorial and may include side effects of prescription medication, a hormone imbalance, or genetic predisposition.

Key Terms

Key terms found in the documentation may include:

BMI >30

BMI >40

Dietary management

Excess abdominal fat

Excessively overweight

Lose 5 to 10 percent of body weight

Morbid obesity

Obesity

Severe obesity

 **CDI ALERT**

BMI can be reported based on documentation by a nurse, dietitian, etc. However, a diagnosis of obesity must be based on physician documentation.

Clinical Tip

Untreated obesity tends to progress and can lead to many common health problems. Common complications include diabetes, cardiovascular disorders, metabolic syndrome, many cancers, osteoarthritis, fatty liver, depression, and obstructive sleep apnea.

Clinician Documentation Checklist

Clinician documentation should indicate the following:

- Obesity
  - morbid or severe
    - drug induced (document drug)
    - due to excess calories
    - familial
    - glandular
- Body mass index (BMI) = weight (kg) divided by the square of the height
- Document associated conditions or resources used
  - dietary consult
  - dietary plan
  - increase in OR time
  - special equipment

Bronchoscopy

Code Axes

Bronchoscopy, rigid or flexible **31622–31649**

Description of Procedure

A bronchoscopy is the examination of the bronchi by means of a fiberoptic scope that can be either flexible or rigid. Rigid bronchoscopies are performed less frequently and are usually used when a wider aperture or channels are required for diagnosing and treating such conditions as:

- Large pulmonary hemorrhages
- Some types of foreign bodies
- Some types of obstructive endobronchial lesions that may require laser debulking and/or stent placement

Flexible fiberoptic scopes are used in most other scenarios.

Like other endoscopic procedures, bronchoscopies can be diagnostic in nature, or when medically indicated, can be therapeutic. Appropriate code selection is dependent upon what, if any, additional procedures or services are documented in the medical record.

Endobronchial ultrasound (sometimes recorded as EBUS in the medical record) is performed to determine the presence of peripheral lesions. Documentation often indicates that a transducer was passed through the bronchoscope to better visualize vascular and nonvascular structures. When documentation indicates that this service was performed, code 31654 is reported additionally.

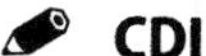

CDI Alert

The documentation should be carefully reviewed to determine what exact procedures were performed. There are times when the procedure performed and listed at the beginning of the operative report will not be the actual procedure described in the body of the report.

Bronchoscopy, with balloon occlusion (31634)

Documentation will indicate that a balloon occlusion was performed to treat an air leak when the documentation states that the physician advanced a balloon catheter through the bronchoscope to the site of the leak and inflated the balloon until the leak is occluded. While keeping the balloon inflated, a sealant such as fibrin is injected. Once the air leak is resolved, the balloon catheter is removed.

An endobronchial valve is a device placed and subsequently removed via the bronchoscope that permits one-way air movement. The valve closes when the patient inhales preventing air flow to the diseased area of the lung. The valve opens during exhalation to allow air to escape from the diseased area of the lung. It is used to treat persistent air leak from the lung into the pleural space.

Key Terms

Balloon occlusion

Endobronchial ultrasound (EBUS)

Endobronchial valve

Transbronchial needle aspiration (TBNA)

Clinician Note

Because some codes may be reported to indicate that additional lobes were treated, the medical record documentation must clearly specify the anatomical location where the procedure or service was performed.

Clinician Documentation Checklist

Clinician documentation should indicate the following:

- Identify the medical condition being treated
- Purpose of bronchoscopy
  - diagnostic
  - therapeutic
- Includes
  - transbronchial needle aspiration (TBNA)
  - endobronchial ultrasound (EBUS)
  - balloon occlusion
  - endobronchial valve
- Anatomical location of procedure

Cataract — Age-related (Senile)

Code Axes

Age-related incipient cataract	**H25.Ø**
Age-related nuclear cataract	**H25.1**
Age-related cataract, Morgagnian type	**H25.2**
Other age-related cataract	**H25.8**
Unspecified age-related cataract	**H25.9**

Note: Conditions classified to chapter 7 include laterality (right, left, bilateral) within the code structure. All ophthalmic conditions should specify the affected eye(s).

Description of Condition

Age-related cataract (H25.--)

Clinical Tip

Cataract is the partial or total opacity of the crystalline lens or lens capsule. Age-related (senile) cataract is slowly progressive partial or total opacity of the lens due to degenerative changes in patients over 55 years of age. Clinical classification of cataract considers the zones of the lens in which the opacity appears: cortical, subcapsular (anterior and posterior poles), and nuclear. Opacities may overlap these zones, encompassing combined clinical classification types. A morgagnian cataract is a mature cataract in which the nucleus moves freely throughout a liquefied cortex. Other causes that contribute to age-related degenerative cataract formation include systemic disease (e.g., diabetes), lifestyle factors (e.g., smoking), exposures (e.g., lead, ultraviolet light), and other intraocular diseases (e.g., glaucoma, retinal defects).

Key Terms

Key terms found in the documentation may include:

- Cataracta brunescens
- Coronary cataract
- Hypermature cataract
- Immature cataract
- Incipient cataract
- Indolent cataract
- Nuclear sclerosis cataract
- Punctate cataract

⇨ I-10 ALERT

ICD-10-CM classification for cataract includes a terminology change in the tabular list from "senile" to "age-related" for cataracts attributed to the effects of the aging process. However, note that the ICD-10-CM alphabetic index refers the coder to "*see* Cataract, senile" to index specific subterm for code assignment.

⇨ I-10 ALERT

Category H25 includes valid codes that are five or six characters in length. The following axes of classification describe those characters:

- Fourth character:
  - Type of age-related cataract (incipient, nuclear, morgagnian, other)
- Fifth character:
  - Location of cataract: point of origin of lens opacification
  - Type (Other: combined forms)
  - Laterality
- Sixth character:
  - Laterality

Senile or age-related

Water clefts

Clinician Note

Specify the nature and location of age-related cataract. Differentiate between opacities originating in the lenticular cortex, lenticular nucleus, and subcapsular poles (anterior or posterior). Document the specific type, as appropriate.

State whether opacification is partial or complete. Document any complications associated with the cataract, including the degree of visual impairment or related ophthalmic (local) conditions and manifestation, such as:

- History of eye surgeries and associated complications
- Myopia
- Glaucoma
- Retinal disease, detachment or defect
- Chronic inflammation or infection (e.g., iridocyclitis, uveitis)

Document any associated or underlying chronic or systemic disease processes. If conditions are inter-related, document the cause-and-effect relationship.

Clinician Documentation Checklist

Clinician documentation should indicate the following:

- Age-related incipient cataract
  - cortical age-related cataract
  - anterior subcapsular polar age-related cataract
  - posterior subcapsular polar age-related cataract
  - other age-related incipient cataract
    - coronary age-related cataract
    - punctate age-related cataract
    - water clefts
- Age-related nuclear cataract
  - cataracta brunescens
  - nuclear sclerosis cataract
- Age-related cataract, morgagnian type
  - age-related hypermature cataract
- Other age-related cataract
  - subtype:
    - combined forms of age-related cataract
    - other age-related cataract
- Unspecified age-related cataract
  - senile cataract

- Identify laterality of eye
  - right
  - left
  - bilateral

Cataract — Complicated

⇨ I-10 ALERT

ICD-10-CM includes a specific subcategory to classify complicated cataract. Subcategory H26.2 includes cataract due to certain ocular disorders or associated with other ophthalmic complications.

Note: Conditions classified to chapter 7 include laterality (right, left, bilateral) within the code structure. All ophthalmic conditions should specify the affected eye(s).

Code Axes

Other cataract	**H26**
Complicated cataract	**H26.2**
Unspecified complicated cataract	**H26.20**
Cataract with neovascularization	**H26.21**
Cataract secondary to ocular disorders	**H26.22**
Glaucomatous flecks	**H26.23**

Description of Condition

Complicated cataract (H26.2--)

Clinical Tip

Complicated cataract in ICD-10-CM includes cataract due to other ocular disorders or cataracts occurring as complications of other certain ophthalmic disorders. Certain ophthalmic diseases have long-term effects on the physiology of the intraocular lens. Complicated cataract often originates at the posterior subcapsular area and progresses to opacify the entire lens if the underlying or precipitating ocular disease remains untreated. Neovascularization occurs when the trabecular meshwork becomes obstructed or ischemic, resulting in deposit buildup on the lens epithelium. Chronic intraocular disease commonly associated with complications of cataract includes recurrent uveitis, glaucoma, retinitis pigmentosa, and retinal detachment or defect.

Key Terms

Key terms found in the documentation for complicated cataract may include:

- Cataracta complicata
- Degenerative cataract
- Glaucomatous flecks
- Glaukomflecken
- Inflammatory cataract
- Neovascularization cataract
- Subcapsular flecks

Clinical Findings

Physical Examination

History and review of systems may include:

Ophthalmoscopy followed by slit-lamp examination. Documentation may indicate well-developed gray, white, or yellow-brown opacities in the lenses. Small cataracts may be described as a dark defect in the red reflex. Documentation indicating a larger cataract may include the obliteration of the red reflex.

Therapeutic Procedures and Services

Surgical removal of the cataract with the placement of an intraocular lens

Clinician Documentation Checklist

Clinician documentation should indicate the following:

- Specify type
  - infantile and juvenile cataract
    - subtype
      - infantile and juvenile cortical, lamellar, or zonular cataract
      - infantile and juvenile nuclear cataract
      - anterior subcapsular polar infantile and juvenile cataract
      - posterior subcapsular polar infantile and juvenile cataract
      - combined forms of infantile and juvenile cataract
      - other infantile and juvenile cataract
      - unspecified infantile and juvenile cataract
        - presenile cataract
  - traumatic cataract
    - identify the external cause
    - subtype
      - localized traumatic opacities
      - partially resolved traumatic cataract
      - total traumatic cataract
      - unspecified traumatic cataract
  - complicated cataract
    - subtype
      - cataract with neovascularization
        - identify associated, such as chronic iridocyclitis
      - cataract secondary to ocular disorders (degenerative) (inflammatory)
        - identify associated ocular disorder
      - glaucomatous flecks (subcapsular)
        - identify underlying glaucoma type
      - unspecified complicated cataract

- cataracta complicata
- drug-induced cataract
  - toxic cataract
  - identify the drug, if applicable
- secondary cataract
  - subtype
    - Soemmering's ring
    - other secondary cataract
    - unspecified secondary cataract
- other specified cataract
  - cataract due to radiation
  - electric cataract
  - glass-blower's cataract
  - heat ray cataract
- Identify laterality of eye
  - right
  - left
  - bilateral

Cataract — Removal of

Code Axes

Extracapsular cataract removal	**66982, 66984**
Intracapsular	**66983**

Description of Procedure

A cataract is opacity of the lens of the eye and can be congenital or degenerative. There are two types of procedures performed to extract the lens. Intracapsular is when the lens is removed in one piece and extracapsular, the more commonly performed service, is when the hard central nucleus is removed in one piece and then the soft cortex is removed in multiple pieces.

Extracapsular cataract removal (66982, 66984)

Intracapsular cataract removal (66983)

Key Terms

Key terms found in the documentation may include:

Extracapsular

Extracapsular cataract extraction (ECCE)

Intracapsular

Intracapsular cataract extraction (ICCE)

Intraocular lens (IOL)

Senile or age related

Clinician Note

State whether opacification is partial or complete. Document any complications associated with the cataract, including the degree of visual impairment or related ophthalmic (local) conditions and manifestations.

Clinical Tip

Dropless cataract surgery: A new cataract procedure known as the dropless cataract procedure is performed when the physician injects (intravitreal) compounded medications (antibiotics and steroids) thus reducing or in some instances preventing the need of medicated eye drops postoperatively. Most payers include the injection in the service; therefore, it should not be billed separately.

CPT Alert

When documentation indicates that a special pupil-stretching device, rings, or hooks are used, code 66982 indicating a complex procedure is supported. Documentation may indicate the use of a device such as a Beehler pupil stretcher or Kuglen hooks.

Clinician Documentation Checklist

Clinician documentation should indicate the following:

- Type of cataract
  - age-related
  - congenital
  - presenile
  - secondary
  - senile
- Conditions and manifestations
  - opacity
    - partial
    - complete
  - complications
    - degree of visual impairment
    - glaucoma
    - diabetes
- Type of removal
  - intracapsular
  - extracapsular
    - pupil stretching device used
  - phacoemulsification
  - dropless procedure
- Location
  - anterior
  - posterior
- Laterality
  - left
  - right

Cellulitis and Acute Lymphangitis

Code Axes

Cellulitis and acute lymphangitis of finger and toe	**LØ3.Ø-**
Cellulitis and acute lymphangitis of other parts of limb	**LØ3.1-**
Cellulitis and acute lymphangitis of face and neck	**LØ3.2-**
Cellulitis and acute lymphangitis of trunk	**LØ3.3-**
Cellulitis and acute lymphangitis of other sites	**LØ3.8-**
Cellulitis and acute lymphangitis, unspecified	**LØ3.9-**

⇨ I-10 ALERT

ICD-10-CM classifies cellulitis (LØ3) and abscess (LØ2) in separate code categories based on whether the infection is encapsulated or contained (abscess, furuncle, carbuncle) or spread throughout the skin, subcutaneous tissues (cellulitis), and lymph channels (lymphangitis).

Infection of the lymph glands or nodes (LØ4) are classified separately.

Description of Condition

Cellulitis and acute lymphangitis (LØ3)

Clinical Tip

Cellulitis describes an infection of the skin and subcutaneous tissues most commonly caused by bacterial infection that spreads to the deeper layers of the dermis from an opening in the skin surface (e.g., open wound or puncture, burn, foreign body penetration). The skin becomes hot, reddened, swollen and painful.

Lymphangitis is an infection of the lymph channels or vessels. In lymphangitis, infection causes the lymph vessels to become inflamed. The abrupt onset of severe swelling is often a clinical indicator of worsening infection and increased risk for septicemia or sepsis. Reddened lines (streaks) may appear, running along the course of the lymphatic vessels in the affected area.

Key terms

Key terms found in the documentation may include:

Finger:

- Felon
- Whitlow

Nail:

- Onychia
- Perionychia
- Paronychia

CDI ALERT

Abscess and cellulitis are classified separately in ICD-10-CM by severity, anatomic site, and laterality. Ensure documentation is specific regarding extent of infection to avoid misrepresentation of severity.

Ensure documentation of site and laterality is thorough and specific to avoid reporting unspecified codes.

Code category LØ3 may indicate a severity progression of infection from localized to adjacent tissues that increases the risk for potentially fatal serious systemic infection (sepsis) from circulating pathogens.

Clinical Findings

Physical Examination

The infected anatomical location is examined and indicates erythema and tenderness. The skin is recorded as hot and red. The borders are described as either indistinct or sharply demarcated. In cases of lymphangitis the findings indicate that there is lymph node enlargement as well as the pain and tenderness.

Diagnostic Procedures and Services

- Laboratory
  - white blood count
  - wound cultures

Therapeutic Procedures and Services

- Antibiotics
- In some instances incision and drainage may be necessary.

> **⇨ I-10 ALERT**
>
> Category LØ3 Cellulitis and lymphangitis, includes valid codes that are four to six characters in length. The following axes of classification describe:
>
> Fourth character:
> Anatomic site or region
>
> Fifth character:
> Type of infection: abscess furuncle or carbuncle
> Anatomic site
>
> Sixth character:
> Anatomic site specificity (further specification of site)
> Laterality

Clinician Note

Differentiate between cellulitis and lymphangitis accurately in the diagnosis. Document the specific anatomic site. For upper limb infections, the axilla is a separately identifiable anatomic site from the upper limb. For paired anatomic sites, specify laterality (right or left).

For example:

Acute lymphangitis of right axilla (LØ3.121)

Acute lymphangitis of the right upper limb (LØ3.122)

Clinician Documentation Checklist

Clinician documentation should indicate the following:

- Identify
  - infectious organism (e.g., bacterial, viral, etc.)
- Document site of cellulitis and acute lymphangitis
  - finger
    - felon
    - whitlow
    - hangnail with lymphangitis of finger
    - infection of nail
    - onychia
    - paronychia
    - perionychia
  - toe
    - hangnail with lymphangitis of toe
    - infection of nail
    - onychia
    - paronychia

- perionychia
- Other parts of limb
  - axilla
  - upper limb
  - lower limb
  - unspecified part of limb
- face
- neck
- trunk
  - abdominal wall
  - back (any part except buttock)
  - chest wall
  - groin
  - perineum
  - umbilicus
  - buttock
  - unspecified part of trunk
- other sites
  - head (any part, except face)
    - scalp
  - other site
- unspecified site

Cerebrovascular Infarction and Hemorrhage

Code Axes

Nontraumatic subarachnoid hemorrhage	**I6Ø**
Nontraumatic intracerebral hemorrhage	**I61**
Other and unspecified nontraumatic intracranial hemorrhage	**I62** **I62.Ø[Ø-3]** **I62.1**
Cerebral infarction due to thrombosis of precerebral arteries	**I63.Ø**
Cerebral infarction due to embolism of precerebral arteries	**I63.1**
Cerebral infarction due to unspecified occlusion or stenosis of precerebral arteries	**I63.2**
Cerebral infarction due to thrombosis of cerebral arteries	**I63.3**
Cerebral infarction due to embolism of cerebral arteries	**I63.4**
Cerebral infarction due to unspecified occlusion or stenosis of cerebral arteries	**I63.5**
Cerebral infarction due to cerebral venous thrombosis, nonpyogenic	**I63.6**
Other and unspecified cerebral infarction	**I63.8, I63.9**

CDI ALERT

Cerebral amyloid angiopathy (CAA) (E85.4/I68.Ø) refers to protein amyloid deposits in the blood vessels of the brain that can cause the blood vessels to crack, allowing blood to leak out causing hemorrhagic strokes.

Description of Condition

A cerebral vascular accident (CVA) is a sudden, focal interruption of the blood to the brain that results in neurologic deficit. Documentation for cerebrovascular accident must identify the type and artery involved:

Type	Location
Occlusion and stenosis Thrombosis Embolism	Precerebral arteries: right, left, or bilateral vertebral artery; basilar artery; right, left, or bilateral carotid artery
Occlusion and stenosis Thrombosis Embolism	Cerebral arteries: right, left, or bilateral middle artery; right, left, or bilateral anterior; right, left, or bilateral posterior artery; right, left, or bilateral cerebellar artery

Nontraumatic subarachnoid hemorrhage (I6Ø.-)

The nontraumatic hemorrhages described in category I6Ø describe bleeding into the subarachnoid space, the area between the arachnoid membrane and the pia mater surrounding the brain. The codes specify where the bleeding is **from**, which includes the following locations:

Anterior communicating artery

Basilar artery

Carotid siphon and bifurcation

Middle cerebral artery

Posterior communicating artery

Vertebral artery

Other intracranial arteries

Unspecified intracranial artery

Key Terms

Key terms found in the documentation may include:

Meningeal hemorrhage

Ruptured cerebral aneurysm

Ruptured (congenital) berry aneurysm

Ruptured (congenital) cerebral aneurysm

Rupture of cerebral arteriovenous malformation

Subarachnoid hemorrhage (nontraumatic) from cerebral artery

Subarachnoid hemorrhage (nontraumatic) from communicating artery

I-10 Alert

ICD-10-CM codes for these categories are much more specific than ICD-9-CM codes and contain many more subcategories representing laterality (where appropriate), specific site of infarction or hemorrhage, and type of disease process, such as thrombosis or embolism.

Nontraumatic intracerebral hemorrhage (I61.-)

An intracerebral hemorrhage involves bleeding inside the brain tissue, and may be caused by a number of conditions, such as hypertension, infections, tumors, blood clotting abnormalities, or arteriovenous malformations. For conditions in this category, the code description includes the terminology of a hemorrhage in a certain location, such as the following:

Brain stem

Cerebellum

Hemisphere (cortical, subcortical, or unspecified)

Intraventricular

Multiple localized

Other and unspecified

Key Terms

Key terms found in the documentation may include:

Cerebral lobe hemorrhage (nontraumatic)

Deep intracerebral hemorrhage (nontraumatic)

Superficial intracerebral hemorrhage (nontraumatic)

CDI Alert

Refer to CT and MRI reports to help clarify the site of the hemorrhage. Physician documentation must be consistent when reporting site, laterality and type of hemorrhage.

Other and unspecified nontraumatic intracranial hemorrhage (I62.-)

Intracranial hemorrhages involve bleeding within the skull and subdural hemorrhages are a result of vein rupture in the subdural space between the dura and arachnoid mater. Conditions in this category are classified according to severity, with designations of acute, subacute, chronic, and unspecified subdural hemorrhages.

CDI ALERT

Refer to CT and MRI reports to help clarify the site of the infarction. Physician documentation must be consistent when reporting site, laterality, and type of infarction.

The mechanism of the hemorrhage is also included in the classification of these conditions. The following diagnoses are described in the cerebral infarction categories:

- Thrombosis
- Embolism
- Unspecified occlusion or stenosis

Cerebral infarction (I63.-)

When a blood vessel that supplies a part of the brain becomes blocked or leakage occurs outside the vessel walls, the condition is known as a cerebral infarction. The loss of blood supply results in tissue death of that area. Cerebral infarctions may be classified to the following locations:

Anterior cerebral artery (right, left, unspecified)

Basilar artery

Carotid artery (right, left, unspecified)

Cerebellar artery (right, left, unspecified)

Middle cerebral artery (right, left, unspecified)

Posterior cerebral artery (right, left, unspecified)

Vertebral artery (right, left, unspecified)

Other cerebral artery

Other precerebral artery

I-10 ALERT

When patients admitted for symptomatic cerebral hemorrhage associated with known cerebral amyloid angiopathy, code I61.9 is assigned as the first-listed diagnosis, followed by the codes for the cerebral amyloid angiopathy I85.4 and I68.0. According to the *ICD-10-CM Official Guidelines for Coding and Reporting*: "When there are two or more interrelated conditions (such as diseases in the same ICD-10-CM chapter or manifestations characteristically associated with a certain disease) potentially meeting the definition of first listed diagnosis, either condition may be sequenced first, unless the circumstances of the admission, the therapy provided, the tabular list, or the alphabetic index indicate otherwise."

Clinical Findings

Symptoms with abrupt onset vary and some reflect infarct or hemorrhage and origin (cerebral/precerebral) or area of brain involved. Stroke severity and progression are often assessed using the standardized scoring scale such as the National Institutes of Health Stroke Scale (NIHSS), Canadian Neurological Scale (CNS), or the Mathew Stroke Scale.

Physical Examination

History and review of systems may include:

- Confusion
- Weakness/paresis
- Hemiplegia/quadriplegia
- Hemisensory loss
- Gaze preference
- Neurological neglect
- Facial droop
- Photophobia
- Stiff neck/pain/chemical meningitis
- Papilledema
- Monocular/binocular blindness
- Blurred vision or visual field defects: homonymous hemianopia

- Eye movement abnormalities (diplopia or nystagmus)
- Anisocoria
- Hyperglycemia
- Dysphagia
- Dysarthria or difficulty understanding speech
- Vertigo
- Ataxia
- Aphasia
- Headache (worst headache of my life, thunderclap)
- Nausea/vomiting
- Syncope
- New onset seizure
- Acute neurological deficit
- Altered loss of consciousness
- Cytotoxic cerebral edema: causes deterioration during the first 48–72 hours after onset
- Hydrocephalus
- Increased intracranial pressure
- Encephalopathy
- Coma/obtunded (GCS ≤ 8)
- Hypertension (systolic BP > 220 mm Hg)
- Fever (indication of neurological deterioration)
- Brain herniation/compression/midline shift
- Decorticate/decerebrate posturing

Diagnostic Procedures and Services

- Laboratory
  - CBC
  - platelet count (<100,000/µl)
  - prothrombin time test (PT)/partial thromboplastin time test (PTT)
  - fasting blood glucose
  - lipid profile
  - homocysteine
  - erythrocyte sedimentation rate (ESR)
  - other tests as warranted for specific dx workup
- Imaging
  - CT: after 24 hours ischemic infarct visible; initial neuroimaging
  - diffusion weighted MRI: follow-up to CT, especially when initial CT is negative
  - gradient echo MRI
  - angiography
  - carotid duplex ultrasonography

- Other
  - ECG
  - swallow study for dysphagia
  - lumbar puncture for subarachnoid hemorrhage (SaH)
  - transesophageal echocardiography to evaluate cardiac etiology

Clinical Tip

Impending or threatened CVA is only reported as a CVA when confirmed, otherwise only the symptoms are reported.

Symptoms that last for one hour or less do not often result in neurologic damage and are classified as transient ischemic attacks (TIA).

Prolonged reversible ischemic neurological deficit ((P)RIND) is a cerebral infarct that lasts between 24 and 72 hours.

⇨ I-10 ALERT

There is no time limit restricting the reporting of sequelae (late effect) codes. Residual conditions may occur months or years following the causal condition. When a patient has had previous cerebral infarctions and presents with a current infarction, coders should refer to medical record documentation to determine if a sequela is the result of the current or previous infarction.

Key Terms

Key terms found in the documentation may include:

Cerebral Infarction due to:
- Embolism
- Hemorrhagic
- Narrowing, obstructing
- Obstruction
- Occlusion and stenosis
- Postoperative
- Thrombosis
- Vasospasm

CVA due to:
- Embolism
- Hemorrhagic
- Narrowing, obstructing
- Obstruction
- Occlusion and stenosis
- Postoperative
- Thrombosis
- Vasospasm

Stroke

Clinician Note
There is no time limit restricting the reporting of sequelae (late effect) codes.

Residual conditions may occur months or years following the causal condition. When a patient has had previous cerebral infarctions and presents with a current infarction, careful attention must be paid to medical record documentation to determine if a sequela is the result of the current or previous infaction.

CDI ALERT

Review documentation carefully to determine whether the cerebral infarction patient had tPA administered in another facility, prior to this encounter. This is important information that affects the specific case, as well as general clinical research efforts.

Clinician Documentation Checklist

Clinician documentation should indicate the following:

- Time of symptom onset
- The symptoms and associated conditions
- How long the symptoms lasted
- History including medical and family history relevant to the encounter
- Type of stroke
  - thrombosis, embolism, other occlusion/stenosis
  - hemorrhagic including site of hemorrhage/infarct, including laterality and cause of hemorrhage (aneurysm, AVM, conversion, treatment)
- Neurology consult
- Procedures performed
  - CT
  - MRI
  - laboratory
  - cardiovascular screening
  - swallow testing
- Evaluation/therapy
  - physical therapy
  - occupational therapy
  - speech
  - nutrition
- Medications provided including tPA
- Discharge summary and discharge disposition

Description of Condition

Cerebral amyloid angiopathy (E85.4/I68.Ø)

Cerebral amyloid angiopathy (CAA) refers to protein amyloid deposits in the blood vessels of the brain that can cause the blood vessels to crack, allowing blood to leak out causing hemorrhagic strokes.

First Listed Diagnosis Note

Admit for symptomatic cerebral hemorrhage associated with known cerebral amyloid angiopathy: As reason for admission was cerebral hemorrhage, code I61.9 is assigned as the first listed diagnosis, followed by the codes for the cerebral amyloid angiopathy I85.4 and I68.Ø. According to Official Coding Guidelines: "When there are two or more interrelated conditions (such as diseases in the same ICD-10-CM chapter or manifestations characteristically associated with a certain disease) potentially meeting the definition of first listed diagnosis, either condition may be sequenced first, unless the circumstances of the admission, the therapy provided, the Tabular List, or the Alphabetic Index indicate otherwise."

Chemotherapy Administration

Code Axes

Injection and intravenous infusion chemotherapy and other highly complex drug or highly complex biologic agent administration	**96401–94617**
Intra-arterial chemotherapy and other highly complex drug or highly complex biologic agent administration	**96420–96425**
Other injection and infusion services	**96440–96542**

Description of Procedure

Chemotherapy is the parenteral administration of nonradionuclide antineoplastic drugs. These drugs can be administered by either injection or infusion. Careful documentation indicating the method of administration as well as the site of the administration (venous, arterial, intrathecal) is required. Documentation must also indicate the substance administered.

Clinical Tip

The following flow chart can be used to determine if the correct code is supported by the medical record documentation.

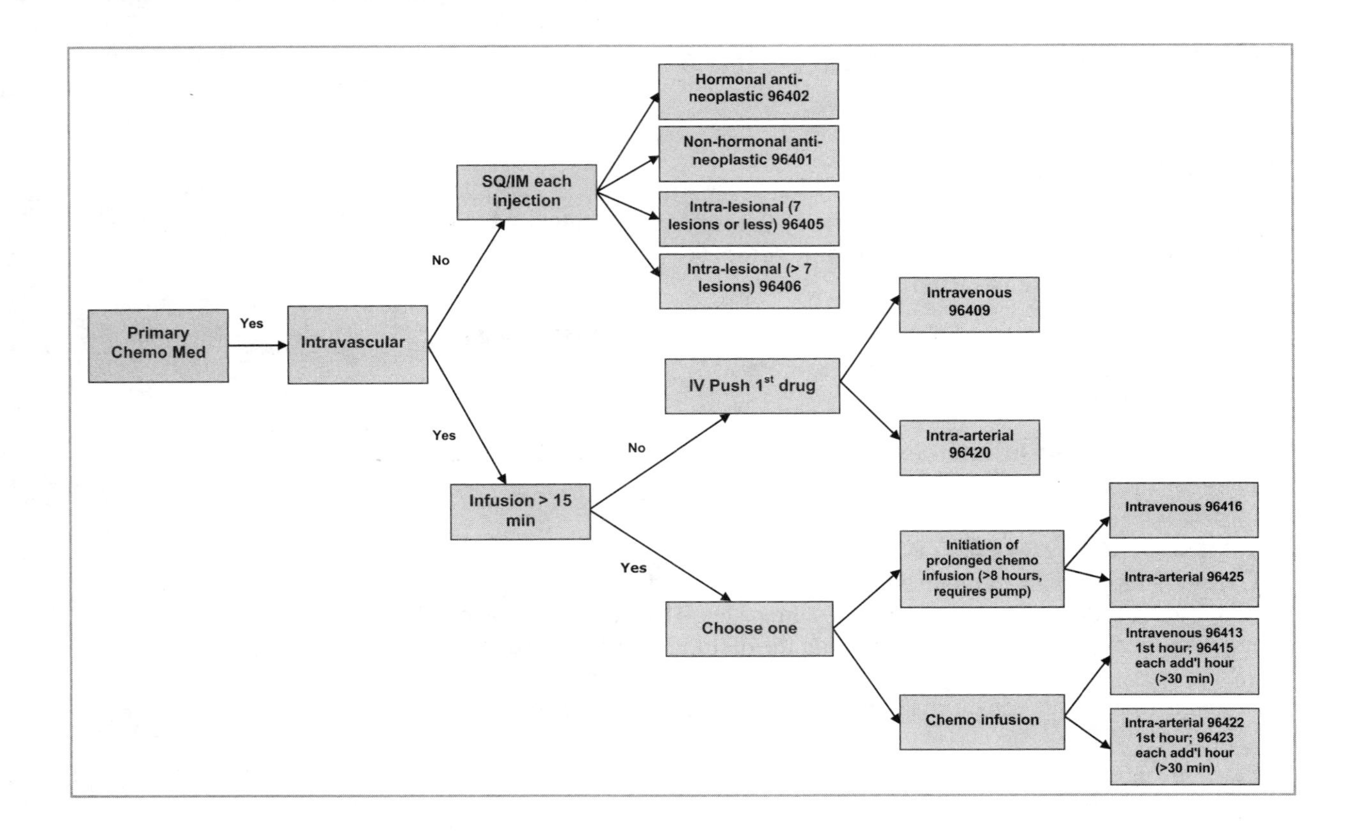
Primary Chemo Med
Yes
Intravascular
No
SQ/IM each injection
Hormonal anti-neoplastic 96402
Non-hormonal anti-neoplastic 96401
Intra-lesional (7 lesions or less) 96405
Intra-lesional (> 7 lesions) 96406
Yes
Infusion > 15 min
No
IV Push 1st drug
Intravenous 96409
Intra-arterial 96420
Yes
Choose one
Initiation of prolonged chemo infusion (>8 hours, requires pump)
Intravenous 96416
Intra-arterial 96425
Chemo infusion
Intravenous 96413 1st hour; 96415 each add'l hour (>30 min)
Intra-arterial 96422 1st hour; 96423 each add'l hour (>30 min)

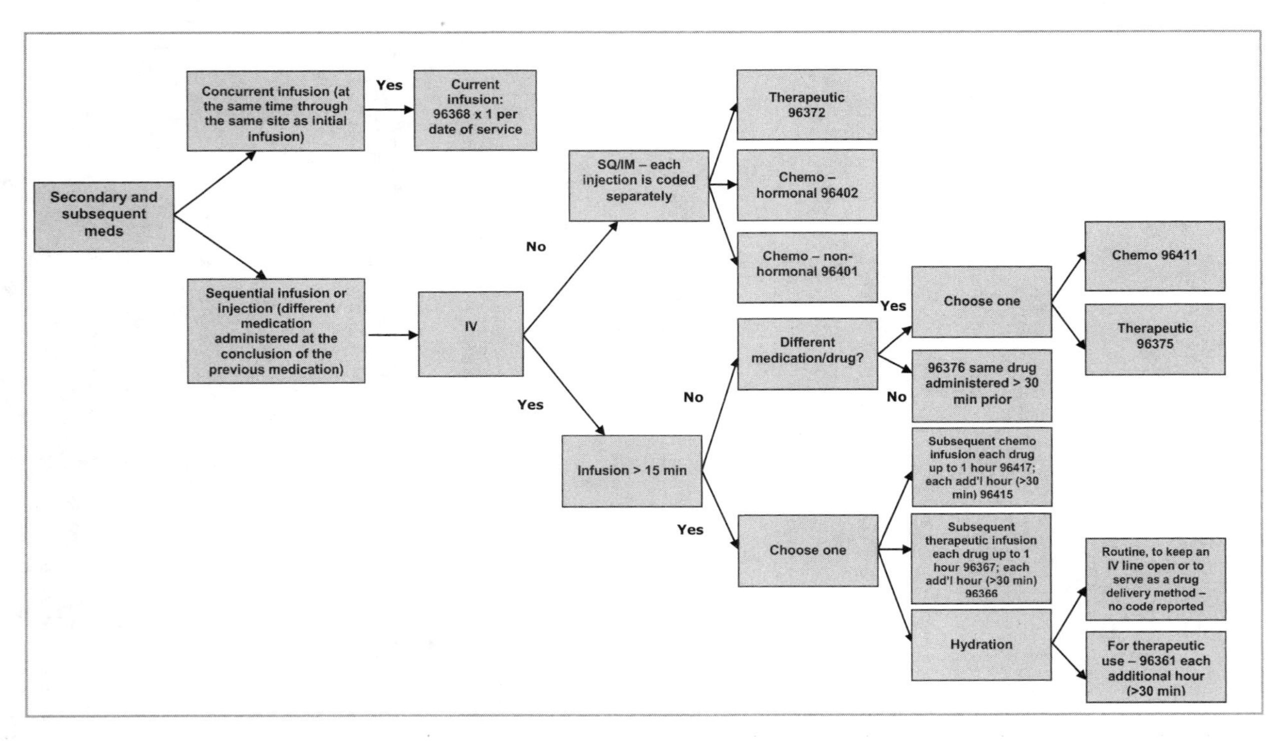
Secondary and subsequent meds
Concurrent infusion (at the same time through the same site as initial infusion)
Yes
Current infusion: 96368 x 1 per date of service
Sequential infusion or injection (different medication administered at the conclusion of the previous medication)
IV
No
SQ/IM – each injection is coded separately
Therapeutic 96372
Chemo – hormonal 96402
Chemo – non-hormonal 96401
Yes
Infusion > 15 min
No
Different medication/drug?
Yes
Choose one
Chemo 96411
Therapeutic 96375
No
96376 same drug administered > 30 min prior
Yes
Choose one
Subsequent chemo infusion each drug up to 1 hour 96417; each add'l hour (>30 min) 96415
Subsequent therapeutic infusion each drug up to 1 hour 96367; each add'l hour (>30 min) 96366
Hydration
Routine, to keep an IV line open or to serve as a drug delivery method – no code reported
For therapeutic use – 96361 each additional hour (>30 min)

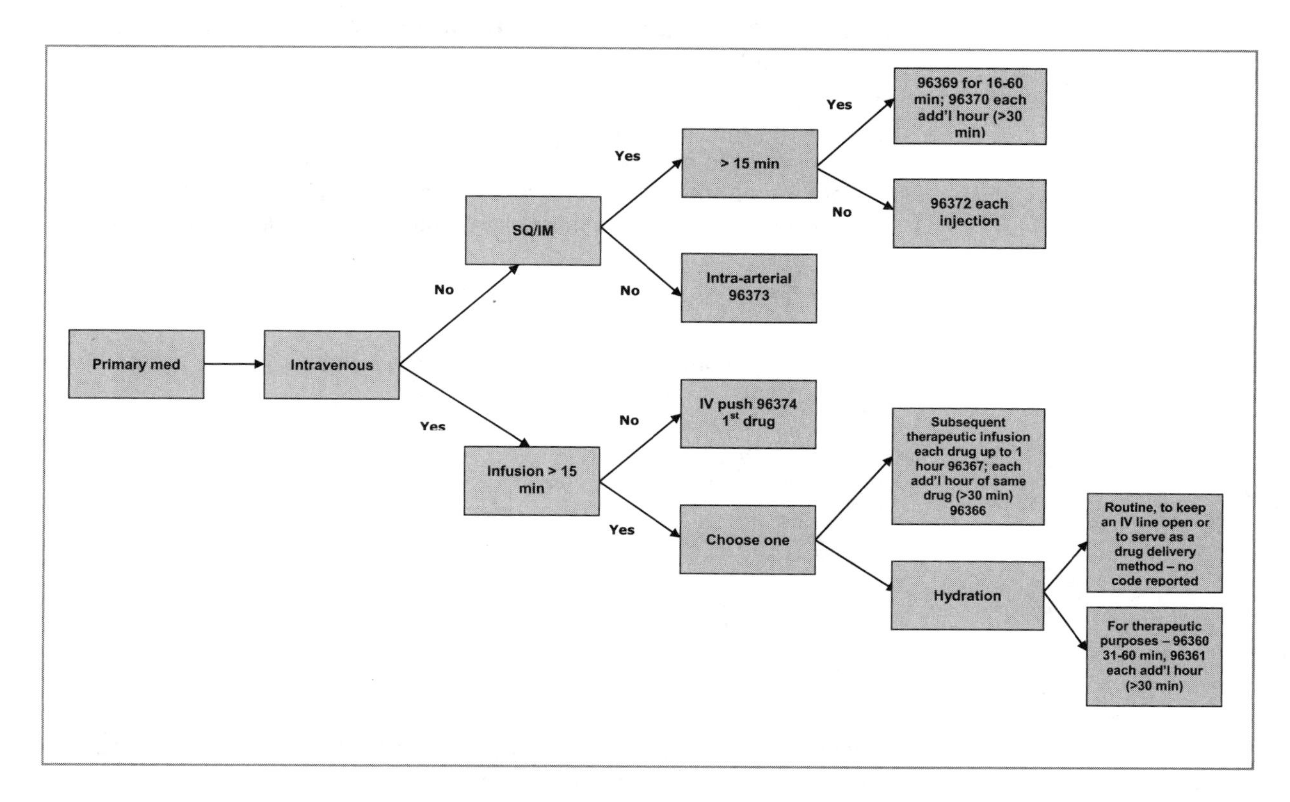
Primary med
Intravenous
No
SQ/IM
Yes
> 15 min
Yes
96369 for 16-60 min; 96370 each add'l hour (>30 min)
No
96372 each injection
No
Intra-arterial 96373
Yes
Infusion > 15 min
No
IV push 96374 1st drug
Yes
Choose one
Subsequent therapeutic infusion each drug up to 1 hour 96367; each add'l hour of same drug (>30 min) 96366
Hydration
Routine, to keep an IV line open or to serve as a drug delivery method – no code reported
For therapeutic purposes – 96360 31-60 min, 96361 each add'l hour (>30 min)

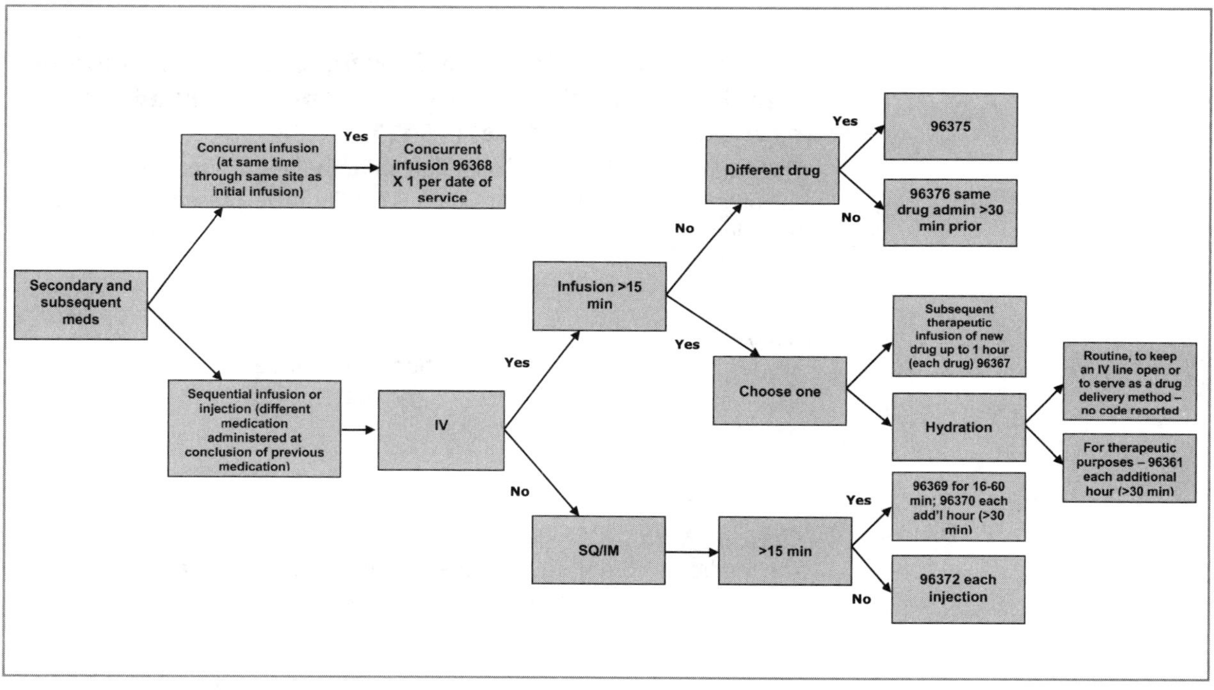
Secondary and subsequent meds
Concurrent infusion (at same time through same site as initial infusion)
Yes
Concurrent infusion 96368 X 1 per date of service
Sequential infusion or injection (different medication administered at conclusion of previous medication)
IV
Yes
Infusion >15 min
No
Different drug
Yes
96375
No
96376 same drug admin >30 min prior
Yes
Choose one
Subsequent therapeutic infusion of new drug up to 1 hour (each drug) 96367
Hydration
Routine, to keep an IV line open or to serve as a drug delivery method – no code reported
For therapeutic purposes – 96361 each additional hour (>30 min)
No
SQ/IM
>15 min
Yes
96369 for 16-60 min; 96370 each add'l hour (>30 min)
No
96372 each injection

Chemotherapy administration, subcutaneous or intramuscular (96401–96402)

Documentation will indicate that the physician or supervised assistant prepares and administers nonhormonal (96401) or hormonal (96402) medication to combat diseases such as malignant neoplasms or microorganisms. These codes apply to medication injected under the skin (subcutaneous) or into a muscle (intramuscular) often in the arm or leg.

Key Terms

Key terms found in the documentation may include:

- IM
- Inj
- Injection
- Sq
- SubQ

Clinician Note

Note any complications that occur during the service.

Chemotherapy administration; intravenous, push technique, single or initial substance/drug (96406)

Chemotherapy administration; intravenous, push technique, each additional substance/drug (List separately in addition to code for primary procedure) (96411)

The drug is administered through intravenous (IV) push technique in which the physician or supervised assistant is continuously present to administer the injection and observe the patient or for an infusion of less than 15 minutes.

Key Terms

Key terms found in the documentation may include:

- IV
- Push

Clinician Note

The medical record should include the disease being treated with the name and dosage of the drug being administered.

Chemotherapy administration, intra-arterial; push technique (96420)

Chemotherapy administration, intra-arterial; infusion technique, up to 1 hour (96422)

Chemotherapy administration, intra-arterial; infusion technique, each additional hour (list separately in addition to code for primary procedure) (96423)

Chemotherapy administration, intra-arterial; infusion technique, initiation of prolonged infusion (more than 8 hours), requiring the use of a portable or implantable pump (96245)

Documentation for these services must indicate that the infusion was intra-arterial. The medical record should identify the vessels used.

Key Terms

Key terms found in the documentation may include:

IA therapy

Clinician Note

The medical record should include the disease being treated with the name and dosage of the drug being administered.

Clinician Documentation Checklist

Clinician documentation should indicate the following:

- The disease being treated
- The treatment phase
  - induction
  - consolidation
  - maintenance
  - intensification
- Substance administered (drugs and dosage)
  - alkylating agents: mechlorethamine, chlorambucil, melphalan
  - antimetabolites: methotrexate, cytarabine
  - plant alkaloids: vincas, vinblastine, podophyllotoxins
  - antibiotics: doxorubicin, bleomycin, mitomycin
  - nitrosoureas: carmustine, lomustine
  - inorganic ions: cisplatin, carboplatin
  - biologic response modification: IFN
  - enzymes: asparaginase
  - hormones: tamoxifen, flutamide
  - high dose infusion interleukin 2

    - aldesleukin
    - interferon gamma
    - antiemetics
        - indicate whether the medication administered is
            - initial/primary medication
            - subsequent or additional medication
- Route of administration
    - injection
    - infusion
    - IV push
- Site of administration
    - venous
    - arterial
    - intrathecal
    - subcutaneous/intramuscular
- Timing
    - concurrent infusion
    - subsequent infusion or injection
- Hydration
    - routine
    - therapeutic
- Administration time
    - start
    - stop
- Additional patient pathology
    - nausea and vomiting
    - dehydration
    - anemia
    - neutropenia
    - pancytopenia
    - fatigue
    - mood changes
    - orthostatic hypotension

Chronic Ischemic Heart Disease

Code Axes

Arteriosclerotic heart disease (ASHD)

ASHD of native coronary artery with and without angina pectoris	**I25.1Ø–I25.119**
ASHD of coronary artery bypass graft(s) and coronary artery of transplanted heart with angina pectoris	**I25.7ØØ–I25.7Ø9**
ASHD of autologous vein coronary artery bypass graft(s) with angina pectoris	**I25.71Ø–I25.719**
ASHD of autologous artery coronary artery bypass graft(s) with angina pectoris	**I25.72Ø–I25.729**
ASHD of nonautologous biological coronary artery bypass graft(s) with angina pectoris	**I25.73Ø–I25.739**
ASHD of native coronary artery of transplanted heart with angina pectoris	**I25.75Ø–I25.759**
ASHD of bypass graft of coronary artery of transplanted heart with angina pectoris	**I25.76Ø–I25.769**
ASHD of other coronary artery bypass graft(s) with angina pectoris	**I25.79Ø–I25.799**
Other and unspecified forms of chronic ischemic heart disease	**I25.8–I25.9**

Clinical Tip

Many patients carry a diagnosis of chronic ischemic heart disease, or more specifically, of atherosclerotic heart disease. The key for correct classification in ICD-10-CM is determining the severity level and whether or not unstable or another form of angina is also present at the time of the encounter. The disease process is similar regardless of whether it is present in a native artery or a bypassed vessel; however, the risk and severity level is higher for bypassed vessels and, if the patient has had any bypass procedures, the status of these vessels should be clearly documented.

Key Terms

Key terms found in the documentation for coronary atherosclerosis may include:

Atherosclerotic cardiovascular disease (ASCVD)

Atherosclerotic heart disease (ASHD)

Atherosclerotic heart disease with angina

Atherosclerotic heart disease with ischemic chest pain

Coronary (artery) atheroma

Coronary (artery) atherosclerosis

⇨ I-10 ALERT

ICD-10-CM codes combine the clinical concepts of coronary atherosclerosis and several different forms of angina. A cause-and-effect relationship may be assumed when a patient has both coronary atherosclerosis and angina (official coding guideline 1.C.9.b). An additional code for the angina is not necessary. Review documentation of angina carefully to ensure correct classification.

CDI ALERT

Refer to cardiac stress test reports, cardiac catheterization reports, and other cardiology results for documentation of coexisting angina. Physician documentation should be consistent throughout the record concerning which of these conditions existed at the time of the encounter.

Coronary (artery) disease (CAD)

Coronary (artery) sclerosis

Clinician Note

According to Medicare coverage guidelines, coronary artery disease with a documented prior MI, a measured left ventricular ejection fraction (LVEF) $\leq$ 0.35, and inducible, sustained VT or VF at EP study supports the medical necessity of an implanted cardiodefibrillator. The MI must have occurred more than 40 days prior to defibrillator insertion. The EP test must be performed more than 4 weeks after the qualifying MI.

Clinical Findings

Physical Examination

History and review of systems may include:

Patients may be asymptomatic. When present, signs and symptoms include stable exertional angina, intermittent claudication, symptoms of unstable angina or infarction, ischemic stroke, or rest pain in limbs. Palpation of extremity pulses is performed. Heart sounds are recorded and any bruits are noted.

Diagnostic Procedures and Services

- Laboratory
  - total cholesterol
  - HDL cholesterol
  - triglycerides
  - glucose
  - lipids
- Imaging
  - CT angiography
  - Ultrasonography
- Other
  - EKG
  - Doppler of extremities when decreased pulses or complaints of pain and cramping

Therapeutic Procedures and Services

Lifestyle changes including patient diet (low fat), desist tobacco use and to increase physical activity.

- Statin use
- ACE inhibitors
- Beta blockers
- Antiplatelet drugs

Clinician Documentation Checklist

Clinician documentation should indicate the following:

- Other acute
  - acute coronary thrombosis without MI
  - Dressler's syndrome
  - other acute ischemic heart disease
  - unspecified acute ischemic heart disease
- Chronic
  - location
    - native vessels
    - bypass graft(s), unspecified
    - bypass graft(s), autologous vein
    - bypass graft(s), autologous artery
    - bypass graft(s), nonautologous biological
    - bypass graft(s) with transplanted heart
    - native vessels of transplanted heart
    - other bypass graft(s)
  - complications/symptoms
    - angina pectoris
    - unstable angina pectoris
    - documented spasm
    - other forms of angina pectoris
    - unspecified angina pectoris
  - types
    - total occlusion of coronary artery
    - due to lipid rich plaque
    - due to calcified coronary lesion
    - other ischemic heart disease
    - ischemic heart disease (chronic) NOS

Chronic Obstructive Pulmonary Disease (COPD)

Code Axes

Chronic obstructive pulmonary disease with acute lower respiratory infection	**J44.Ø**
Chronic obstructive pulmonary disease with (acute) exacerbation	**J44.1**
Chronic obstructive pulmonary disease, unspecified	**J44.9**

Clinical Tip

Chronic obstructive pulmonary disease is an umbrella term that contains other conditions, but there are two primary types of COPD: one involves chronic bronchitis, which is usually manifested with a chronic cough and mucous production. The other type of COPD is emphysema (discussed above), which involves lung destruction over time.

Key Terms

Key terms found in the documentation may include:

Asthma with chronic obstructive pulmonary disease
Chronic airflow limitation
Chronic asthmatic (obstructive) bronchitis
Chronic bronchitis with emphysema
Chronic emphysematous bronchitis
Chronic obstructive airway disease
Chronic obstructive asthma
Chronic obstructive bronchitis
Chronic obstructive lung disease
Chronic obstructive respiratory disease
Chronic obstructive tracheobronchitis
COPD

⇨ I-10 ALERT

Ensure that the underlying infection is documented appropriately; an additional code is necessary for proper classification.

Description of Condition

Chronic obstructive pulmonary disease with acute lower respiratory infection (J44.Ø)

Clinical Tip

An acute exacerbation of COPD is not the same thing as a superimposed infection, although the exacerbation may be triggered by the infection. Ensure that documentation is clear concerning the infectious process.

Chronic obstructive pulmonary disease with (acute) exacerbation (J44.1)

Clinical Tip

An acute exacerbation of COPD is defined as a decompensation of the disease, with increased symptoms such as wheezing and shortness of breath. Treatment typically consists of easing symptoms and returning the patient to their baseline respiratory status.

Key Terms

Key terms found in the documentation may include:

Decompensated COPD

Decompensated COPD with acute exacerbation

⇨ I-10 ALERT

If the COPD exacerbation is in the setting of an acute bronchitis, the Excludes 2 note under J44.1 indicates both J44.Ø and J44.1 may be reported together when appropriate.

Clinical Findings

Physical Examination

Indicators include dyspnea, poor exercise tolerance, chronic cough with or without sputum, wheezing, decreased breath sounds, respiratory failure, or cor pulmonale. A diagnosis is confirmed when the patient has symptoms of COPD and has a postbronchodilator FEV1/FVC ratio of less than 0.70.

Diagnostic Procedures and Services

- Imaging
  - chest x-ray
  - chest CT
- Other
  - spirometry
  - pulse oximetry

Therapeutic Procedures and Services

Treatment depends upon the severity and may include:

- Nebulizer
- Inhaler
  - albuterol
  - levalbuterol
  - salmeterol (Serevent)
  - formoterol (Foradil, Perforomist)
  - arformoterol (Brovana)
  - indacaterol (Arcapta)
  - tiotropium (Spiriva)
  - aclidinium (Tudorza)
  - corticosteriods
- Oxygen

- Medications
  - beta2-agonist bronchodilators
  - anticholinergic drugs
  - theophylline
  - antibiotics

Clinician Documentation Checklist

Clinician documentation should indicate the following:

- Identification of
  - exposure to environmental tobacco smoke
  - history of tobacco use
  - occupational exposure to environmental tobacco smoke
  - tobacco dependence
  - tobacco use
- Includes
  - asthma with chronic obstructive pulmonary disease
  - chronic asthmatic (obstructive) bronchitis
  - chronic emphysematous bronchitis
  - chronic bronchitis
    - with airway obstruction
    - with emphysema
  - chronic obstructive
    - asthma
    - bronchitis
    - tracheobronchitis
  - identify type of asthma
- Type of COPD
  - COPD with acute lower respiratory infection
    - identify the infection
  - COPD with (acute) exacerbation
    - decompensated COPD
    - decompensated COPD with (acute) exacerbation
  - unspecified
    - chronic obstructive airway disease
    - chronic obstructive lung disease

Colectomies and Enterectomies

Code Axes

Enterectomy, resection of small intestine	**44120–44128**
Colectomy, partial	**44140–44147, 44160**
Colectomy, total, abdominal, without proctectomy	**44150–44151**
Colectomy, total, abdominal, with proctectomy	**44155–44158**

Description of Procedure

An enterectomy is the removal of a portion of the small bowel. A colectomy is the removal of a portion of the large bowel. Careful documentation indicating the anatomical site and the amount of intestine removed is critical for correct code assignment.

These services can be performed as treatment for both diseases and congenital abnormalities. Additionally, it may be necessary to remove multiple segments and to anastomose the intestine multiple times.

Enterectomy, resection of small intestine; single resection and anastomosis (44120)

Enterectomy, resection of small intestine; each additional resection and anastomosis (List separately in addition to code for primary procedure) (44121)

Key Terms

Key terms found in the documentation may include:

Anastomosis

Resection

Clinical Tip

These procedures are commonly performed for the following conditions and when documented, will support the medical necessity of the service:

- A blockage in the intestine caused by scar tissue or congenital (from birth) deformities.
- Bleeding, infection, or ulcers caused by inflammation of the small intestine. Three conditions that may cause inflammation are regional ileitis, regional enteritis, and Crohn's disease.
- Cancer
- Carcinoid tumor
- Injuries to the small intestine

- Meckel's diverticulum
- Noncancerous (benign) tumors
- Precancerous polyps (nodes)

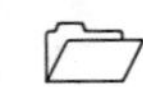

CPT ALERT

When significant additional time and effort is documented, it is appropriate to append modifier 22 and submit a cover letter along with the operative report.

Colectomy, partial (44140–44147)

Codes within this range represent the removal of a segment of the large bowel. They are differentiated by other procedures that may be performed during the same surgical session or the anatomical approach.

Key Terms

Key terms found in the documentation may include:

Cecostomy
Coloproctostomy
Colostomy
Ileostomy

Clinician Documentation Checklist

Clinician documentation should indicate the following:

- The disease or condition being treated
- Procedure
  - enterectomy
    - resection–single
    - resection–multiple
    - anastomosis
    - enterostomy
  - colectomy
    - resection–single
    - resection–multiple
    - anastomosis
    - colostomy
    - ileostomy
    - loop ileostomy
    - coloprotostomy
    - rectal mucosectomy

Coma

Code Axes

Unspecified coma	**R40.20**
Coma scale, eyes open	**R40.21**
Coma scale, best verbal response	**R40.22**
Coma scale, best motor response	**R40.23**
Glasgow coma scale, total score	**R40.24**

Key Terms

Key terms found in the documentation for coma may include:

Comatose

Unconsciousness NOS

Clinical Tip

In table format, the Glasgow coma scale appears as below:

Criteria Type & Points	1	2	3	4	5	6
Eyes Open	Never	To pain	To sound	Spontaneous	N/A	N/A
Best Verbal Response	None	Incompre-hensible words	Inappropriate words	Confused conversation	Oriented; converses normally	N/A
Best Motor Response	None	Extension to painful stimuli	Abnormal flexion to painful stimuli	Flexion withdrawal from painful stimuli	Localizes painful stimuli	Obeys com-mands

Generally, brain injury is classified according to the Glasgow coma scale (GCS) score:

- Severe, with GCS < 9
- Moderate, GCS 9–12
- Minor, GCS ≥ 13

Clinical Tip

In order to produce a valid score, one value (and code) from each subcategory (R40.21-, R40.22-, R40.23-) should be assigned. A seventh character designating when the scores were taken (e.g., in the field (EMT), at the hospital ED, at the time of hospital admission) should be assigned to each of the component Glasgow coma scale (GCS) score codes; all three should match. If only the GCS total score is documented in the medical record, a code from subcategory R40.24- may be assigned.

⇨ I-10 ALERT

The ICD-10-CM classification for coma is vastly improved and expanded. The classification is based on the Glasgow coma scale, which provides a neurologically objective way to measure the conscious state of a person for an initial as well as a subsequent assessment. A patient is assessed against the criteria of the scale and the resulting points provide a patient score between 3 (indicating deep unconsciousness) and 15 (fully awake).

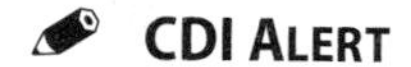

CDI ALERT

The detail of the Glasgow coma scale score may be found in emergency department or trauma records. In some facilities, the ICU will track GCS over time.

> ⇨ **I-10 ALERT**
>
> New guidelines in 2017 allow the coma scale to be used to evaluate the status of the central nervous system for other nontrauma conditions, including monitoring patients in the intensive care unit regardless of medical condition. In these circumstances the coma scale code will be sequenced after the diagnosis code.

The GCS score codes should be reported in conjunction with traumatic brain injury (TBI) codes, or acute cerebrovascular disease or sequelae of cerebrovascular disease codes. They should never be sequenced as principal or first-listed diagnoses.

Clinical Findings

Physical Examination

History and review of systems may include:

- Neurological examination
  - decreased consciousness
  - stimuli to arouse a patient that is briefly or not at all
  - eye abnormality including dilation, pinpoint or unequal (One or both pupils may be fixed in midposition.)
  - confusion or inappropriate responses
  - limited or no response to pain
- Respiratory
  - possible abnormal breathing patterns including Cheyne-Stokes or Biot's respirations
- Cardiac
  - tachycardia
  - cardiac arrest
  - hypotension
- Other
  - nausea
  - vomiting
  - ataxia

Therapeutic Procedures and Services

- Immediate stabilization of airway and circulation
- Supportive measures including control of intracranial pressure (ICP)
- Treatment of underlying conditions

Clinician Note

Coordination of benefits is often required for payment from third-party payers so the documentation should indicate how the injury occurred (e.g., auto accident, fall from ladder at work, fall when riding a bike).

Congenital Malformations of Great Arteries

Code Axes

Patent ductus arterious	Q25.Ø
Coarctation of aorta	Q25.1
Atresia of aorta	Q25.2
Supravalvular aortic stenosis	Q25.3
Other congenital malformation of aorta	Q25.4
Atresia of pulmonary artery	Q25.5
Stenosis of pulmonary artery	Q25.6
Other congenital malformation of pulmonary artery	Q25.7-
Other congenital malformation of other great arteries	Q25.8
Congenital malformation of great arteries, unspecified	Q25.9

Description of Condition

Coarctation of aorta (Q25.1)

This condition is the narrowing of the aortic lumen resulting in upper extremity hypertension, left ventricular hypertrophy, and malperfusion of the abdominal organs and lower extremities.

Key Terms

Key terms found in the documentation may include:

Coarctation of aorta

Clinical Findings

Physical Examination

History and review of systems may include:

- Headache
- Chest pain
- Fatigue
- Intracranial hemorrhage

Diagnostic Procedures and Services

- Imaging
  - echocardiogram
  - chest x-ray

  - chest CT
  - chest MRI
  - cardiac catheterization
- Other
  - electrocardiogram
  - extremity blood pressure measurements

Therapeutic Procedures and Services

- Surgical repair

Clinician Documentation Checklist

Clinician documentation should indicate the following:

- Aorta
  - patent ductus arteriosus
    - patent ductus botalli
    - persistent ductus arteriosus
  - coarctation of aorta
    - preductal
    - postductal
  - supravalvular aortic stenosis
    - absence of aorta
    - aneurysm of sinus of Valsalva (ruptured)
    - aplasia of aorta
    - congenital aneurysm of aorta
    - congenital malformation of aorta
    - congenital dilatation of aorta
    - double aortic arch (vascular ring of aorta)
    - hypoplasia of aorta
    - persistent convolutions of aortic arch
    - persistent right aortic arch
- Pulmonary artery
  - atresia
  - stenosis
    - supravalvular
  - coarctation
  - arteriovenous malformation
    - arteriovenous aneurysm
  - other
    - aberrant
    - agenesis
    - aneurysm
    - anomaly
    - hypoplasia

- Other congenital malformation of other great arteries
- Unspecified congenital malformation of great arteries

Great Veins

- Vena cava
  - stenosis (inferior) (superior)
  - persistent left superior vena cava
- Pulmonary
  - total anomalous pulmonary venous connection (TAPVR)
    - subdiaphragmatic
    - supradiaphragmatic
  - partial anomalous pulmonary venous connection (venous return)
  - unspecified
- Portal
  - anomalous portal venous connection
  - portal vein-hepatic artery fistula
- Other congenital malformations of great veins
  - absence of vena cava (inferior) (superior)
  - azygos continuation of inferior vena cava
  - persistent left posterior cardinal vein
  - scimitar syndrome
- Unspecified

Coumadin Toxicity

Code Axes

Poisoning, adverse effect of and underdosing of anticoagulants	**T45.51**
Poisoning by anticoagulants, accidental (unintentional)	**T45.511**
Poisoning by anticoagulants, intentional self-harm	**T45.512**
Poisoning by anticoagulants, assault	**T45.513**
Poisoning by anticoagulants, undetermined	**T45.514**
Adverse effect of anticoagulants	**T45.515**
Underdosing of anticoagulants	**T45.516**

Clinician Note
Laboratory studies to evaluate the patient's anticoagulation status are necessary for treatment and monitoring and, therefore, it is necessary to document this therapeutic treatment. Documentation should also indicate any adverse effects when present.

I-10 ALERT

ICD-10-CM has combined several different components of poisoning classifications, and has sequenced the poisoning, adverse effect, and new underdosing codes together in subcategories for each type of drug. No additional external cause code is required. The type of encounter is also classified in these codes, whether initial or subsequent encounter, or sequela.

Poisoning by anticoagulants, [all types] (T45.511–T45.514)

Clinical Tip
Although most poisonings are accidental, other examples of poisonings include errors in drug prescriptions and intentional overdoses of drugs. In addition, it is important to note that even if the drug in question was taken correctly, if it was taken in combination with another properly prescribed and administered drug, the resulting effect is classified as a poisoning. The same concept applies if the drug was taken in combination with alcohol; the resulting affect is a poisoning.

Clinician Note
Ensure that all other conditions are appropriately coded, such as specific drug reactions or complications of poisonings and adverse effects.

CDI ALERT

The documentation must clearly indicate the type of drug reaction, whether it was an adverse reaction, a poisoning, or an underdosing. If the issue involved a poisoning, the intent (accidental, self-harm, etc.) should also be documented in the medical record. It is important to determine what is meant by documentation indicating a drug "toxicity," because it could mean either a poisoning or an adverse effect.

Adverse effect of anticoagulants (T45.515)

Clinical Tip
An adverse effect of a drug is defined as an unintended consequence of a drug ingestion that was correctly prescribed and properly administered. It is important to note that the code representing the specific adverse effect (tachycardia, nausea and vomiting, etc.) should be reported first, followed by the adverse effect code.

Clinician Note
Ensure that all other conditions are appropriately coded, such as specific drug reactions or complications of poisonings and adverse effects.

Clinical Tip

An anticoagulant prevents blood from clotting; therefore, bleeding is a common adverse effect. When coagulopathy causing bleeding is due to anticoagulant therapy that is properly prescribed and administered, the nature of the adverse effect (manifestation) is reported first, followed by the code T45.515 with the appropriate seventh character to identify anticoagulation medication.

A prolonged PT/PTT or elevated INR is an expected result of anticoagulation therapy. This increases the risk for bleeding; when this level is excessive, requires treatment to lower or extends care, but has no overt bleeding condition, this is reported with R79.1 as the adverse effect manifestation, followed by T45.515 with the appropriate seventh character.

First Listed Diagnosis Note

Admit to reverse anticoagulation prior to a procedure: The reason/condition for the procedure is the first listed diagnosis, followed by Z51.81 for drug monitoring, Z79.Ø1 for long-term anticoagulant use and the code for the condition under treatment/prophylaxis by the medication.

Admit due to skin necrosis due to anticoagulation therapy: Gangrene I96 will be the first listed diagnosis as the nature of the adverse effect (manifestation) followed by T45.515 with the appropriate seventh character.

Underdosing of anticoagulants (T45.516)

Clinical Tip

Underdosing is a new concept in ICD-10-CM and is defined as a circumstance in which a patient has taken less of a medication than is prescribed by a provider or a manufacturer's instruction. Taking less of a drug than prescribed can cause breakthrough symptoms of the underlying condition or may cause other problems. The clinical effects of underdosing of a drug should be classified separately.

Clinician Note

Ensure that all other conditions are appropriately coded, such as specific drug reactions or complications of poisonings, adverse effects, and underdosings.

 **CDI ALERT**

Although it may appear counterintuitive to have an underdosing circumstance classified together with drug poisonings and adverse effects, the circumstances surrounding any encounter involving either prescribed or over the counter drugs must be documented clearly. Ensure that clinicians are aware that this classification axis is now available.

Clinical Findings

Physical Examination

History and review of systems may include:

- Ecchymoses
- Subconjunctival hemorrhage
- Epistaxis
- Vaginal bleeding
- Bleeding gums
- Hematuria

Diagnostic Procedures and Services

- Laboratory
  - prothrombin elevated

Therapeutic Procedures and Services

- Blood transfusion may be necessary (packed red cells)
- Medication
  - vitamin K

Clinician Documentation Checklist

Clinician documentation should indicate the following:

- Identify the medical condition being treated
- Adverse effect was a result of
  - accidental poisoning
  - intentional self-harm
  - assault
  - undetermined
  - under dosing

Critical Care Services

Code Axes

Critical Care **99291–99292**

Description of Procedure

These services are rendered for the care of a patient who has an illness or injury to one or more vital organ systems such that there is the high probability of imminent or life-threatening deterioration to the patient's condition. These services are based upon the time spent involved in activities directly related to the patient's care and need not be strictly spent at the bedside but rather on a patient's floor or unit.

Critical care, evaluation and management of the critically ill or critically injured patient (99291–99292)

Clinician Documentation Tip

The Clinician documentation must indicate the time spent providing the critical care services, the procedures and services performed, and the nature of the condition requiring the service. Note that there are a number of procedures bundled into critical care services and, therefore, not separately reported. See the CPT® manual or payer guidelines for a list of these services.

Clinician Documentation Checklist

Clinician documentation should indicate the following:

- Identify illness or injury reason for encounter
- Type of vital organ failure
  - central nervous system failure
  - circulatory failure
  - shock
  - renal
  - hepatic
  - metabolic
  - respiratory
- Start/stop time spent providing critical care services
- Procedures performed

Crohn's Disease

⇨ I-10 ALERT

Combination codes include information related not only to site of the disease, but to specific complication.

Code Axes

Note: Sixth characters for subcategories K5Ø.Ø1, K5Ø.11, K5Ø.81, and K5Ø.91 include that for rectal bleeding, intestinal obstruction, fistula, abscess, and other and unspecified complications.

Crohn's disease of small intestine without complications	**K5Ø.ØØ**
Crohn's disease of small intestine with complications	**K5Ø.Ø1**
Crohn's disease of large intestine without complications	**K5Ø.1Ø**
Crohn's disease of large intestine with complications	**K5Ø.11**
Crohn's disease of both small and large intestine without complications	**K5Ø.8Ø**
Crohn's disease of both small and large intestine with complications	**K5Ø.81**
Crohn's disease, unspecified, without complications	**K5Ø.9Ø**
Crohn's disease, unspecified, with complications	**K5Ø.91**

CDI ALERT

Ensure that if any of the following complications are present they are clearly documented in the medical record: rectal bleeding, intestinal obstruction, fistula, or abscess. Any other complications that are indicated as being due to Crohn's disease should also be documented.

Clinical Tip

Crohn's disease is similar to other inflammatory bowel diseases including irritable bowel syndrome and ulcerative colitis and is usually differentiated by location and severity. While Crohn's disease can affect the mucus membranes of the digestive tract from the mouth to the anus, it most commonly affects the ileum (small bowel) and the cecum. Ulcerative colitis primarily affects the large bowel. Additionally, some experts use the following three endoscopic findings as evidence of Crohn's:

Aphthous ulcers: Small, discrete aphthous ulcers (canker sores) appear in the early stages of the disease and progress to involve the entire wall of the bowel; may grow to several centimeters.

Cobblestoning: Normal tissues in between the ulcers indicate the typical cobblestone appearance.

Discontinuous lesions: Areas of inflammation are scattered between normal bowel "skip areas."

Ulcerative colitis and Crohn's disease are very similar. The table below describes some of the differences.

Ulcerative Colitis	Crohn's Disease
Limited to colon	Entire GI tract (mouth to anus)
Continuous inflammation	Inflammation with intermittent inflammation
Inner most lining	All layers within bowel walls

Key Terms

Key terms found in the documentation may include:

CD

Crohn's disease

Crohn's disease of colon, large bowel, or rectum

Granulomatous colitis

Regional enteritis

Regional ileitis or colitis

Terminal ileitis

Clinical Findings

Physical Examination

- Check for bowel sounds
- Abdominal palpation for pain, tenderness, and distention

Diagnostic Procedures and Services

- Laboratory
  - stool guaiac: positive if active bleeding
  - CBC: may indicate blood loss anemia or elevated WBCs
  - pathology examination of tissue biopsies characterized by transmural (full-thickness) inflammation
- Imaging
  - colonoscopy
  - EGD
  - ERCP
  - small bowel endoscopy
  - upper GI series
  - barium enema

Therapeutic Procedures and Services

- Medications
  - loperamide
  - metronidazole
  - ciprofloxacin (in cases of present fistulas)
  - antispasmodics
  - 5-ASA
- Dietary restrictions
- Antibiotics in instances of fulminant disease or abscess
- Surgical intervention

Clinician Note

Fistulas and abscesses are common complications of Crohn's disease. Carefully review clinical documentation and, if present, assign the appropriate code from category K5Ø as well as the appropriate code indicating the specific type of fistula/abscess.

Clinician Documentation Checklist

Clinician documentation should indicate the following:

- Includes
  - granulomatous enteritis
- Identify
  - manifestations such as pyoderma gangrenosum
  - part of intestinal tract involved
    - small intestine
      - ♦ Crohn's disease of duodenum
      - ♦ Crohn's disease of ileum
      - ♦ Crohn's disease of jejunum
      - ♦ regional ileitis
      - ♦ terminal ileitis
    - large intestine
      - ♦ Crohn's disease of colon
      - ♦ Crohn's disease of large bowel
      - ♦ Crohn's disease of rectum
      - ♦ granulomatous colitis
      - ♦ regional colitis
    - both small and large intestine
    - unspecified part
      - ♦ Crohn's disease
      - ♦ regional enteritis
  - associated
    - without complications
    - with complications
      - ♦ rectal bleeding
      - ♦ intestinal obstruction
      - ♦ fistula
      - ♦ abscess
      - ♦ other complication
      - ♦ unspecified complications

Cutaneous Abscess, Furuncle, and Carbuncle

Code Axes

Cutaneous abscess, furuncle and carbuncle of face	**LØ2.Ø-**
Cutaneous abscess, furuncle and carbuncle of neck	**LØ2.1-**
Cutaneous abscess, furuncle and carbuncle of trunk	**LØ2.2-**
Cutaneous abscess, furuncle and carbuncle of buttock	**LØ2.3-**
Cutaneous abscess, furuncle and carbuncle of limb	**LØ2.4-**
Cutaneous abscess, furuncle and carbuncle of hand	**LØ2.5-**
Cutaneous abscess, furuncle and carbuncle of foot	**LØ2.6-**
Cutaneous abscess, furuncle and carbuncle of other sites	**LØ2.8-**
Cutaneous abscess, furuncle and carbuncle, unspecified	**LØ2.9-**

I-10 Alert

ICD-10-CM classifies cellulitis (LØ3) and abscess (LØ2) in separate code categories based on whether the infection is encapsulated or contained (abscess, furuncle, carbuncle) or spread throughout the skin, subcutaneous tissues (cellulitis) and lymph channels (lymphangitis).

Infection of the lymph glands or nodes (LØ4) is classified separately.

Description of Condition

Cutaneous abscess, furuncle and carbuncle (LØ2)

Clinical Tip

A cutaneous abscess is a collection of pus resulting from an acute or chronic localized skin infection. Pus is the byproduct of tissue damage, fluid, and white blood cells formed by the body's immune response to fight off pathogens (e.g., infection, foreign substances).

A furuncle (boil) is a painful nodule formed by circumscribed inflammation of the skin and subcutaneous tissue that encloses a central core, usually the base of a hair follicle.

Furuncles may be caused by *Staphylococcus* or other bacteria. Accumulation of pus and tissue results in pressure, causing pain that is relieved by drainage.

Carbuncle, furuncle, and abscess are localized, contained pockets of infection. A carbuncle is a collection of pus contained in a cavity or sac, often associated with a hair follicle or groups of hair follicles that form a hardened, circumscribed lump deep in the skin tissues. Carbuncles are commonly associated with *Staphylococcus aureus* infection

A carbuncle is often described as a collection of lesions or boils.

CDI Alert

Abscess and cellulitis are classified separately in ICD-10-CM by severity, anatomic site, and laterality. Ensure documentation is specific regarding extent of infection to avoid misrepresentation of severity.

Documentation of site and laterality should be thorough and specific to avoid reporting unspecified codes.

Code category LØ3 may indicate a severity progression of infection from localized (LØ2) to adjacent tissues that increases the risk for potentially fatal serious systemic infection (sepsis) from circulating pathogens.

I-10 ALERT

Category LØ2 Cutaneous abscess, furuncle and carbuncle, includes valid codes that are five or six characters in length. The following axes of classification describe:

- Fourth character:
  - Anatomic site or region
- Fifth character:
  - Type of infection: abscess furuncle or carbuncle
  - Anatomic site
- Sixth character:
  - Anatomic site specificity (further specification of site)
  - Laterality

Key terms

Key terms found in the documentation may include:

Boil

Folliculitis

Furunculosis

Documentation Tip

Specify the nature of the localized infection. Differentiate between abscess, furuncle, and carbuncle. Document the specific anatomic site. For upper limb infections, the axilla is a separately identifiable anatomic site from the upper limb. For paired anatomic sites, specify laterality (right or left).

For example:

Cutaneous abscess of right axilla	(LØ2.411)
Cutaneous abscess of the right upper limb	(LØ2.412)

Clinical Findings

Physical Examination

- Examination of skin for localized infection
- Examination of neck, breasts, face, and buttocks for furuncles
- Examination for carbuncles: may be accompanied by fever and prostration
  - usually described as 1 to 3 cm in size

Diagnostic Procedures and Services

- Laboratory
  - culture for infective agent
  - gram stain

Therapeutic Procedures and Services

- Incision and drainage
- Antibiotics when signs of systemic infection

Clinician Documentation Checklist

Clinician documentation should indicate the following:

- Identification of
  - infectious organism (e.g., bacterial)
- Furuncle includes
  - boil
  - folliculitis
  - furunculosis
- Document site of cutaneous abscess, furuncle, and carbuncle
  - face
  - neck

- trunk
  - abdominal wall
  - back (any part except buttock)
  - chest wall
  - groin
  - perineum
  - umbilicus
  - unspecified part
- buttock
  - gluteal region
- limb
  - axilla
  - upper limb
  - lower limb
  - unspecified part of limb
- hand
- foot
- other sites
  - head (any part, except face)
  - other site
- unspecified site

• Identify the laterality of axilla, upper and lower limb, hand, and foot
  - right
  - left

Cystoscopies, Urethroscopies and Cystourethroscopies

Code Axes

Endoscopy—cystoscopy, urethroscopy, cystourethroscopy **52000–52356**

Description of Procedure

These codes represent the endoscopic examination of the urethra, bladder, and ureteric openings into the bladder through an endoscope. Documentation should specify if the procedure is diagnostic or therapeutic, and if therapeutic, what procedures or services were performed.

Clinician documentation should include the following key terms as they apply in order to determine correct code assignment.

Key Term	Code
Biopsy	
Urethra and bladder	52204
Ureter or renal pelvic	52354
Dilation	
Bladder	52260–52265
Intrarenal	52343, 52346
Ureteral	52341, 52344
Urethral	52281, 52285
Ureteropelvic	52342, 52345
Diverticulum	
Bladder	52305
Excision	
Urethra and bladder	
Minor lesions	52224
Small bladder tumor	52234
Medium bladder tumor	52235
Large bladder tumor	52240
Ureteral or renal pelvic tumor	52355
Fulguration	
Bladder neck	52214
Lesions	
Bladder and urethra	52214–52250, 52285
Ureter	52300, 52301

Key Term	Code
Lesions (Continued)	
Periurethral glands	52214
Prostatic fossa	52214
Trigone	52214
Ureteral or renal pelvic lesion	52354
Urethra	52214
Injection	
Chemodenervation, bladder	52287
Radiocontrast, radiologic study, bladder	52281
Into urethral/bladder stricture	52283
Subureteric implant material	52327
Insertion	
Guidewire	52334
Stent	
Urethra	52282
Ureter	52332
Lithotripsy	
Ureter and Pelvis	52353, 52356
Manipulation	
Ureteral calculus	52330, 52352
Pyeloscopy	52351
Radioactive substance	52250
Removal	
Calculus	
Urethra or bladder	52310–52315
Ureter and pelvis	52320–52325, 52352
By litholapaxy	52317–52318
Foreign Body	52310–52315
Stent	
Ureteral	52310–52315, 52356
Sphincterotomy	52277
Tumor	
Bladder	52234–52240
Ureteral or renal pelvic	52355
Ureter Surgery	
Meatotomy	52290
Ureterocele	52300–52301
Urethral syndrome	52285
Ureteroscopy	52351
Urethrotomy	52270–52276

CDI ALERT

Documentation should be reviewed to determine why the procedure was performed (e.g., for removal of foreign body, biopsy, excision of tumor, etc.).

Depression — Major

Code Axes

Major depressive disorder, single episode, mild	**F32.Ø**
Major depressive disorder, single episode, moderate	**F32.1**
Major depressive disorder, single episode, severe without psychotic features	**F32.2**
Major depressive disorder, single episode, severe with psychotic features	**F32.3**
Major depressive disorder, single episode, in partial remission	**F32.4**
Major depressive disorder, single episode, in full remission	**F32.5**
Other depressive episodes	**F32.8**
Major depressive disorder, single episode, unspecified	**F32.9**
Major depressive disorder, recurrent, mild	**F33.Ø**
Major depressive disorder, recurrent, moderate	**F33.1**
Major depressive disorder, recurrent, severe without psychotic features	**F33.2**
Major depressive disorder, recurrent, severe with psychotic symptoms	**F33.3**
Major depressive disorder, recurrent, in remission, unspecified	**F33.4Ø**
Major depressive disorder, recurrent, in partial remission	**F33.41**
Major depressive disorder, recurrent, in full remission	**F33.42**
Other recurrent depressive disorders	**F33.8**
Major depressive disorder, recurrent, unspecified	**F33.9**

Description of Condition

Major depressive disorder (F32.-, F33.-)

Major depressive disorder is a disabling condition which impacts social, interpersonal and physical functioning. It is characterized by a combination of traits: pervasive, persistent depressed mood, loss of interest or pleasure in usually enjoyable activities and reduced energy.

Key Terms

Key terms found in the documentation may include:

Depressive disorder, recurrent, severe, without psychotic symptoms

Masked depression (single episode)

MDD

Psychogenic depression, single episode

Reactive depression

QUERY NOTE

Excludes 1 note at F31 and F32, F33 indicates that bipolar disorder (depression/hypomania) cannot be reported with major depressive disorder. When both are documented, query for clarification. Additionally, for some types of major depressive disorders such as psychotic, the physician should be queried when documentation does not indicate if the episode is single or recurrent.

Clinical Findings

Physical Examination

History and review of systems may include:

- Interview of patient with no physical findings
- Fatigue
- Sleeping problem
- Loss of appetite or over eating
- Depressed mood that is frequent, persistent, and sad
- Frequent or persistent intense feeling of guilt
- Suicidal thoughts
- Inability to feel pleasure or take interest in things
- Difficulty in concentrating and focusing
- Impaired judgment, planning, or problem-solving
- Low self-esteem
- Pessimism
- Feelings of loneliness
- Unassertiveness
- Difficulty handling conflict
- Social withdrawal

Therapeutic Procedures and Services

- Psychotherapy
- Antidepressant medication
  - tricyclic antidepressants (TCA)
  - amitriptyline
  - amoxapine
  - desipramine (Norpramin)
  - doxepin
  - imipramine (Tofranil)
  - nortriptyline (Pamelor)
  - protriptyline (Vivactil)
  - trimipramine (Surmontil)

- Selective serotonin reuptake inhibitors (SSRI)
  - Brintellix
  - Lexapro
  - Luvox
  - Paxil
  - Prozac
  - Zoloft
  - Viibryd

Clinician Note
Documentation should specify whether this is a single episode or recurrent, the current degree of depression, the presence of psychotic features or symptoms, and remission status (i.e., partial, full) when applicable.

Clinician Documentation Checklist

Clinician documentation should indicate the following:

- Type of mood disorder
  - manic episode
  - bipolar disorder
  - major depressive disorder
  - persistent mood (affective) disorder
    - cyclothymic
    - dysthymic
- Frequency of occurrence
  - single episode
  - recurrent episode
  - part of bipolar disorder
- Level of severity
  - hypomanic: for bipolar
  - depressed
  - mild
  - moderate
  - mixed: for bipolar
  - severe
- Psychotic symptoms or features
  - presence of psychotic symptoms or features
    - if present, the level of severity is severe
  - absence of psychotic symptoms or features

Diabetes Mellitus

Code Axes

Note: Subclassifications exist for subcategories EØ8, EØ9, E1Ø, E11, and E13 to represent manifestations including hyperosmolarity, ketoacidosis, kidney complications (e.g., CKD), ophthalmic complications (e.g., retinopathy, cataract), neurological complications (e.g., neuropathy, amyotrophy), circulatory complications (e.g., peripheral angiography, gangrene), skin complications (e.g., dermatitis, foot ulcer), oral complications (e.g., periodontal disease), hypoglycemia, hyperglycemia, other and unspecified complications.

Diabetes mellitus due to underlying condition	**EØ8.-**
Drug or chemical induced diabetes mellitus	**EØ9.-**
Type 1 diabetes mellitus	**E1Ø.-**
Type 2 diabetes mellitus	**E11.-**
Other specified diabetes mellitus	**E13.-**

I-10 ALERT

Each of the five subcategories for diabetes mellitus follows the same format, with combination codes for the most commonly diagnosed diabetic complications.

CDI ALERT

Ensure that the type of diabetes is clearly documented as it is essential for appropriate classification purposes.

Description of Condition

Diabetes mellitus due to underlying condition (EØ8.-)

Diabetes or glucose intolerance due to an underlying condition other than genetics or environmental conditions is found in category EØ8.

Key Terms

Key terms found in the documentation may include:

Cystic fibrosis-related diabetes (CFRD)

Malnutrition-related diabetes (MRDM) (MMDM)

Clinical Tip

Although rarer than type 1 or type 2 diabetes, it is important to be able to track and classify the type of diabetes due to other underlying conditions. Examples of this type of condition include: chronic pancreatitis; cystic fibrosis; hemochromatosis pancreatic cancers; liver diseases, including hepatitis C; carcinoid tumors of the lungs, intestines or stomach; celiac disease and other autoimmune diseases and malnutrition.

Clinician Note

Many payers, including Medicare, have quality measures in place to determine that quality and cost effective care is provided to the patient. It is imperative that the diabetes and any associated conditions or complications be documented in the medical record. Documentation should include statements that demonstrate the condition and therapy was monitored, evaluated, assessed/addressed, and/or treated on the current encounter.

I-10 ALERT

Although a drug or chemical causing a diabetic condition can technically be considered an "underlying condition," there is a separate subcategory for those diabetic conditions caused by drugs or chemicals (EØ9).

I-10 ALERT

It is uncommon for a provider to document "Borderline Diabetes Mellitus". According to the official ICD-10-CM Official Coding Guidelines when the documentation contains a statement such as "borderline" the diagnosis at the time of discharge is coded as confirmed unless the classification provides a specific entry (e.g., borderline diabetes). The ICD-10-CM index contains the main term "Borderline," subterm "diabetes mellitus," referencing code R73.Ø9. For this reason, documentation in this instance would not support a code from the EØ8 through E11 categories.

Drug or chemical induced diabetes mellitus (EØ9.-)

Diabetes due to drug or chemical ingestion is found in category EØ9. Poisoning would be reported for overdose or substance taken improperly; adverse effect indicates it was properly prescribed and taken but which resulted in an adverse reaction.

Key Terms

Key terms found in the documentation may include:

Steroid induced diabetes

Clinical Tip

Some drugs and chemicals, whether considered therapeutic or not, can have unintended consequences and can cause diabetic conditions.

Examples of drugs known to cause diabetes include: hormone supplements, antihypertensive diuretics and beta blockers, antipsychotics and some antidepressants, some anticonvulsants, antiretrovirals, and immunosuppressives.

Clinician Note

Many payers, including Medicare, have quality measures in place to determine that quality and cost effective care is provided to the patient. It is imperative that the diabetes and any associated conditions or complications be documented in the medical record. Documentation should include statements that demonstrate the condition and therapy was monitored, evaluated, assessed/addressed, and/or treated on the current encounter.

⇨ I-10 ALERT

If the diabetic condition is due to a drug or chemical poisoning, the code for that poisoning should be sequenced first, with the EØ9 code sequenced as a manifestation. If it is due to an adverse reaction to a drug properly administered, the code for the drug with adverse effect (T36–T5Ø) should be assigned as a secondary condition to identify the drug itself; the manifestation (EØ9) will be sequenced first.

CDI ALERT

Diabetes described as "out of control," "inadequately controlled," or "poorly controlled" is reported as the specified type of diabetes with hyperglycemia, fourth character 6. When another diabetic complication is present and the diabetes is stated as poorly controlled, etc., both complications are reported. The exception is diabetes with ketoacidosis: report only the code for diabetes with ketoacidosis as it is inherently uncontrolled.

Type 1 diabetes mellitus (E1Ø.-)

Type 1 diabetes mellitus results from autoimmune destruction of insulin-producing beta cells of the pancreas resulting in little or no insulin production; it is a chronic condition characterized by hyperglycemia; insulin must be taken daily. Triggers can interact with genetic susceptibility at any age to produce type 1 diabetes. Type 1.5 diabetes mellitus has characteristics of both type 1 and type 2 but is autoimmune and manifests in adults, thus it is known as latent autoimmune diabetes of adulthood. Since diabetes type 1.5 is not recognized in ICD-10-CM, query if the diabetes is type 1 or type 2.

Key Terms

Key terms found in the documentation for type 1 diabetes may include:

Diabetes due to autoimmune process

Diabetes due to immune mediated pancreatic islet beta-cell destruction

Idiopathic diabetes

Juvenile onset diabetes

Ketosis-prone diabetes

Latent autoimmune diabetes of adults (Type 1.5)

Slow onset type 1 diabetes

⇨ I-10 ALERT

Codes for typical diabetic type 1 conditions are now presented with more combination code choices, for the most commonly reported diabetic complications. Subcategory codes for hyperosmolarity are not found in this subgroup of codes.

Clinician Note
Many payers, including Medicare, have quality measures in place to determine that quality and cost effective care is provided to the patient. It is imperative that the diabetes and any associated conditions or complications be documented in the medical record. Documentation should include statements that demonstrate the condition and therapy was monitored, evaluated, assessed/addressed, and/or treated on the current encounter.

I-10 ALERT

Codes for typical diabetic type 2 conditions are now presented with more combination code choices, for the most commonly reported diabetic complications.

Type 2 diabetes mellitus (E11.-)

Type 2 diabetes mellitus is a metabolic disorder that involves high blood glucose in the context of insulin resistance and relative insulin deficiency. Unlike type 1 diabetics, those with type 2 diabetes have insulin produced in the pancreas, but it is either in small quantities or their bodies are resistant to it. It is caused by an interaction of lifestyle choices and genetics. This is a chronic condition but can be maintained by anti-diabetic medications, insulin, or diet regimen.

CDI ALERT

The age documented in the medical record is not used to select the type of diabetes mellitus unless other documentation is noted. When the documentation does not indicate the type of diabetes the clinician should be queried. If not, the appropriate code from category E11 (diabetes mellitus type 2) is reported.

Key Terms
Key terms found in the documentation for type 2 diabetes may include:

Diabetes due to insulin secretory defect

Diabetes NOS

DMII

Insulin resistant diabetes

I-10 ALERT

If the documentation in a medical record does not indicate the type of diabetes but does indicate that the patient uses insulin, a code from category E11 Type 2 diabetes mellitus, should be assigned. Code Z79.4 or Z79.84 should also be assigned to indicate that the patient uses insulin or hypoglycemic drugs. Code Z79.4 should not be assigned if insulin is given temporarily to bring a type 2 patient's blood sugar under control during an encounter.

Clinician Note
Many payers, including Medicare have quality measures in place to determine that quality and cost effective care is provided to the patient. It is imperative that the diabetes and any associated conditions or complication be documented in the medical record. Documentation should include statements that demonstrate the condition and therapy was monitored, evaluated, assessed/addressed, and/or treated on the current encounter.

Other specified diabetes mellitus (E13.-)

There are several other types of diabetes that are caused by various other mechanisms. One type involves the body's tissue receptors not responding to insulin, even when insulin levels are normal, which is what differentiates it from type 2 diabetes. In other cases, genetic mutations (autosomal or mitochondrial) can lead to defects in pancreatic beta cell function. Diseases associated with excessive secretion of insulin-antagonistic hormones can cause diabetes; this condition is typically resolved once the hormone excess is removed.

I-10 ALERT

Ensure that the medical record documentation does not specify a diabetic disease process that could be classified in one of the other four subcategories of diabetes mellitus codes.

⇨ I-10 ALERT

The ICD-10-CM Official Coding Guidelines state that when documentation indicates postpancreatectomy diabetes mellitus (lack of insulin due to the surgical removal of all or part of the pancreas), code E89.1 Postprocedural hypoinsulinemia should be reported. Report a code from subcategory Z90.41 Acquired absence of pancreas, and a code from category E13 as additional codes.

Key Terms

Key terms found in the documentation for other specified diabetes may include:

Diabetes mellitus due to genetic defects in insulin action

Diabetes mellitus due to genetic defects of beta-cell function

Postpancreatectomy diabetes mellitus

Postprocedural diabetes mellitus

Secondary diabetes mellitus NEC

Clinical Findings

The table listed below will help differentiate between type1 and type 2 diabetes mellitus.

Finding	Type 1	Type 2
Age of onset	Most commonly 30 years or younger	Most commonly over 30 years
Obesity	Not associated	Associated
Propensity to ketoacidosis	Yes, usually requires insulin	Variable
Associated with HLA-D	Yes	No
Islet pathology	Insulitis	Normal appearing islets
Prone to develop associated complications	Yes	Yes
Hyperglycemia responds to antihyperglycemic drugs	No	Yes

Signs and symptoms include hyperglycemia, urinary frequency, polyuria, and polydipsia. Patients with type 1 diabetes mellitus typically present symptomatic. Patients with type 2 diabetes mellitus are often asymptomatic and the condition is found during routine testing.

Diagnostic Procedures and Services

- Laboratory
  - fasting plasma/serum glucose
  - hemoglobin A1C
  - urine testing for proteinuria and microalbuminuria
  - serum creatinine
  - lipid profile
- Imaging
  - fundoscopy for ophthalmologic disorders
- Other
  - diabetic foot screening
  - Therapeutic Procedures and Services
- Home blood sugar monitoring
- Dietary restrictions (concentrated sugars)
- Insulin

Clinician Note

Many payers, including Medicare have quality measures in place to determine that quality and cost effective care is provided to the patient. It is imperative that the diabetes and any associated conditions or complications be documented in the medical record. Documentation should include statements that demonstrate the condition and therapy was monitored, evaluated, assessed/addressed, and/or treated on the current encounter.

Clinician Documentation Checklist

Clinician documentation should indicate the following:

- Type 1
  - juvenile onset
  - ketosis-prone
  - idiopathic
  - brittle
  - due to autoimmune process
  - due to immune mediated pancreatic islet beta-cell destruction
- Type 2
  - due to insulin secretory defect
  - insulin resistant
  - insulin use, if any
- Drug or chemical induced
  - the drug
  - insulin use, if any
- Due to underlying condition
  - underlying conditions
    - Cushing syndrome
    - cystic fibrosis
    - malignant neoplasm
    - malnutrition
    - pancreatitis and other diseases of pancreas
  - insulin use, if any
- Other specified causes
  - due to genetic defects of beta-cell function
  - due to genetic defects in insulin action
  - postpancreatectomy
  - postprocedural
  - secondary
- Associated complications
  - ketoacidosis
    - without coma
    - with coma
  - hyperosmolarity

- — without nonketotic hyperglycemic-hyperosmolar coma
- — with coma

- Kidney
  - With diabetic nephropathy
    - — intercapillary glomerulosclerosis
    - — intracapillary glomerulosclerosis
    - — Kimmelstiel-Wilson disease
  - with diabetic chronic kidney disease
    - — stage of chronic kidney disease
  - with other diabetic kidney complication
    - — renal tubular degeneration
- Ophthalmic
  - with or without macular edema
    - — unspecified diabetic retinopathy
    - — mild nonproliferative diabetic retinopathy
    - — moderate nonproliferative diabetic retinopathy
    - — severe nonproliferative diabetic retinopathy
    - — proliferative diabetic retinopathy
  - with diabetic cataract
  - with other diabetic ophthalmic complication
- Neurological
  - mononeuropathy
  - polyneuropathy
    - — diabetic neuralgia
  - autonomic (poly) neuropathy
  - diabetic gastroparesis
  - amyotrophy
- Circulatory
  - peripheral angiopathy
    - — with gangrene
    - — without gangrene
- Diabetes mellitus in pregnancy, childbirth, and puerperium
  - type
    - — pre-existing diabetes mellitus, type1
    - — pre-existing diabetes mellitus, type2
    - — gestational diabetes mellitus
    - — diet controlled
    - — insulin controlled
    - — trimester

Drug Dependence

(Opioid F11, Cannabis F12, Sedative F13, Cocaine F14, Other Stimulant F15, Hallucinogen F16, Inhalant F18, Other Psychoactive Substance F19)

Code Axes

Drug/substance dependence, uncomplicated	**F1[1-6, 8-9].2Ø** **F1[1, 3-6, 9].2Ø**
Drug/substance dependence, in remission	**F1[1-6, 8-9].21**
Drug/substance dependence with intoxication, uncomplicated	**F1[1-6, 8-9].22Ø** **F11.22Ø**
Drug/substance dependence with intoxication delirium	**F1[1-6, 8-9].221**
Drug/substance dependence with intoxication with perceptual disturbance	**F1[1, 3-5, 9].222** **F1[1, 3-5, 9].222**

Note: F16.2 Hallucinogen is not reported in this subcategory.

Drug/substance dependence with intoxication, unspecified	**F1[1-6, 8-9].229** **F1[1, 3, 4].229**
Drug/substance dependence with withdrawal	**F1[1, 4, 5].23**
Drug/substance dependence with withdrawal, uncomplicated	**F1[3, 9].23Ø**
Drug/substance dependence with withdrawal delirium	**F1[3, 9].231**
Drug/substance dependence with withdrawal with perceptual disturbance	**F1[3, 9].232**
Drug/substance dependence with withdrawal, unspecified	**F1[3, 9].239**
Drug/substance dependence with drug-induced mood disorder	**F1[1, 3-6, 8-9].24**
Drug/substance dependence with drug-induced psychotic disorder with delusions	**F1[1- 6, 8-9].25Ø**
Drug/substance dependence with drug-induced psychotic disorder with hallucinations	**F1[1-6, 8-9].251**
Drug/substance dependence with drug-induced psychotic disorder, unspecified	**F1[1, 3-6, 8-9].259**
Drug/substance dependence with drug-induced persisting amnestic disorder	**F1[3, 9].26**
Drug/substance dependence with drug-induced persisting dementia	**F1[3, 8-9].27**
Drug/substance dependence with other drug-induced disorder, anxiety disorder	**F1[2-6, 8-9].28Ø** **F1[2-6, 8-9].28Ø**

Drug/substance dependence with opioid-induced sexual dysfunction **F1[1, 3-5, 9].281**

Drug/substance dependence with drug-induced sleep disorder **F1[1, 3-5, 9].282**

Drug/substance dependence with hallucinogen persisting perception disorder (flashbacks) **F16.283**

Note: this subcategory pertains to Hallucinogen drugs only.

Drug/substance dependence with other drug-induced disorder **F1[1-6, 8-9].288**
F1[1, 3-6, 8-9].288

Drug/substance dependence with unspecified drug-induced disorder **F1[1-6, 8-9].29**
F1[1, 3, 8].29

Description of Condition

Drug dependence (F11.2, F12.2, F13.2, F14.2, F15.2, F16.2, F18.2, F19.2)

Drug/substance dependence is a chronic disorder characterized by use of large amounts of or frequent use of a drug/substance or multiple drugs/substances in which the individual becomes physically and mentally dependent upon to function. Long-term consequences are physical, psychological, and behavioral. Criterion denoting dependence is increased tolerance and continued use despite impairment of health, social life, and job performance. Cessation results in withdrawal symptoms, including early seizures.

CDI ALERT

When a blood test gives evidence of the presence of alcohol/drugs without documentation of substance use, abuse, or dependence and the information is provider-documented and has clinical significance for the encounter and/or meets criteria as an additional diagnosis, report the appropriate code from category R78.[Ø-6].

Key Terms

Key terms found in the documentation may include:

Chronic drug dependence

Drug addiction

Drug dependence

Inhalant dependence

Clinical Findings

Physical Examination

Signs and symptoms reveal intoxication followed by withdrawal from the drug when discontinued. This may be either minor or severe.

Findings of physical withdrawal include:

- Sweating
- Racing heart
- Palpitations
- Muscle tension
- Tightness in the chest
- Difficulty breathing

- Tremor
- Nausea, vomiting, or diarrhea
- Grand mal seizures
- Heart attacks
- Strokes
- Hallucinations
- Delirium tremens (DT)

Emotional withdrawal symptoms include:

- Anxiety
- Restlessness
- Irritability
- Insomnia
- Headaches
- Poor concentration
- Depression
- Social isolation

Diagnostic Procedures and Services

- Laboratory
  - drug screening
  - hepatitis panel
  - laboratory panel
  - CBC
  - HIV screening
  - chemistry panel
- Other
  - EKG

Clinician Note

The provider must state the pattern of harmful usage (dependence, abuse or use) and its current clinical state (uncomplicated, intoxication, remission, etc.) and indicate the relationship to any identified mental, behavioral, or physical disorder or its relevance to the patient's status or encounter including its clinical significance. The specific drug(s) or substance should be identified and documented and in cases of legal medication indicated if it had been prescribed for that individual. Classification should be made according to the most important drug/substance or class of drug/substance used or causing the presenting disorder.

⇨ I-10 ALERT

According to ICD-10-CM Official Coding Guidelines, when documentation indicates the presence of use, abuse, and dependence of the same substance, only one code is reported. The following reporting hierarchy is used when assigning the ICD-10-CM codes:

- If both use and abuse are documented, assign only the code for abuse.
- If both abuse and dependence are documented, the code for dependence only is reported.
- If use, abuse, and dependence are all documented, the code for dependence only is reported
- If both use and dependence are documented, the code for dependence only is reported

Clinician Documentation Checklist

Clinician documentation should indicate the following:

Psychoactive Substance

- Name of substance
  - alcohol
    - blood alcohol level
  - anxiolytics, cannabis, cocaine, hallucinogens, hypnotics, inhalants, nicotine, opioids, sedatives, volatile solvents
  - polysubstance
- Level of substance use
  - use
  - abuse
  - dependence
- Any additional description of use
  - intoxication
  - remission
  - withdrawal
- Associated psychoactive-induced disorders
  - anxiety
  - delirium
  - delusions
  - hallucinations
  - mood disorder
  - perception disturbance
  - persisting amnestic disorder
  - persisting dementia
  - psychotic disorder
  - sexual dysfunction
  - sleep disorder

Nonpsychoactive Substance Abuse

- Name of nonpsychoactive substance
  - antacids
  - herbal/folk remedies
  - laxatives
  - steroids/hormones
  - vitamins
  - other

Drug/Substance Abuse

(Opioid F11, Cannabis F12, Sedative F13, Cocaine F14, Other Stimulant F15, Hallucinogen F16, Inhalant F18, Other Psychoactive Substance F19)

Code Axes

Drug/substance abuse, uncomplicated	**F1[1-6, 8-9].1Ø**
Drug/substance abuse with intoxication, uncomplicated	**F1[1-6, 8-9].12Ø**
Drug/substance abuse with intoxication, delirium	**F1[1-6, 8-9].121**
Drug/substance abuse with intoxication with perceptual disturbance	**F1[1-2, 4-6, 9].122** **F11.122**
Drug/substance abuse with intoxication, unspecified	**F1[1-6, 8-9].129**
Drug/substance abuse with drug-induced mood disorder	**F1[1, 3-6, 8-9].14**
Drug/substance abuse with drug-induced psychotic disorder with delusions	**F1[1-6, 8-9].15Ø**
Drug/substance abuse with drug-induced psychotic disorder with hallucinations	**F1[1-6, 8-9].151**
Drug/substance abuse with other drug-induced psychotic disorder, unspecified	**F1[1-6, 8-9].159**
Drug/substance abuse with drug-induced persisting amnestic disorder	**F19.16**
Note: Psychoactive substance abuse only for this subcategory.	
Drug/substance abuse with drug-induced persisting dementia	**F1[8-9].17**
Note: Only psychoactive substance and inhalant abuse are in this subcategory.	
Drug/substance abuse with other drug-induced disorder, anxiety disorder	**F1[2-6, 8-9].18Ø**
Drug/substance abuse with other drug-induced disorder, sexual dysfunction	**F1[1, 3-5, 9].181**
Drug/substance abuse with drug-induced sleep disorder	**F1[1, 3, 4-5, 9].182**
Drug/substance abuse with drug-induced persisting perception disorder (flashbacks)	**F16.183**
Note: Hallucinogen drug abuse only for this subcategory.	
Drug/substance abuse with other drug-induced disorder	**F1[1-6, 8-9].188**
To use this code, the other drug-related disorder must be specified and not found in any other subcategory.	
Drug/substance abuse with unspecified drug-induced disorder	**F1[1-6, 8-9].19**

Description of Condition

Drug/substance abuse (F11.1, F12.1, F13.1, F14.1, F15.1, F16.1, F18.1, F19.1)

Drug/substance abuse is characterized by recurring misuse of a drug in excess with identifiable harmful and dysfunctional behaviors and negative consequences for health, psycho-social state, and employment. It lacks the criteria of dependency. Time frame for consideration of abuse would be persisting for at least one month or has occurred repeatedly within a 12 month period.

Key Terms

Key terms found in the documentation may include:

Drug Use Disorder of:

- Barbiturate abuse (F13.1-)
- Cannabis abuse (F12.1-)
- Cocaine abuse (F14.1-)
- Crack (cocaine) abuse (F14.1-)
- Hallucinogen abuse (F16.1-)
- Heroin abuse (F11.1-)
- Hypnotic abuse (F13.1-)
- Opioid abuse (F11.1-)
- Other stimulant abuse (F15.1-)
- Sedative abuse (F13.1-)

⇨ I-10 ALERT

According to ICD-10-CM Official Coding Guidelines, when documentation indicates the presence of use, abuse, and dependence of the same substance, only one code is reported. The following reporting hierarchy is used when assigning the ICD-10-CM codes:

- If both use and abuse are documented, assign only the code for abuse.
- If both abuse and dependence are documented, the code for dependence only is reported.
- If use, abuse, and dependence are all documented, the code for dependence only is reported.
- If both use and dependence are documented, the code for dependence only is reported.

Clinical Findings

Physical Examination

Signs and symptoms reveal intoxication of the drug, which can differ depending upon the type of substance. Examples may be euphoria, hyperactivity, and sedation. Documentation may indicate flushing or itching of skin. GI complaints including nausea, vomiting, decreased bowel sounds, and constipation may be recorded.

Diagnostic Procedures and Services

- Laboratory
  - drug screen
- Other
  - EKG

Clinician Note

The provider must state the pattern of harmful usage (dependence, abuse, or use) and its current clinical state (uncomplicated, intoxication, remission, etc.) and indicate the relationship to any identified mental, behavioral, or physical disorder or its relevance to the patient's status or encounter including its clinical significance. The specific drug(s) or substances should be identified and documented and in cases of legal medication indicated if it had been prescribed for that individual. Classification should be made according to the most important drug/substance or class of drug/substance used or causing the presenting disorder.

First Listed Diagnosis Note

Final diagnosis: Drug-seeking with Narcotic Abuse, including past prescription abuse, abdominal pain somatic complaint without organic evidence: The appropriate code from category F11 (F11.1Ø) will be the first listed diagnosis, followed by Z76.5 Person feigning illness (with obvious motivation).

Clinician Documentation Checklist

Clinician documentation should indicate the following:

Psychoactive Substance

- Name of substance
  - alcohol
    - blood alcohol level
  - anxiolytics, cannabis, cocaine, hallucinogens, hypnotics, inhalants, nicotine, opioids, sedatives, volatile solvents
  - polysubstance
- Level of substance use
  - use
  - abuse
  - dependence
- Any additional description of use
  - intoxication
  - remission
  - withdrawal
- Associated psychoactive-induced disorders
  - anxiety
  - delirium
  - delusions
  - hallucinations
  - mood disorder
  - perception disturbance
  - persisting amnestic disorder
  - persisting dementia
  - psychotic disorder

  - sexual dysfunction
  - sleep disorder

Nonpsychoactive Substance Abuse

- Name of nonpsychoactive substance
  - antacids
  - herbal/folk remedies
  - laxatives
  - steroids/hormones
  - vitamins
  - other

Drug/Substance Use

(Opioid F11, Cannabis F12, Sedative F13, Cocaine F14, Other Stimulant F15, Hallucinogen F16, Inhalant F18, Other Psychoactive Substance F19)

Code Axes

Drug/substance use, unspecified, uncomplicated	F1[1-6, 8-9].90
Drug/substance use, unspecified with intoxication, uncomplicated	F1[1-6, 8-9].920
Drug/substance use, unspecified with intoxication, delirium	F1[1-6, 8-9].921
Drug/substance use, unspecified with intoxication with perceptual disturbance	F1[1-2, 4-5, 9].922
Drug/substance use, unspecified with intoxication, unspecified	F1[1-6, 8-9].929
Drug/substance use, unspecified with withdrawal	F1[1, 5].93
Drug/substance use, unspecified with withdrawal, uncomplicated	F1[3, 9].930
Drug/substance use, unspecified with withdrawal delirium	F1[3, 9].931
Drug/substance use, unspecified with withdrawal with perceptual disturbance	F1[3, 9].932
Drug/substance use, unspecified with withdrawal, unspecified	F1[3, 9].939
Drug/substance use, unspecified with drug-induced mood disorder	F1[1, 3-6, 8-9].94
Drug/substance use, unspecified with drug-induced psychotic disorder with delusions	F1[1-6, 8-9].950
Drug/substance use, unspecified with drug-induced psychotic disorder with hallucinations	F1[1-6, 8-9].951
Drug/substance use, unspecified with drug-induced psychotic disorder, unspecified	F1[1-6, 8-9].959
Drug/substance use, unspecified with drug-induced persisting amnestic disorder	F1[3, 9].96
Drug/substance use, unspecified with other drug-induced persisting dementia	F1[3, 8-9].97
Drug/substance use, unspecified with other drug-induced disorders, anxiety disorder	F1[2-6, 8-9].980
Drug/substance use, unspecified with drug-induced sexual dysfunction	F1[1, 3-5, 9].981

Drug/substance use, unspecified with other drug-induced sleep disorder	**F1[1, 3-5, 9].982**
Drug/substance use, unspecified with other drug-induced disorder	**F1[1-6, 8-9].988**
Drug/substance use, unspecified with unspecified drug-induced disorder	**F1[1-6, 8-9].99**

Description of Condition

Drug/substance use (F11.9, F12.9, F13.9, F14.9, F15.9, F16.9, F18.9, F19.9)

Harmful drug or substance use is characterized by mental, behavioral, and physical disorders due to drug/substance use when dependency or abuse is not documented. Drug/substance use without negative consequences documented, e.g., uncomplicated, is reported with subcategory F1[1-6, 8-9].9Ø. Provider should document the specified drug(s) or substances, when known.

Key Terms

Key terms found in the documentation may include:

Drug intoxication, unknown usage

Drug use with clinical manifestation/state

Clinician Note

The provider must state the pattern of harmful usage (dependence, abuse, or use) and its current clinical state (uncomplicated, intoxication, remission, etc.) and indicate the relationship to any identified mental, behavioral, or physical disorder or its relevance to the patient's status or encounter including its clinical significance. The specific drug(s) or substances should be identified and documented and in cases of legal medication indicated if it had been prescribed for that individual. Classification should be made according to the most important drug/substance or class of drug/substance used or causing the presenting disorder.

Clinician Documentation Checklist

Clinician documentation should indicate the following:

Psychoactive Substance

- Name of substance
  - alcohol
    - blood alcohol level
  - anxiolytics, cannabis, cocaine, hallucinogens, hypnotics, inhalants, nicotine, opioids, sedatives, volatile solvents
  - polysubstance
- Level of substance use
  - use
  - abuse

  - dependence
  - Any additional description of use
  - intoxication
  - remission
  - withdrawal
- Associated psychoactive-induced disorders
  - anxiety
  - delirium
  - delusions
  - hallucinations
  - mood disorder
  - perception disturbance
  - persisting amnestic disorder
  - persisting dementia
  - psychotic disorder
  - sexual dysfunction
  - sleep disorder

Nonpsychoactive Substance Abuse

- Name of nonpsychoactive substance
  - antacids
  - herbal/folk remedies
  - laxatives
  - steroids/hormones
  - vitamins
  - other

Electrocardiogram

Code Axes

Electrocardiogram	**93000–93010**

Description of Procedure

An electrocardiogram is the recording of the electrical activity of the heart on a moving strip of paper that detects and records the electrical potential of the heart during contraction. These may be performed as part of a routine physical examination or due to cardiac symptoms or monitor cardiac conditions.

Electrocardiogram, routine ECG with at least 12 leads; with interpretation and report (93000)

Electrocardiogram, routine ECG with at least 12 leads; tracing only, without interpretation and report (93005)

Electrocardiogram, routine ECG with at least 12 leads; interpretation and report only (93010)

Key Terms

Key terms found in the documentation may include:

ECG
EKG

Clinician Note

Careful documentation is necessary to identify the medical necessity of the procedure, otherwise it is considered routine screening and noncovered by most third-party payers. The following list identifies those conditions which frequently support the medical necessity:

- Acid-base disorders
- Arteriovascular disease including coronary, central, and peripheral disease
- Cardiac hypertrophy
- Cardiac rhythm disturbances
- Chest pain or angina pectoris
- Conduction abnormalities
- Drug cardiotoxicity
- Electrolyte imbalance
- Endocrine abnormalities
- Heart failure

- Hypertension
- Myocardial ischemia or infarction
- Neurological disorders affecting the heart
- Palpitations
- Paroxysmal weakness
- Pericarditis
- Pulmonary disorders
- Sudden lightheadedness
- Structural cardiac conditions
- Syncope
- Temperature disorders

A preoperative EKG may be reasonable and necessary under one of the following conditions:

- In the presence of pre-existing heart disease such as angina, congestive heart failure, coronary artery disease, dysrhythmias, or prior myocardial infarction
- In the presence of known comorbid conditions that may affect the heart, such as chronic pulmonary disease, diabetes, peripheral vascular disease, or renal impairment
- When the pending surgical procedure requires a general or regional anesthetic

CDI Alert

When reporting the interpretation and report of an EKG, the physician's findings should be clearly documented in the medical record documentation, even when within normal limits. Some payers may require that measurement of all intervals and axis, rhythm and heart rate, as well as an interpretation be recorded and signed by the provider. A notation of "within normal limits" or WNL may not be sufficient.

Clinician Documentation Checklist

Clinician documentation should indicate the following:

- Identify the reason for the test
  - routine screening
  - preoperative EKG
  - monitor cardiac symptoms or cardiac conditions
  - conditions that often support medical necessity
    - acid-base disorders
    - arteriovascular disease including coronary, central, and peripheral disease
    - cardiac hypertrophy
    - cardiac rhythm disturbances
    - chest pain or angina pectoris
    - conduction abnormalities
    - drug cardiotoxicity
    - electrolyte imbalance
    - endocrine abnormalities
    - heart failure
    - hypertension
    - myocardial ischemia or infarction

- neurological disorders affecting the heart
- palpitations
- paroxysmal weakness
- pericarditis
- pulmonary disorders
- sudden lightheadedness
- structural cardiac conditions
- syncope
- temperature disorders

- With interpretation
- Without interpretation

Embolectomy/Thrombectomy

Code Axes

Arterial, with or without catheter **34001–34203**

Venous, direct or with catheter **34401–34490**

Description of Procedure

These procedures represent the removal of blood clots or other foreign material from various vessels. The codes are differentiated by arterial and venous procedures as well as the specific vessel. Terms such as anatomical location, embolectomy, or thrombectomy provide guidance.

Key Terms

Key terms found in the documentation may include:

Atheroembolism

Atherosclerosis

Occlusion

Steal syndrome

Stenosis

Vessel injury

Clinical Tip

Documentation will indicate that the artery is isolated and dissected from other critical structures and that it may be clamped above and below the clot. If a catheter is required, it is threaded past the clot and a small balloon found at its tip is inflated.

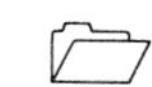

CPT ALERT

When documentation indicates that an angioscopy was performed during therapeutic intervention it should be reported in addition to the code for the primary procedure.

Clinician Documentation Checklist

Clinician documentation should indicate the following:

- The medical condition being treated
- Anatomic location
  - artery or vein
    - — neck
    - — thorax
    - — arm
    - — abdomen
    - — leg
- Type of procedure
  - embolectomy
  - thrombectomy
  - catheter

EMG (Electromyography)

Code Axes

Needle electromyography	95860–95887

CDI Alert

Carefully review the medical record documentation to determine if the complete procedure, technical component, or interpretation only was performed as this can affect modifier assignment.

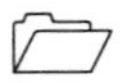

CPT Alert

When a cervical paraspinal or lumbar paraspinal muscle is tested, there is no corresponding limb study documented on the same day report code 95887.

Description of Procedure

Needle electromyography (EMG) records the electrical properties of muscle using an oscilloscope. Recordings, which may be amplified and heard through a loudspeaker, are made during needle insertion, with the muscle at rest, and during contraction. Documentation should clearly indicate the site of the study (e.g., extremity, paraspinal areas, cranial nerve) and if other nerve conduction studies are performed in conjunction with the EMG.

Needle electromyography (95860–95864)

Needle electromyography (95867–95870)

These code ranges represent an EMG when no nerve conduction studies are performed in conjunction with the EMG in the same day. Document the specific nerves being tested and, when appropriate, if the procedure is unilateral or bilateral.

Needle electromyography, each extremity, with related paraspinal areas, when performed with nerve conduction, amplitude and latency/velocity study (95885–95887)

Documentation supporting this series of codes will indicate that other nerve conduction studies were performed during the same encounter.

Clinician Documentation Checklist

Clinician documentation should indicate the following:

- The medical condition or symptoms being treated
  - pain
  - weakness
  - numbness
  - neuropathies
  - dystrophies
  - carpal tunnel syndrome
- Procedure
  - complete procedure (technical and professional)
  - technical component only
  - interpretation (professional) component only
- Nerves being tested

- Number of nerves being tested
  - unilateral
  - bilateral
  - paraspinal
- Other nerve conduction studies

Emphysema

> **⇨ I-10 ALERT**
>
> When emphysema is documented as being present with chronic bronchitis, refer to classification rules at category J44 Other chronic obstructive pulmonary disease. Review documentation carefully to ensure proper classification.

Code Axes

Unilateral pulmonary emphysema [MacLeod's syndrome]	**J43.Ø**
Panlobular emphysema	**J43.1**
Centrilobular emphysema	**J43.2**
Other emphysema	**J43.8**
Emphysema, unspecified	**J43.9**
Compensatory emphysema	**J98.3**

Clinical Tip
Emphysema is one of several conditions that comprises chronic obstructive pulmonary disease (COPD). Primarily found in tobacco smokers, the lung tissue around the small alveoli are destroyed, thus making them unable to hold their shape on exhalation.

Description of Condition

Unilateral pulmonary emphysema [MacLeod's syndrome] (J43.Ø)

> **⇨ I-10 ALERT**
>
> As with many pulmonary conditions in ICD-10-CM, a coding instructional note at this category indicates that any exposure to tobacco smoke or smoking behavior should be coded in addition to the code(s) for the conditions themselves.

Clinical Tip
MacLeod's syndrome is a rare disorder that is typically diagnosed in childhood, associated with postinfectious bronchiolitis obliterans. The affected lung tissue does not grow normally and consequently is somewhat smaller than the nonaffected lung. The primary radiographic appearance is that of pulmonary hyperlucency. It is an x-linked disorder, meaning that it primarily affects males.

Key Terms
Key terms found in the documentation for unilateral pulmonary emphysema may include:

- Swyer-James-MacLeod syndrome
- Unilateral hyperlucent lung syndrome
- Unilateral pulmonary artery functional hypoplasia
- Unilateral transparency of lung

Clinical Tip
Documentation may include terms such as pink puffer (a descriptor for a patient with COPD and severe emphysema, who has a pink complexion and dyspnea) or blue bloater (a descriptor to indicate the appearance of a patient with COPD who has symptoms of chronic bronchitis). Verify with the physician before assigning a code for emphysema.

Panlobular emphysema (J43.1)

Clinical Tip

Panlobular emphysema is the type that involves the entire lung lobule, from the bronchiole to the alveoli, which has expanded. This type of emphysema most commonly involves the lower lobes.

Key Terms

Key terms found in the documentation for panlobular emphysema may include:

Panacinar emphysema

Centrilobular emphysema (J43.2)

Clinical Tip

In this type of emphysema only the proximal and central portions of the bronchiole have expanded. This type of emphysema most commonly involves the upper lobes.

Other and unspecified emphysema (J43.8, J43.9)

Clinical Tip

An emphysematous bleb is caused by damaged alveoli in the lung tissue that can no longer perform oxygen exchange. The air becomes trapped in the adjacent tissue, forming a bleb, and scar tissue accumulates around it.

Key Terms

Key terms found in the documentation may include:

Bullous emphysema

Emphysema NOS

Emphysematous bleb

Vesicular emphysema

Compensatory emphysema (J98.3)

Clinical Tip

Compensatory emphysema is a nonobstructive process in which the unaffected lung tissue adapts and enlarges, due to another portion of the lung being damaged or removed. It does not involve the same destructive lung tissue pattern as the other types of emphysema.

Key Terms

Key terms found in the documentation for other and unspecified emphysema may include:

Bullous emphysema

Emphysema NOS

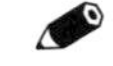

CDI ALERT

Ensure that the appropriate type of emphysema is documented in the medical record.

Emphysematous bleb

Vesicular emphysema

Clinical Findings

Physical Examination

Patients present with complaints of cough and shortness of breath, which is usually upon exertion. Documentation indicates wheezing and increased expiratory phase of breathing. There are decreased heart and lung sounds. The chest may appear larger in the anteroposterior diameter (barrel chest). Neck vein distention may be present in signs of advanced disease.

Diagnostic Procedures and Services

- Laboratory
  - antitrypsin levels to detect possible deficiency
- Imaging
  - echocardiogram
  - chest x-ray
- Other
  - pulmonary function tests
  - EKG

Clinician Documentation Checklist

Clinician documentation should indicate the following:

- Exposure to environmental tobacco smoke
- History of tobacco use
- Occupational exposure to environmental tobacco smoke
- Tobacco dependence
- Tobacco use
- Type
  - unilateral pulmonary (MacLeod's syndrome)
    - Swyer syndrome
    - unilateral emphysema
    - unilateral hyperlucent lung
    - unilateral pulmonary artery functional hypoplasia
    - unilateral transparency of lung
  - panlobular
    - panacinar
  - centrilobular
  - other

- unspecified
  - bullous
  - emphysematous bleb
  - vesicular

Encephalopathy

Code Axes

Anoxic encephalopathy	**G93.1**
Metabolic encephalopathy	**G93.41**
Toxic encephalopathy	**G92**
Other encephalopathy	**G93.49**
Encephalopathy, unspecified	**G93.4Ø**

Description of Condition

Encephalopathy is a generalized, or global, alteration in brain function that is typically acute (or subacute) in onset and due to a systemic underlying cause that is usually reversible and resolves when the underlying cause is corrected. Common causes of encephalopathy include fever, infection, dehydration, electrolyte imbalance, acidosis, organ failure, sepsis, hypoxia, drugs, poisons, or toxins.

Anoxic encephalopathy (G93.1)

Anoxic or hypoxic encephalopathy is brain damage due to lack of oxygen.

Clinical Tip

Common causes are cardiopulmonary arrest, prolonged seizures with inadequate breathing, prolonged asthma attacks or exacerbations of COPD.

Key Terms

Key terms found in the documentation may include:

Anoxic brain damage
Anoxic encephalopathy

Metabolic encephalopathy (G93.41)

Potentially reversible encephalopathy due to metabolic causes; most commonly due to infections, fever, dehydration, electrolyte imbalance, acidosis, hypoxia, and organ failure. Metabolic encephalopathy often presents acutely and rapidly and with fluctuating levels of consciousness/alertness.

Clinical Tip

Septic encephalopathy is a clinical term that expresses brain dysfunction as a manifestation of severe sepsis. Metabolic encephalopathy often presents acutely and rapidly and with fluctuating levels of consciousness/alertness.

Key Terms

Key terms in the documentation may include:

Metabolic encephalopathy

Septic encephalopathy

First Listed Diagnosis Note

Admit for encephalopathy due to dehydration: The patient was admitted with mental status changes and diagnostic workup revealed metabolic encephalopathy due to dehydration. Treatment of the metabolic encephalopathy was directed towards reversing the dehydration. However, metabolic encephalopathy may be designated as the first listed diagnosis as it was documented as the condition established after study to be chiefly responsible for the admission of the patient to the hospital for care.

Admit for severe sepsis with septic encephalopathy: Patient was admitted with severe fever, tachycardia, and mental status changes and was documented as having severe *Escherichia coli* sepsis with septic encephalopathy. According to Official Coding Guidelines, the coding of severe sepsis requires a minimum of two codes: first a code for the underlying systemic infection A41.51, followed by a code from subcategory R65.2 Severe sepsis. An additional code is assigned for the associated acute organ dysfunction; in this case septic encephalopathy G93.41.

CDI Alert

Documentation of the results of blood tests, spinal fluid examination, imaging studies, electroencephalograms, and similar diagnostic studies may be used to differentiate the various causes of encephalopathy and is necessary for reporting specificity.

Toxic encephalopathy (G92)

Toxic encephalopathy is defined as brain tissue degeneration due to a toxic substance and is identified with drugs, poisonings, and chemical substances. Toxic-metabolic can be found in organ failure or intoxication.

Clinical Tip

Toxic and toxic-metabolic encephalopathy generally refer to the effects of drugs, toxins, poisons, and medications, but this term may also be used clinically to refer to encephalopathy caused by fever, sepsis, or other toxic conditions. Review documentation carefully and query if documentation is insufficient to assign the most specific code.

CDI Alert

The instructional note under G92 states to code first (T51–T65) to identify the toxic agent. Note that T51–T65 identifies substances that are primarily nonmedicinal, including alcohol, organic solvents, carbon monoxide, smoke, venomous animals and plants and tobacco.

For encephalopathy due to drugs, the alphabetic index instructs to see also the Table of Drugs and Chemicals.

Key Terms

Key terms found in the documentation may include:

Toxic encephalopathy

Toxic encephalitis

Toxic metabolic encephalopathy

First Listed Diagnosis Note

Admit for toxic encephalopathy due to lead poisoning: Patient was admitted with mental status changes, which after evaluation was determined to be toxic encephalopathy due to accidental toxic lead exposure that occurred while he was removing lead contaminated paint in his home. Toxic encephalopathy should not be sequenced as the first listed diagnosis, as there is an instructional note under code/category G92 instructing to code first the underlying toxic agent. Code T56.ØX1A Toxic effect of lead and its compounds, accidental (unintentional), initial encounter, would be assigned as the first listed diagnosis, with code G92 assigned as an additional code.

QUERY NOTE

When encephalopathy is documented and the etiology is not identified or clear, query for the underlying cause based on information within the record.

Other encephalopathy (G93.49)

This code is reported when the type of encephalopathy is identified but does not have an alphabetic index entry nor is it an inclusion term in the tabular list for a particular code (e.g., Encephalopathy due to significant burns, multifactorial).

Key Terms

Key terms found in the documentation may include:

Encephalopathy due to (specified; does not fit into any of the index classifications)

CDI ALERT

When a cause cannot be identified, then G93.4Ø Encephalopathy, unspecified, will be reported. When a type of encephalopathy is identified or specified, but does not fit into any of the classifications, G93.49 Other encephalopathy, Encephalopathy NEC, would be reported.

Encephalopathy, unspecified (G93.4Ø)

This code should rarely be reported. Documentation within the record should provide information with which clarification can be queried for specificity.

First Listed Diagnosis Note

Admit for acute mental status changes with a final diagnosis of encephalopathy due to unknown cause: Patient was transferred to another acute care facility for further diagnostic evaluation and treatment. In this case, G93.4Ø Encephalopathy, unspecified, would be reported as the first listed diagnosis.

CDI ALERT

The term encephalopathy is vague, and should generally be preceded by terminology describing the reason, cause, or medical condition of the patient that led to the brain disease or malfunction.

Clinical Findings

Physical Examination

History and review of systems may include:

- Altered mental status
- Dementia
- Seizures
- Tremors
- Muscle twitching
- Poor coordination

Diagnostic Procedures and Services

- Laboratory
  - complete blood count
  - electrolyte level
  - ammonia
  - glucose
  - liver functions

    - drug screening
    - lead level
    - blood cultures
    - creatinine
- Imaging
    - head CT
    - head MRI
    - Doppler ultrasound
- Other
    - EEG

Clinician Note
For more precise documentation and correct coding, the clinician should make a clinical distinction between encephalopathy and delirium. The diagnostic term encephalopathy is preferred for describing mental status alteration when it is due to toxic or metabolic states. The term delirium is usually classified as a mental disorder or a symptom and is more appropriately documented in psychiatric conditions unrelated to underlying systemic conditions.

Clinician Documentation Checklist

Clinician documentation should indicate the following:

- Other disorders of brain
    - anoxic brain damage
    - toxic encephalopathy
        - includes:
            - toxic encephalitis
            - toxic metabolic encephalopathy
        - identification of the toxic agent
    - benign intracranial hypertension
    - postviral fatigue syndrome
        - benign myalgic encephalomyelitis
    - other and unspecified encephalopathy
        - metabolic encephalopathy
            - septic encephalopathy
        - other encephalopathy
        - unspecified encephalopathy
    - compression of brain
        - Arnold-Chiari type 1 compression of brain
        - compression of brain (stem)
        - herniation of brain (stem)
    - cerebral edema
    - Reye's syndrome

  - also identification of, if salicylates-induced
- other specified disorders of brain
  - temporal sclerosis
    - hippocampal sclerosis
    - mesial temporal sclerosis
  - brain death
  - other disorders of brain
    - postradiation encephalopathy
- unspecified disorder of brain

- Other disorders of brain in diseases
  - the underlying disease

Endoscopy — Lower GI

Code Axes

Colonoscopy	**45378–45398**
Flexible sigmoidoscopy	**45330–45350**

Description of Procedure

These codes represent the examination of the colon by flexible fiberoptic endoscope. Since code selection is based upon the portion of the intestine being examined as well as any other services and procedures performed during the surgical encounter, it is critical that the documentation be clear and complete. As with any other endoscopic procedures, this procedure can be performed for either diagnostic or therapeutic purposes.

A flexible sigmoidoscopy is reported when the documentation indicates that the provider examined only the lower one third of the intestine and documentation does not include notation that the splenic flexure was examined. Report a colonoscopy when the entire colon, including the cecum is examined according to the documentation. When the documentation does not indicate that the cecum is examined, report the appropriate colonoscopy code with modifier 52 Reduced services.

Key Terms

Key terms found in the documentation may include:

Colo

Colo with bx

Colo w/polypectomy

Flex sig

Flex sig w/bx

Flex sig w/polypectomy

Clinical Tip

Control of bleeding that is the result of a biopsy or polypectomy is considered part of the main service and is not reported separately; however, it should be clearly documented.

Clinician Documentation Checklist

Clinician documentation should indicate the following:

- Type of sedation provided
- Quality of bowel preparation
- Clearly indicate the anatomical structures examined
  - colonoscopy
    - examination of cecum or terminal ileum (or small bowel proximal to an anastomosis)

- sigmoidoscopy
  - examination of sigmoid colon (may include a portion of descending colon)
- The medical condition being treated
- Flexible sigmoidoscopy
  - biopsy
  - removal of foreign body
  - removal of tumor
  - control of bleeding
  - submucosal injection
  - decompression
  - snare technique used
  - ablation
  - balloon dilation
  - ultrasound examination
  - fine needle aspiration
  - placement of stent
  - band ligation
- Colonoscopy
  - removal of foreign body
  - biopsy
  - mucosal injection
  - control of bleeding
  - ablation
  - removal of tumor-hot biopsy forceps
  - removal of tumor-snare technique
  - balloon dilation
  - stent placement
  - ultrasound
  - fine needle aspiration
  - decompression
  - band ligation
- Summary of findings and recommendations

Endoscopy — Upper GI

Code Axes

Esophagoscopy	**43180–43232**
Esophagogastroduodenoscopy	**43233–43259**

Description of Procedure

These codes represent the examination of the esophagus and stomach by endoscope. Code selection is dependent upon the anatomical structures examined.

An esophagoscopy is the examination of the stomach with either a rigid or flexible endoscope. Documentation should indicate that the esophagus from the cricopharyngeus muscle to gastroesophageal junction was visualized. When the documentation indicates that the esophagus, stomach, duodenum, and/or jejunum are visualized, an esophagogastroduodenoscopy is supported.

Like other endoscopic procedures, these can be performed for either diagnostic or therapeutic reasons. The table below helps identify key terms in the documentation and cross-walks to the code that is supported by those terms.

Physician documentation should include the following key terms as they apply in order to determine correct code assignment.

Key Term	Esophagus Only	EGD
Brushing and washings	43191, 43197, 43200	43235
Submucosal injections	43192, 43201	43236
Biopsy	43193, 43198, 43202	43239
Diverticulectomy	43180	
Injection varices	43204	43243
Band varices	43205	43244
Foreign body removal	43194, 43215	43247
Lesion removal or destruction		
hot biopsy or bipolar	43216	43250
snare	43217	43251
ablation	43229	43270
Insertion		
tube or stent	43212	43266
intraluminal tube or catheter		43241
Percutaneous gastrostomy tube		43246

Key Term	Esophagus Only	EGD
Dilation		
balloon less than 30 mm	43195, 43220	43249
balloon greater than 30 mm	43214	43233
balloon or dilator, retrograde		43213
over guidewire	43196, 43226	43248
gastric/duodenal stricture		43245
Control of bleeding	43227	43255
Ultrasound examination		
intramural or transmural fine needle aspiration/biopsy	43232	43238, 43242
transmural injection of diagnostic or therapeutic substance		43253
esophagus only	43231	
esophagus, stomach or duodenum, and adjacent structures		43237
esophagus, stomach and either duodenum or jejunum distal to anastomosis of surgical altered stomach		43259
Drainage of pseudocyst		43240
Mucosal resection	43211	43254
Optical endomicroscopy	43206	43252
Thermal energy for gastroesophageal reflux		43257
Esophagogastric fundoplasty		43210

Key Terms

Key terms found in the documentation may include:

EGD

Esophagoscopy

Clinician Documentation Checklist

Clinician documentation should indicate the following:

- The medical condition being treated
- The type of sedation including medications
- The anatomical structures examined including esophagus (cricopharyngeus muscle [upper esophageal sphincter]), the stomach, and the duodenum. If duodenum is not deliberately examined, the clinical reason should be described.
  - washings
  - biopsy
  - ultrasound examination and aspiration, etc. performed
  - removal of foreign body
  - destruction of lesion including instrumentation used
  - control of bleeding
  - injection varices

  - insertion of tube, stent or intraluminal tube or catheter
  - placement of percutaneous gastrostomy tube
  - dilation including type of instrumentation
  - drainage of pseudocyst
  - mucosal resection
  - optical endomicroscopy
  - thermal energy
  - esophagogastric fundoplasty
- Summary of findings and recommendations

Epilepsy and Recurrent Seizures

Code Axes

Localization-related (focal) (partial) idiopathic epilepsy and epileptic syndromes with seizures of localized onset	**G40.0**
Localization-related (focal) (partial) symptomatic epilepsy and epileptic syndromes with simple partial seizures	**G40.1**
Localization-related (focal) (partial) symptomatic epilepsy and epileptic syndromes with complex partial seizures	**G40.2**
Generalized idiopathic epilepsy and epileptic syndromes	**G40.3**
Absence epileptic syndrome	**G40.A**
Juvenile myoclonic epilepsy (impulsive petit mal)	**G40.B**
Other generalized epilepsy and epileptic syndromes	**G40.4**
Epileptic seizures related to external causes	**G40.5**
Other epilepsy and recurrent seizures	**G40.8**
Epilepsy, unspecified	**G40.9** **G40.911** **G40.919**

⇨ I-10 ALERT

There is an additional classification axis for the presence of status epilepticus. Sixth characters are found throughout the subcategory representing this condition.

Clinical Tip

The following definitions should be used for all subclassifications related to epilepsy and epileptic syndromes:

Status epilepticus: Typically defined as one continuous, unremitting seizure lasting longer than 30 minutes, or recurrent seizures without regaining consciousness between seizures for greater than 30 minutes. The condition is always considered a medical emergency.

Intractable epilepsy: There is not a universal definition for this complication, but it appears that most agree that a definition of drug-resistant epilepsy is a failure of adequate trials of two tolerated and appropriately chosen and used antiepileptic drug (AED) schedules.

CDI ALERT

Ensure that not only is the type of epilepsy or recurrent seizure documented, but that the details related to status epilepticus and intractable epilepsy are also present in the medical record.

Key Terms

Key terms found in the documentation for intractable epilepsy may include:

Focal epilepsy

Pharmacoresistant (pharmacologically) resistant epilepsy

Poorly controlled epilepsy

Refractory (medically) epilepsy

Treatment resistant epilepsy

Description of Condition

Localization-related (focal) (partial) idiopathic epilepsy and epileptic syndromes with seizures of localized onset (G4Ø.Ø-)

Clinical Tip

Localization-related epilepsy also referred to as a focal or partial syndrome, is either symptomatic (i.e., the cause is known) or cryptogenic, which means there is a presumed focal structural cause that cannot be identified historically or be seen with current imaging techniques. Localization-related epilepsy arises from an epileptic focus, a small portion of the brain that serves as the irritant driving the epileptic response.

Key Terms

Key terms found in the documentation for localization-related epilepsy may include:

Benign childhood epilepsy with centrotemporal EEG spikes

Childhood epilepsy with occipital EEG paroxysms

Localization-related idiopathic epilepsy and epileptic syndromes with seizures of localized onset

Clinician Note

Many types of procedures are used to treat specific forms of epilepsy. For example, vagus nerve stimulation and stereotaxic depth electrode implantation are used to treat focal epilepsy. However, medical necessity must be clearly indicated by the type of epilepsy the patient has. Careful attention to the documentation indicating the specific type of epilepsy is, therefore, crucial in supporting the medical necessity of these procedures.

Localization-related (focal) (partial) symptomatic epilepsy and epileptic syndromes with simple partial seizures (G4Ø.1-)

Clinical Tip

Simple partial seizures (SPS) are those that are not associated with any impairment of consciousness. The seizures may also include experiences of unusual feelings or sensations.

Key Terms

Key terms found in the documentation for localization-related epilepsy with simple partial seizures may include:

Attacks without alteration of consciousness

Epilepsia partialis continua [Kozhevnikov]

Simple partial seizures developing into secondarily generalized seizures

Clinician Note

Many types of procedures are used to treat specific forms of epilepsy. For example, vagus nerve stimulation and stereotaxic depth electrode implantation are used to treat focal epilepsy. However, medical necessity must be clearly indicated by the type of epilepsy the patient has. Careful attention to the documentation indicating the specific type of epilepsy is, therefore, crucial in supporting the medical necessity of these procedures.

Localization-related (focal) (partial) symptomatic epilepsy and epileptic syndromes with complex partial seizures (G4Ø.2-)

Clinical Tip

Complex partial seizures (CPS) usually start in a small area of the temporal lobe or frontal lobe of the brain, but quickly involve other areas of the brain that affect alertness and awareness. Some CPS seizures (typically starting in the temporal lobe) begin with a simple partial seizure. Also called an aura, this warning seizure often includes an odd feeling in the stomach. Then the person loses awareness and stares blankly. Complex partial seizures starting in the frontal lobe tend to be shorter and are also more likely to include automatisms like bicycling movements of the legs or pelvic thrusting.

Key Terms

Key terms found in the documentation for localization-related epilepsy with complex partial seizures may include:

Attacks with alteration of consciousness, often with automatisms

Complex partial seizures developing into secondarily generalized seizures

Clinician Note

Many types of procedures are used to treat specific forms of epilepsy. For example, vagus nerve stimulation and stereotaxic depth electrode implantation are used to treat focal epilepsy. However, medical necessity must be clearly indicated by the type of epilepsy the patient has. Careful attention to the documentation indicating the specific type of epilepsy is, therefore, crucial in supporting the medical necessity of these procedures.

CDI ALERT

MERRF (Myoclonic epilepsy with ragged-red fibers) syndrome (E88.42) is related to this (G4Ø.3) classification subcategory. If present in the medical record, it should clearly be documented as a part of the epilepsy classification.

Generalized idiopathic epilepsy and epileptic syndromes (G4Ø.3-)

Clinical Tip

Generalized epilepsies arise from many independent foci (multifocal epilepsies) or from epileptic circuits that involve the whole brain. One third of all epilepsies are classified as idiopathic generalized epilepsy (IGE), which are genetically determined and affect otherwise normal people of both sexes and all races. They involve typical absences, myoclonic jerks, and generalized tonic-clonic seizures, alone or in varying combinations and severity. The condition is usually life-long, although some are age-related. A major advance in recent epileptology is the recognition of different epileptic syndromes that allows an accurate diagnosis and management of seizure disorders. This is important because the short- and long-term treatment strategies are entirely different for each disorder.

Clinician Note
Many types of procedures are used to treat specific forms of epilepsy. For example, vagus nerve stimulation and stereotaxic depth electrode implantation are used to treat focal epilepsy. However, medical necessity must be clearly indicated by the type of epilepsy the patient has. Careful attention to the documentation indicating the specific type of epilepsy is, therefore, crucial in supporting the medical necessity of these procedures.

Absence epileptic syndrome (G4Ø.A-)

Clinical Tip
This condition is idiopathic generalized epilepsy that affects children between the ages of 10 and 17 years of age, typically beginning at or near puberty. It involves recurrent absence seizures, which are brief episodes of unresponsive staring, sometimes with minor motor features such as eye blinking or subtle chewing. Some patients go on to develop generalized tonic-clonic seizures, but for some, the prognosis is favorable with no decline in cognition or any other neurological defects, and the seizures spontaneously cease with age.

Key Terms
Key terms found in the documentation for absence epileptic syndrome may include:

Absence epileptic syndrome

Childhood absence epilepsy (pyknolepsy)

Juvenile absence epilepsy

Clinician Note
Many types of procedures are used to treat specific forms of epilepsy. For example, vagus nerve stimulation and stereotaxic depth electrode implantation are used to treat focal epilepsy. However, medical necessity must be clearly indicated by the type of epilepsy the patient has. Careful attention to the documentation indicating the specific type of epilepsy is, therefore, crucial in supporting the medical necessity of these procedures.

Juvenile myoclonic epilepsy (impulsive petit mal) (G4Ø.B-)

Clinical Tip
This condition involves idiopathic generalized epilepsy that develops in patients aged 8 to 20 years and continues for the rest of their lives. Patients have normal cognition and are otherwise neurologically intact. Myoclonic jerks (quick little jerks of the arms, shoulder, or occasionally the legs) are the most common type of seizure, although generalized tonic-clonic seizures and absence seizures may occur as well. Sleep deprivation is a common triggering mechanism for this type of seizure.

Key Terms

Key terms found in the documentation for juvenile myoclonic epilepsy may include:

Janz syndrome

Clinician Note

Many types of procedures are used to treat specific forms of epilepsy. For example, vagus nerve stimulation and stereotaxic depth electrode implantation are used to treat focal epilepsy. However, medical necessity must be clearly indicated by the type of epilepsy the patient has. Careful attention to the documentation indicating the specific type of epilepsy is, therefore, crucial in supporting the medical necessity of these procedures.

Other generalized epilepsy and epileptic syndromes (G40.4-)

Clinical Tip

Generalized epilepsies arise from many independent foci (multifocal epilepsies) or from epileptic circuits that involve the whole brain.

Key Terms

Key terms found in the documentation for other generalized epilepsy and epileptic syndromes may include:

Epilepsy with grand mal seizures on awakening
Epilepsy with myoclonic absences
Epilepsy with myoclonic-astatic seizures
Doose syndrome epilepsy
Drop attacks
Grand mal seizure NOS
MAE
Nonspecific atonic epileptic seizures
Nonspecific clonic epileptic seizures
Nonspecific myoclonic epileptic seizures
Nonspecific tonic epileptic seizures
Nonspecific tonic-clonic epileptic seizures
Symptomatic early myoclonic encephalopathy

Clinician Note

Many types of procedures are used to treat specific forms of epilepsy. For example, vagus nerve stimulation and stereotaxic depth electrode implantation are used to treat focal epilepsy. However, medical necessity must be clearly indicated by the type of epilepsy the patient has. Careful attention to the documentation indicating the specific type of epilepsy is, therefore, crucial in supporting the medical necessity of these procedures.

Epileptic seizures related to external causes (G4Ø.5-)

Clinical Tip

Seizures may be caused by an exposure to several external causes, such as lead or carbon monoxide, or from alcohol or drugs taken internally, such as antidepressants. The seizure disorder may also be triggered by environmental factors, such as stress, lack of sleep, or hormonal changes related to the menstrual cycle. In some patients, lights flashing at a certain speed can trigger seizures.

Key Terms

Key terms found in the documentation for epileptic seizures related to external causes may include:

Epileptic seizures related to alcohol

Epileptic seizures related to drugs

Epileptic seizures related to hormonal changes

Epileptic seizures related to sleep deprivation

Epileptic seizures related to stress

⇨ I-10 ALERT

Combination codes are available in ICD-10-CM that indicate seizure activity due to a number of external causes. These codes are differentiated by the presence of intractability and status epilepticus as are the other codes in the epilepsy subcategories. Additional codes should be assigned for drug adverse effects, and to clearly classify the type of epilepsy, if documented.

Other epilepsy and recurrent seizures (G4Ø.8-)

Clinical Tip

Lennox-Gastaut syndrome is a generalized epilepsy that is characterized by a developmental delay or childhood dementia, mixed generalized seizures, and EEG demonstrating a pattern of approximately 2 Hz "slow" spike-wave. Onset typically occurs between the ages of 2 and 18, and different types of seizures may be associated with the condition, such as astatic seizures (drop attacks), tonic seizures, tonic-clonic seizures, atypical absence seizures, and sometimes, complex partial seizures.

West's syndrome is a rare epileptic disorder that affects infants, with a triad of infantile spasms, a characteristic EEG pattern called hypsarrhythmia, and developmental regression. Patients are generally between the third and the twelfth month of age, most often around five months of age. The syndrome is typically caused by an organic brain dysfunction whose origins may be prenatal, perinatal (caused during birth), or postnatal.

Landau–Kleffner syndrome (LKS) is a neurological syndrome that involves the sudden or gradual development of aphasia (the inability to understand or express language) and an abnormal electroencephalogram (EEG). Patients are typically between the ages of 3 and 7 years old and because this syndrome appears during such a critical period of language acquisition in a child's life, speech production may be affected just as severely as language comprehension.

Key Terms

Key terms found in the documentation for Lennox-Gastaut syndrome may include:

Lennox syndrome

⇨ I-10 ALERT

This is a residual subcategory that includes all types of epileptic seizures that are not included in the previous subcategories in G4Ø.-. Also included here are epilepsies and epileptic syndromes that are undetermined as to whether they are focal or generalized.

Key terms found in the documentation for West's syndrome may include:

Epileptic spasms
Generalized flexion epilepsy
Infantile epileptic encephalopathy
Infantile myoclonic encephalopathy
Infantile spasms
Jackknife convulsions
Massive myoclonia
Salaam spasms or attacks

Key terms found in the documentation for Landau–Kleffner syndrome may include:

Acquired epileptic aphasia
Aphasia with convulsive disorder
Infantile acquired aphasia

Clinical Findings

Physical Examination

The history and review of systems may include:

- Seizures
  - Bitten tongue
  - Incontinence
  - Lost consciousness
- Generalized seizures
  - followed by postictal state

Clinical indicators on physical examination that may indicate the cause of a seizure include:

- Fever and stiff neck
- Papilledema
- Asymmetry of muscle strength
- Hyperreflexia
- Skin lesions

Diagnostic Procedures and Services

- Laboratory
  - glucose
  - BUN
  - electrolytes
  - creatinine
  - liver function
- Imaging
  - head CT

  - head MRI
- Other
  - EEG

Clinician Note

Many types of procedures are used to treat specific forms of epilepsy. For example, vagus nerve stimulation and stereotaxic depth electrode implantation are used to treat focal epilepsy. However, medical necessity must be clearly indicated by the type of epilepsy the patient has. Careful attention to the documentation indicating the specific type of epilepsy is, therefore, crucial in supporting the medical necessity of these procedures.

Clinician Documentation Checklist

Clinician documentation should indicate the following:

- Type
  - localization-related (focal) (partial) idiopathic epilepsy and epileptic syndromes with seizures of localized onset
    - includes
      - benign childhood epilepsy with centrotemporal EEG spikes
      - childhood epilepsy with occipital EEG paroxysms
  - localization-related (focal) (partial) symptomatic epilepsy and epileptic syndromes with simple partial seizures
    - includes
      - attacks without alteration of consciousness
      - epilepsia partialis continua (Kozhevnikov)
      - simple partial seizures developing into secondarily generalized seizures
      - Bravais Jacksonian epilepsy
  - localization-related (focal) (partial) symptomatic epilepsy and epileptic syndromes with complex partial seizures
    - includes
      - attacks with alteration of consciousness, often with automatisms
      - complex partial seizures developing into secondarily generalized seizures
  - generalized idiopathic epilepsy and epileptic syndromes
    - MERRF (myoclonic epilepsy with ragged red fibers) syndrome, if applicable
  - absence epileptic syndrome
    - includes
      - childhood absence epilepsy (pyknolepsy)
      - juvenile absence epilepsy
  - Juvenile myoclonic epilepsy (impulsive petit mal)

- other generalized epilepsy and epileptic syndromes
  - includes
    - epilepsy with grand mal seizures on awakening
    - epilepsy with myoclonic absences
    - epilepsy with myoclonic-astatic seizures
    - grand mal seizure
    - nonspecific atonic epileptic seizures
    - nonspecific clonic epileptic seizures
    - nonspecific myoclonic epileptic seizures
    - nonspecific tonic epileptic seizures
    - nonspecific tonic-clonic epileptic seizures
    - symptomatic early myoclonic encephalopathy
- epileptic seizures related to external causes
  - associated epilepsy and recurrent seizures
  - includes
    - epileptic seizures related to alcohol
    - epileptic seizures related to drug
      - identify the drug
    - epileptic seizures related to hormonal changes
    - epileptic seizures related to sleep deprivation
    - epileptic seizures related to stress
- other specified epilepsy and recurrent seizures
  - includes
    - epilepsies and epileptic syndromes undetermined as to whether they are focal or generalized
    - Landau-Kleffner syndrome
    - infant benign myoclonic epilepsy
  - subtype
    - Lennox-Gastaut syndrome
    - epileptic spasms
      - infantile spasms
      - salaam attacks
      - West's syndrome
    - other epilepsy
    - other seizures
- unspecified epilepsy

- Identification of the above type of epilepsy and seizures as:
  - not intractable
  - intractable
    - includes
      - pharmacoresistant (pharmacologically resistant)
      - treatment resistant

    - refractory (medically)
    - poorly controlled
  - with status epilepticus
  - without status epilepticus

Facet Joint Injections

Code Axes

Injection(s), diagnostic or therapeutic agent, paravertebral facet (zygapophyseal) joint (or nerves innervating that joint) with image guidance (fluoroscopy or CT), cervical or thoracic	**64490–64492**
Injection(s), diagnostic or therapeutic agent, paravertebral facet (zygapophyseal) joint (or nerves innervating that joint) with image guidance (fluoroscopy or CT), lumbar or sacral	**64493–64495**

CDI ALERT

The documentation should be carefully reviewed to determine what exact procedures were performed. There are times when the procedure performed listed at the beginning of the operative report will not be the actual procedure described in the body of the report.

Description of Procedure

Facet joint injections should be reported using the appropriate codes from range 64490–64495. Correct code selection is dependent upon:

- Level of the spine injected
- Number of levels reported
- Whether the service was performed unilaterally or bilaterally

Single level: A single level injection occurs when the physician administers one or more substances to a level using one or more needles. A physician may insert a needle and attach a small tube through which the first substance is administered via a syringe. The physician may then change out the syringe and administer a second substance. However, only one needle puncture is performed.

In another method, the physician inserts the needle, administers a substance, and then removes the needle and makes a second puncture with a new needle and syringe to administer an additional substance. Despite the fact that there are two puncture sites, only a single level is being treated.

Multiple levels: When the physician documentation clearly indicates that multiple levels of the spine were injected, add-on codes 64491–64492 and 64494–64495, respectively, are reported.

Bilateral injections: Modifier 50 should be appended when the documentation states that injections were made on the same level but on different sides. Add-on codes 64491–64492 or 64494–64495 are not appropriate when the documentation indicates that the injections were performed bilaterally.

Anesthetic/steroids: Examine the documentation for the name and dosage of the anesthetic agent and/or steroid agent administered. List the appropriate HCPCS Level II code separately.

Clinician Note

Documentation must indicate if the procedure was performed unilaterally or bilaterally. This supports the use of modifier 50 when documentation indicates that the injection was performed bilaterally.

Clinical Tip

Medicare considers facet joint blocks to be reasonable and necessary for chronic pain (persistent pain for three (3) months or greater) suspected to originate from the facet joint. Facet joint block is one of the methods used to document/confirm suspicions of posterior element biomechanical pain of the spine. Hallmarks of posterior element biomechanical pain are as follows:

- The pain does not have a strong radicular component.
- There is no associated neurological deficit and the pain is aggravated by hyperextension, rotation, or lateral bending of the spine, depending on the orientation of the facet joint at that level.
- A paravertebral facet joint represents the articulation of the posterior elements of one vertebra with its neighboring vertebrae; it is further noted that there are two (2) facet joints at each level, left and right.

During a paravertebral facet joint block procedure, a needle is placed in the facet joint or along the medial branches that innervate the joints under fluoroscopic guidance and a local anesthetic and/or steroid is injected. After the injection(s) has been performed, the patient is asked to indulge in the activities that usually aggravate his/her pain and to record his/her impressions of the effect of the procedure. Temporary or prolonged abolition of the pain suggests that the facet joints are the source of the symptoms and appropriate treatment may be prescribed in the future. Some patients have long-lasting relief with local anesthetic and steroid; others require a denervation procedure for more permanent relief. Before proceeding to a denervation treatment, the patient should experience at least a 50 percent reduction in symptoms for the duration of the local anesthetic effect.

Diagnostic or therapeutic injections/nerve blocks may be required for the management of chronic pain. It may take multiple nerve blocks targeting different anatomic structures to establish the etiology of the chronic pain in a given patient. It is standard medical practice to use the modality most likely to establish the diagnosis or treat the presumptive diagnosis. If the first set of procedures fails to produce the desired effect or to rule out the diagnosis, the provider should proceed to the next logical test or treatment indicated. For the purpose of this paravertebral facet joint block, an anatomic region is defined per CPT as cervical/thoracic (64490, 64491, 64492) or lumbar/sacral (64493, 64494, 64495).

CDI ALERT

Medical record documentation should contain information regarding the preoperative evaluation leading to suspicion of the presence of facet joint pathology, as well as the provider's postoperative conclusions. In addition, the anatomical area of the spine and the exact location of the injection site should be clearly notated, as well as the specific name and dosage of the anesthetic agent and/or steroid administered.

Clinician Documentation Checklist

Clinician documentation should indicate the following:

- Medical condition being treated
- Anatomic region
  - cervical/thoracic
  - lumbar/sacral
- Exact location of the injection
- Name and dosage of medication
  - anesthetic agent
  - steroid administered

- Level of spine injected
  - single level
  - second level
  - third or additional levels
- Number of levels injected
  - single
  - multiple
- Laterality
  - unilateral
  - bilateral
- Imaging guidance
  - fluoroscopy
  - CT

Foodborne Intoxication and Infection

Code Axes

ICD-10-CM codes for bacterial foodborne intoxication (i.e., bacterial food poisoning) are located in category AØ5 with the exceptions of *Clostridium difficile* (AØ4.7), *E. coli* (AØ4.Ø-4), *Salmonella* with gastroenteritis (AØ2.Ø), listeriosis (A32.89) and *Norovirus* enteritis (AØ8.11).

Salmonella with gastroenteritis	**AØ2.Ø**
E. coli intestinal infection	**AØ4.[Ø-4]**
Campylobacter enteritis	**AØ4.5**
Clostridium difficile enterocolitis	**AØ4.7**
Bacterial foodborne intoxication	**AØ5.[Ø-5, 8]**
Unspecified bacterial foodborne intoxication	**AØ5.9**
Other form of Listeriosis	**A32.89**
Norovirus enteritis	**AØ8.11**

⇨ I-10 ALERT

ICD-10-CM includes a new concept in category AØ5: bacterial foodborne intoxications. A foodborne intoxication involves a toxin caused by a microorganism in the food causing the illness. There are eight codes for foodborne intoxications in ICD-10-CM, differentiated by toxin.

Description of Condition

Food poisoning is foodborne infection, intoxication or toxin-mediated infection due to ingested bacterium that produces toxins or virus or parasite which causes intestinal illness (dysentery). The food or water is either contaminated externally (e.g., Salmonella) or the bacterium is present in the food and produces an exotoxin as a byproduct (e.g., Botulism).

(AØ5) Other bacterial foodborne intoxications, not elsewhere classified, including that due to staphylococcal intoxication (AØ5.Ø), botulism food poisoning (AØ5.1), foodborne Clostridium perfringens intoxication (AØ5.2), Vibrio parahaemolyticus intoxication (AØ5.3), Bacillus cereus intoxication (AØ5.4), Vibrio vulnificus intoxication (AØ5.5), and other and unspecified foodborne intoxications (AØ5.8, AØ5.9)

Toxins are produced by harmful microorganisms, the result of a chemical contamination, or are naturally part of a plant or seafood. When these toxins are ingested and invade the gastrointestinal tract, they are considered bacterial foodborne intoxications. Viruses and parasites do not cause foodborne intoxications.

Key Terms

Key terms found in the documentation may include:

Botulism (AØ5.1)

Classical foodborne intoxication due to *Clostridium botulinum* (AØ5.1)

Enteritis necroticans (AØ5.2)

Pig-bel (AØ5.2)

(AØ2.Ø) Salmonella enteritis, (AØ4.[Ø-4]) E. coli intestinal infection, (AØ4.5) Campylobacter enteritis, (AØ4.7) Clostridium difficile enterocolitis, (A32.89) Other forms of Listeriosis, and (AØ8.11) Norovirus enteritis represents foodborne intoxications

Key Terms

Key terms found in the documentation may include:

C difficile enterocolitis

E. coli (EHEC)

E. coli (EIEC) (EPEC) (ETEC) (EAEC/EAgEC)

(STEC) other Shiga toxin producing *E. coli*

Clinical Findings

The following clinical information may primarily be found in *E. coli* and *Salmonella.*

Physical Examination

History and review of systems may include:

- Copious, watery diarrhea
- Fever
- Ingestion of potentially tainted food
- Contact with an ill person
- GI bleeding with little stool

Diagnostic Procedures and Services

- Laboratory
  - stool culture
  - blood culture
  - serum electrolytes
  - BUN
  - creatinine

Therapeutic Procedures and Services

- Oral or IV hydration
- Antidiarrheal medication, if appropriate
- Antiemetics
- Antibiotics, if appropriate

Clinician Documentation Checklist

Clinician documentation should indicate the following:

- Listeriosis
  - cutaneous
  - meningitis
  - meningoencephalitis
  - sepsis
  - oculoglandular
  - endocarditis

Fracture Care

Code Axes

Fracture care codes are contained in the musculoskeletal subsection of the CPT® manual and are classified according to the anatomical location.

Description of Procedure

There are numerous types of fracture care. Clear and concise documentation is required for the procedures to be reported appropriately. Codes are categorized by the type of reduction and the method of stabilization (fixation or immobilization) and may be either open or closed.

Documentation for fractures should include the type and location of the fracture performed to correct it, including percutaneous skeletal fixation when applicable.

It should be noted that careful documentation is required as it is sometimes difficult to differentiate between the type of fracture and the type of treatment. For example, a closed fracture may require closed or open treatment while an open fracture requires open treatment. When documenting fracture care include:

- The site of the fracture
- If the treatment was open or closed
- If manipulation was performed (reduction)
- Type of fixation if any

 **CDI ALERT**

Internal fixation involves wires, pins, screws, and plates placed through the skin or within the fractured area to stabilize and immobilize the injury. It is often described as open reduction with internal fixation (ORIF).

Key Terms

Manipulation

Open treatment

Percutaneous fixation

Reduction

Skeletal traction

Clinician Note

Terms such as open, closed, pins, or wires provide the guidance needed to ensure correct code assignment.

Fracture of Femur

Code Axes

Fracture of unspecified part of neck of femur **S72.ØØ**

Unspecified intracapsular fracture of femur **S72.Ø1**

Fracture of epiphysis (separation) (upper) of femur **S72.Ø2**
(Displaced and non-displaced)

Midcervical fracture of femur **S72.Ø3**
(Displaced and non-displaced)

Fracture of base of neck of femur **S72.Ø4**
(Displaced and non-displaced)

Unspecified fracture of head of femur **S72.Ø5**

Articular fracture of head of femur **S72.Ø6**
(Displaced and non-displaced)

Other fracture of head and neck of femur **S72.Ø9**

Unspecified trochanteric fracture of femur **S72.1Ø**

Fracture of greater trochanter of femur **S72.11**
(Displaced and non-displaced)

Fracture of lesser trochanter of femur **S72.12**
(Displaced and non-displaced)

Apophyseal fracture of femur **S72.13**
(Displaced and non-displaced)

Intertrochanteric fracture of femur **S72.14**
(Displaced and non-displaced)

Subtrochanteric fracture of femur **S72.2**
(Displaced and non-displaced)

Classification Note

Many diverse types of care can be provided to patients with fracture injuries; ICD-10-CM allows the easy classification of each type of visit in a seventh-character format. Many fracture classifications include seventh-character definitions similar to the one below, which is related to hip fractures (category S72))

Character	Description
A	initial encounter for closed fracture
B	initial encounter for open fracture type I or II
C	initial encounter for open fracture type IIIA, IIIB, or IIIC
D	subsequent encounter for closed fracture with routine healing
E	subsequent encounter for open fracture type I or II with routine healing

⇨ I-10 ALERT

The number of codes representing hip fractures has expanded significantly, from 18 in ICD-9-CM to 69 in ICD-10-CM. Part of the expansion is due to laterality issues (right, left, unspecified), but many of the codes are also differentiated by whether or not the fracture was displaced. Codes are also available to classify hip articular and apophyseal fractures as well.

Character	Description
F	subsequent encounter for open fracture type IIIA, IIIB, or IIIC with routine healing
G	subsequent encounter for closed fracture with delayed healing
H	subsequent encounter for open fracture type I or II with delayed healing
J	subsequent encounter for open fracture type IIIA, IIIB, or IIIC with delayed healing
K	subsequent encounter for closed fracture with nonunion
M	subsequent encounter for open fracture type I or II with nonunion
N	subsequent encounter for open fracture type IIIA, IIIB, or IIIC with nonunion
P	subsequent encounter for closed fracture with malunion
Q	subsequent encounter for open fracture type I or II with malunion
R	subsequent encounter for open fracture type IIIA, IIIB, or IIIC with malunion
S	sequela

It is essential that the type of encounter be clearly documented, along with timeframes, history of initial injury and prior treatment, and current encounter treatment plan. Initial encounter is defined as the period of time in which the patient is receiving active treatment for the fracture (surgical treatment, emergency department encounter, and evaluation and treatment by a new physician). When the patient is receiving subsequent care for encounters after the patient has completed active treatment of the fracture and it is routine care for the fracture during the healing or recovery phase, a seventh character for subsequent encounter should be reported. Examples of fracture aftercare are: cast change or removal, removal of external or internal fixation device, medication adjustment, and follow-up visits following fracture treatment. If a code is not specified as open or closed, it should be classified as closed; if not specified as displaced or nondisplaced, it should be classified as displaced.

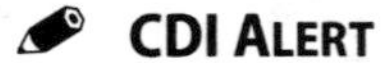

CDI ALERT

Ensure that each fracture site is described in its entirety, including the specific site (including laterality) and whether or not it is displaced. The circumstances of the encounter should be clearly documented, such as initial encounter for closed fracture, etc.

Other official guidelines related to fractures that affect documentation include:

- Fractures in patients with known osteoporosis whose injury would not usually break a normal, healthy bone should not be classified with a traumatic injury code, but with a combination code from category M8Ø Osteoporosis with current pathological fracture.
- When malunion or nonunion complications of fractures are present, the injury is classified with an injury code, but with the appropriate seventh character. All other complications should be classified separately with the appropriate complication codes.
- The reason and provision of fracture aftercare should be clearly documented and should not be classified to a separate aftercare (Z code) code. The appropriate injury seventh character is to be used instead.

Clinician Note

Careful review of medical record documentation is necessary because the type of fracture (severity) may or may not support the medical necessity of the service provided. Additionally, coordination of benefits is often required for payment from third-party payers for fracture codes so the documentation should indicate how the fracture occurred (auto accident, fall from ladder at work, fall when riding a bike).

Clinician Documentation Checklist

Clinician documentation should indicate the following:

The 7th character in fractures is based on the Gustilo classification. The following information is important to assign the appropriate 7th character:

- Episode of care: initial, subsequent, sequela
  - initial encounter: patient is receiving active treatment for the fracture
    - examples: surgical treatment, emergency department encounter, evaluation by new physician
  - subsequent encounter: patient has completed active treatment for the condition
    - examples: cast change/removal, medication adjustment, follow-up visits
  - sequela: complication or condition that arises as a direct result of a condition
    - example: scar from a burn. (The scar would be coded separately, but the burn would be assigned the S seventh character as the injury responsible for the scar.)
- Open or closed fracture
  - if open, type I or type II (Gustilo classification)
  - if open, type IIIA, IIIB, or IIIC
- Healing
  - routine healing
  - delayed healing
  - malunion
  - nonunion

Fracture — Nontraumatic of Spine/Vertebra

Code Axes

Fatigue fracture of vertebra, site unspecified	M48.4Ø
Fatigue fracture of vertebra, cervical regions	M48.41, M48.42, M48.43
Fatigue fracture of vertebra, thoracic regions	M48.44, M48.45
Fatigue fracture of vertebra, lumbosacral regions	M48.46, M48.47, M48.48
Collapsed vertebra, NEC, site unspecified	M48.5Ø
Collapsed vertebra, NEC, cervical regions	M48.51, M48.52, M48.53
Collapsed vertebra, NEC, thoracic regions	M48.54, M48.55
Collapsed vertebra, NEC, lumbosacral regions	M48.56, M48.57, M48.58
Age-related osteoporosis with current pathological fracture, vertebra(e)	M8Ø.Ø8
Other osteoporosis with current pathological fracture, vertebra(e)	M8Ø.88
Pathological fracture in neoplastic disease, vertebrae	M84.58
Pathological fracture in other disease, other site	M84.68
Personal history of (healed) osteoporosis fracture	Z87.31Ø

I-10 ALERT

Codes for nontraumatic fractures have been vastly expanded in ICD-10-CM, with specific codes related to cause and type of fracture (collapsed vertebra, etc.). These codes require the addition of seventh characters that specify the episode of care, such as that for initial or subsequent encounter, or that for sequela (late effect) of the fracture.

CDI ALERT

Any nontraumatic fracture must be documented specifically, including the type, cause, and age of fracture (new versus old). Specificity of site is also necessary in order to classify these cases appropriately.

Description of Condition

Fatigue fracture of vertebra (M48.4-)

Clinical Tip

A fatigue fracture is one that results from excessive activity rather than from a specific injury. This type of fracture is most commonly found in people who have engaged in unaccustomed, repetitive, vigorous activity. It is important to note that this type of fracture is not a result of a disease process and is typically found in younger patients than that involving a disease. These fractures may also be referred to as stress fractures, but the mechanism causing the fracture should be indicated.

Key Terms

Stress fracture

I-10 ALERT

The category for collapsed vertebra(e) should only be used when the underlying cause of the fracture has not been documented.

CDI ALERT

Ensure that the underlying cause of any stress or fatigue fracture is clearly documented for appropriate classification.

Clinician Note
When documentation indicates that an admission or encounter is for a procedure aimed at treating an underlying condition, the code for the underlying condition (such as a vertebral fracture) should be the first listed diagnosis. It is not necessary to indicate any signs or symptoms such as pain or neuropathy that may also be documented.

Collapsed vertebra, NEC (M48.5-)

Key Terms
Key terms found in the documentation for collapsed vertebra may include:

Collapsed vertebra NOS

Compression fracture

Wedging of vertebra NOS

Clinician Note
Review the medical record for terms such as osteoporosis, fatigue fracture, pathological fracture, stress fracture, or traumatic fracture. If present, query the physician to determine if a more specific type of vertebral fracture code is appropriate.

CDI Alert

Review documentation carefully for mention of collapsed vertebra(e) underlying cause. For patients under the age of 50, the condition is most often due to trauma; for patients over age 60, a common cause for females is postmenopausal (age-related) osteoporosis. In elderly patients, other common causes include malignancy and/or infection, and may be the presenting clinical symptom in multiple myeloma patients.

Age-related osteoporosis with current pathological fracture, vertebra(e) (M8Ø.Ø8-)

Clinical Tip
Osteoporosis, or a weakened state of bone density, may be caused by a number of conditions. Primary osteoporosis, which includes that designated as "age-related," may relate to a lower level of estrogen in postmenopausal women; men with decreased testosterone levels are also at risk for increased bone loss.

Key Terms
Key terms found in the documentation for age-related osteoporosis with current pathological fracture may include:

Involutional osteoporosis with current pathological fracture

Osteoporosis NOS with current pathological fracture

Osteoporosis with current fragility fracture

Osteoporotic fracture

Postmenopausal osteoporosis with current pathological fracture

Senile osteoporosis with current pathological fracture

Clinician Note
Documentation should be reviewed to determine if any major osseous defect is present as this should be reported separately. Look for terms such as bone loss or bone fragility. However, before assigning a code from M89.7- verify that this is indeed a major osseous defect.

I-10 Alert

Codes in the subcategory for age-related osteoporosis are differentiated by the presence of a current pathological fracture and then by site, including laterality. Seventh characters are required that represent the episode of care, whether initial or subsequent, or whether healing has been routine or delayed, whether any nonunion or malunion has occurred, or whether any sequela (late effect) conditions are present.

⇨ I-10 ALERT

Codes in the subcategory for other osteoporosis are differentiated by the presence of a current pathological fracture and then by site, including laterality. Seventh characters are required that represent the episode of care, whether initial or subsequent, or whether healing has been routine or delayed, whether any nonunion or malunion has occurred, or whether any sequela (late effect) conditions are present.

CDI ALERT

Ensure that the underlying cause of the pathological fracture is documented. If it is not due to age-related osteoporosis but an osteoporotic condition is present, it should be classified to subcategory M8Ø.8-. Any condition that is drug-induced should also be classified with an additional code from the T36–T5Ø code range.

⇨ I-10 ALERT

Codes for pathological fracture in the setting of neoplastic disease are differentiated by site, including laterality. Seventh characters are required that represent the episode of care, whether initial or subsequent, or whether healing has been routine or delayed, whether any nonunion or malunion has occurred, or whether any sequela (late effect) conditions are present. To appropriately capture the full diagnosis, additional codes should be assigned for the neoplastic disease process.

Other osteoporosis with current pathological fracture, vertebra(e) (M8Ø.88-)

Clinical Tip

Osteoporosis that is not age-related may be related to several other conditions, such as rheumatoid arthritis, hyperparathyroidism, Cushing's disease, chronic kidney disease, multiple myeloma or other malignancy, or drugs such as anti-epileptics, glucocorticoids, or lithium.

Key Terms

Key terms found in the documentation for other osteoporosis with current pathological fracture may include:

Drug-induced osteoporosis with current pathological fracture

Idiopathic osteoporosis with current pathological fracture

Osteoporosis of disuse with current pathological fracture

Post-oophorectomy osteoporosis with current pathological fracture

Postsurgical malabsorption osteoporosis with current pathological fracture

Post-traumatic osteoporosis with current pathological fracture

Clinician Note

Documentation should be reviewed to determine if any major osseous defect is present as this should be reported separately. Look for terms such as bone loss or bone fragility. However, before assigning a code from M89.7- verify that this is indeed a major osseous defect.

Pathological fracture in neoplastic disease, vertebrae (M84.58-)

Clinical Tip

The majority of bony metastases involves the axial skeleton (skull, vertebral column, ribs, and sternum), the proximal femur and the proximal humerus. Patients with bony lesions are at increased risk for pathological fracture and treatment typically consists of providing pain relief and stability of the area involved.

Clinical Findings

The following are specific to fatigue or stress fractures but may apply to other listed diagnosis within this topic.

Physical Examination

History and review of systems may include:

- History of back pain associated with a specific activity
- Pain with palpation of the affected site
- Localized swelling of the area
- Leg alignment

- Motor function
- Flexibility

Diagnostic Procedures and Services

- Imaging
  - x-ray
  - ultrasound
  - MRI
  - CT scan
  - scintigraphy

Therapeutic Procedures and Services

- Physical therapy
- Restricted activity and rest
- Medication
  - analgesics
  - NSAIDs

Clinician Note

The pathological fracture due to neoplastic disease should not be reported when documentation indicates bone loss but not a fracture of the bone.

The affected bone may be upper or lower end, but if the portion of the bone is at the joint, the clinician should designate the site as the bone, not the joint.

CDI ALERT

If a pathological fracture is documented for a case involving a neoplastic disease process, query the physician to determine whether the fracture is due to bony metastasis. These cases are classified to subcategory M84.5-, with an additional code for the neoplastic process.

Clinician Documentation Checklist

Clinician documentation should indicate the following:

- Osteoporosis with pathologic fracture
  - excludes: acute traumatic fractures
  - history of healed pathologic fracture
- Osteoporosis without pathologic fracture
  - history of healed pathologic fracture
- Age-related osteoporosis
  - postmenopausal
  - senile
  - involutional
- Other osteoporosis
  - idiopathic
  - drug-induced
  - postsurgical malabsorption
  - post-traumatic
  - disuse

Gastroenteritis (Viral, Bacterial, Protozoal)

⇨ I-10 ALERT

Viral infections are the most common cause of gastroenteritis but bacteria, parasites, and food-borne illnesses are also common causes. CDC statistics indicate that deaths from gastroenteritis have increased dramatically. In 2007, the most recent statistics available from the CDC, 17,000 people died from gastroenteritis; overwhelmingly, these people were older and the most common infections were Clostridium difficile and norovirus.

Code Axes

The majority of the ICD-10-CM viral, bacterial, protozoal, and gastroenteritis codes are in categories AØ2 through AØ9:

Salmonella enteritis	**AØ2.Ø**
Shigellosis	**AØ3.Ø** **AØ3.[1-3, 8-9]**
Other bacterial intestinal infections	**AØ4**
Other protozoal intestinal diseases	**AØ7**
Viral and other specified intestinal infections	**AØ8** **AØ8.Ø** **AØ8.1[1, 9]** **AØ8.2** **AØ8.3[1-2, 9]** **AØ8.[4, 8]**
Infectious gastroenteritis and colitis, unspecified	**AØ9**

Description of Condition

(AØ4) Other bacterial intestinal infections, including specific codes for various types of Escherichia coli (E. coli) infections (AØ4.Ø–AØ4.4), enteritis due to Campylobacter (AØ4.5), Yersinia enterocolitica (AØ4.6), Clostridium difficile (AØ4.7), and other and unspecified bacterial intestinal infections (AØ4.8, AØ4.9)

E. coli is one of the most commonly reported causes of human infections, particularly of the urinary and digestive tracts. The infections are classified to the following groups:

Enteropathogenic (AØ4.Ø): These bacteria are typically ingested through contaminated drinking water or through meat. The *E. coli* bacteria interfere with signal transduction of cells in the colon.

Enterotoxigenic (AØ4.1): This type of bacteria is ingested through contaminated water or food and invades the intestinal mucosa.

Enteroinvasive (AØ4.2): This strain of *E. coli* causes dysentery-like diarrhea by invading and multiplying on epithelial cells in the colon and then destroying those cells. It is transmitted solely by infected humans.

Enterohemorrhagic (AØ4.3): This is one of the most serious strains of the bacteria, causes bloody diarrhea, and, if left untreated, can cause hemolytic uremic syndrome, which can be fatal. It releases toxins into the lumen of the GI tract. The sources are mostly from water or food, such as raw meat, unpasteurized milk, fruits, and vegetables.

Documentation Tip

It is important to translate the terms the physician documents to the correct main term in the index. For example, if the physician documents the term gastroenteropathy the ICD-10-CM index includes entries related to this section and has a "see also" instructional note indicating that the main term gastroenteritis should also be referenced.

Key Terms

Key terms found in the documentation may include:

Bacterial dysentery

Bacterial enteritis

Diffusely adherent *E. coli* (enteropathogenic)

E. coli 0157:H7 (enterohemorrhagic)

Enterotoxigenic *E. Coli* (ETEC)

Pseudomembranous colitis (*C. difficile*)

Travelers' diarrhea

CDI ALERT

Ensure that the organism responsible for the gastroenteritis (if known) is documented. If the organism is presumed, suspected, etc., documentation should indicate the signs, symptoms, manifestations, clinical scenario, work-up, and treatment that support the probable diagnosis.

Clinical Tip

Another serious form of bacterial intestinal infection is that caused by *Clostridium difficile*, which is typically found as a result of extended antibiotic use: antibiotic associated diarrhea (AAD). It causes severe diarrhea when competing bacteria in the gut have been destroyed by antibiotics. The bacterium releases toxins that cause the diarrhea, bloating, and abdominal pain. The antibiotics most commonly associated with AAD include the following:

- Clindamycin (e.g., Cleocin)
- Fluoroquinolones (e.g., levofloxacin [Levaquin])
- Ciprofloxacin (Cipro, Cipro XR, Proquin XR)
- Penicillins
- Cephalosporins

(AØ8) Viral and other specified intestinal infections, including rotaviral enteritis (AØ8.Ø), acute gastroenteropathy due to Norwalk agent and other small round viruses (AØ8.1-), adenoviral enteritis (AØ8.2), calicivirus (AØ8.31), astrovirus (AØ8.32), and other and unspecified viral intestinal infections (AØ8.39, AØ8.4)

CDI ALERT

The term enteritis relates to an inflammation of the small bowel and can be caused by a number of factors including but not limited to bacterial infection, viral infection, and immune responses. Medical documentation should be reviewed to determine if bacterial or viral infection is the cause of the inflammation before a code from this chapter of the ICD-10-CM system is assigned.

Key Terms

Key terms found in the documentation may include:

Coxsackie virus enteritis

Echovirus enteritis

Enterovirus enteritis

Norovirus

Norwalk-like agent

Small round virus (SRV) gastroenteropathy

Torovirus enteritis

Clinical Findings

Physical Examination

History and review of systems may include:

- Copious, watery diarrhea
- Ingestion of potentially tainted food
- Contact with an ill person
- GI bleeding with little stool
- Fever
- Nausea
- Vomiting
- Abdominal pain

Diagnostic Procedures and Services

- Laboratory
  - stool culture
  - blood culture
  - serum electrolytes
  - BUN
  - creatinine

Therapeutic Procedures and Services

- Oral or IV hydration
- Antidiarrheal medication, if appropriate
- Antiemetics
- Antibiotics, if appropriate

Clinician Documentation Checklist

Clinician documentation should indicate the following:

- Suspected cause
  - viral
  - bacterial
    - *Salmonella*
    - *Staphylococcus*
    - *Escherichia coli*
    - *Clostridium*
    - *Shigella*
    - *Campylobacter jejuni*
    - *Yersinia*
  - parasitic

- food poisoning
- drug reactions
- food allergies
- colitis
- short bowel syndrome
- obstructing tumors
- ingestion of toxins
- In the absence of a specific organism, indicate signs, symptoms, manifestations, etc.
  - duration of illness
  - location of pain
  - stools
    - frequency
    - blood/mucous
  - primary symptoms
    - diarrhea
    - nausea
    - vomiting
    - abdominal cramps
    - fever
    - malaise
- Associated pathology
  - dehydration
  - hypokalemia
  - acidosis
  - metabolic alkalosis
  - hyponatremia
- Therapies
  - hydration
  - medications
  - antibiotics
  - antiemetics
  - antimotility agents
  - antispasmodics

Glaucoma

Code Axes

Glaucoma suspect	**H40.0**
Open-angle glaucoma	**H40.1**
Primary angle-closure glaucoma	**H40.20**
Acute angle-closure glaucoma	**H40.21**
Glaucoma secondary to eye trauma	**H40.3**
Glaucoma secondary to eye inflammation	**H40.4**
Glaucoma secondary to other eye disorders	**H40.5**
Glaucoma secondary to drugs	**H40.6**
Other glaucoma	**H40.8**
Unspecified glaucoma	**H40.9**
Glaucoma in diseases classified elsewhere	**H42**

I-10 ALERT

ICD-10-CM classifications for glaucoma include combination codes with the stage of disease specified in the seventh character for certain categories requiring reporting of disease stage.

Multiple codes should be reported, as appropriate to report the type of glaucoma, the affected eye and stage (when required).

Note: Conditions classified to chapter 7 include laterality (right, left, bilateral) within the code structure. All ophthalmic conditions should specify the affected eye(s).

Description of Condition

CDI ALERT

Ensure that the type of glaucoma is documented and the laterality of the affected eye or eyes (right, left, bilateral).

Ensure documentation of type, severity and status of disease is complete and specific.

Glaucoma (H40.----)

Clinical Tip

Glaucoma is an eye disease that gradually causes peripheral vision degradation caused by an increase in intraocular pressure (IOP) from abnormal aqueous humor outflow from the anterior chamber or decreased aqueous humor production by the ciliary body. If untreated, increased pressure leads to optic nerve damage and blindness. Prognosis and treatment depends on the type of disease, the underlying cause and whether the disease is a primary or secondary condition.

Borderline glaucoma is a condition indicative of the clinical signs and symptoms associated with glaucoma, such as borderline high IOP with associated visual field deficits.

Open angle glaucoma is an increase in IOP due to free access of the aqueous humor to the trabecular network in the angle of the anterior chamber causing progressive "tunnel vision," photophobia, and poor night vision Heredity, trauma, and chronic intraocular disease are contributing factors.

Acute closed angle glaucoma entails a sudden onset of severe eye pain and visual disturbances. The severe rise in IOP due to aqueous obstruction necessitates immediate intervention to preserve sight.

Therapies vary according to the type and severity of glaucoma, and include topical, systemic and numerous surgical procedures to reduce intraocular pressure.

Key Terms

Key terms found in the documentation for glaucoma vary depending on the type of disease, and may include:

- Acute angle-closure glaucoma:
  - Acute angle closure attack (crisis)
- Anatomic narrow angle:
  - Angle closure suspect
  - Primary angle closure suspect
- Glaucoma suspect:
  - Borderline glaucoma
  - Ocular hypertension
  - Pre-glaucoma
- Primary open angle glaucoma:
  - Chronic simple glaucoma
- Aqueous misdirection:
  - Malignant glaucoma

Clinical Tip

Borderline open angle glaucoma: level of risk (low or high) should be specifically documented to report appropriate severity level.

Ensure complete documentation that specifies the underlying causal condition as required by ICD-10-CM coding conventions for the following types of glaucoma:

H40.3 Glaucoma secondary to eye trauma

Documentation must specify nature of trauma.

H40.4 Glaucoma secondary to eye inflammation

Documentation must specify type and nature of inflammatory disorder.

H40.5 Glaucoma secondary to other eye disorders

Documentation must specify underlying eye disorder.

H40.6 Glaucoma secondary to drugs

Documentation must specify the causal drug or agent and intent (e.g., poisoning, overdose, adverse effect of drug in therapeutic use, underdosing, assault).

H42 Glaucoma in disease classified elsewhere

(This code cannot be reported alone or sequenced first.)

Documentation must specify the underlying causal disease.

Indeterminate stage of disease (seventh character 4) is not interchangeable with unspecified disease stage (seventh character 0). An indeterminate stage of disease should only be reported if the stage of disease cannot be clinically determined.

⇨ I-10 ALERT

Subcategory H40 includes valid codes that are five or six characters in length. Code H42 is a valid three-digit manifestation code that requires the associated underlying disease to be sequenced first.

The following axes of classification in category H40 describe:

- Fifth character:
  - Type of glaucoma (suspect, angle closure, primary, secondary, other)
- Sixth character:
  - Laterality (right, left, bilateral, unspecified)
- Seventh character (where required):
  - Disease stage

Clinical Findings

Physical Examination

History and review of systems may include:

- Visual examination
  - optic nerve changes on ophthalmoscopy
  - typical visual field defects
  - elevated intraocular pressure (IOP)
- Family history of glaucoma

Therapeutic Procedures and Services

- Decrease IOP
  - laser
  - medication
  - surgery

CDI ALERT

Specify laterality of affected eye for all ophthalmic conditions.

Clinician Documentation Checklist

Clinician documentation should indicate the following:

- Specifiy laterality of affected eye
  - right
  - left
  - bilateral
- Document the stage of disease as
  - mild
  - moderate
  - severe
  - indeterminate
- Document the specific type of glaucoma, underlying cause and significant findings, such as:
  - glaucoma suspect
    - open angle (specify high or low risk)
    - anatomic narrow angle (primary angle closure suspect)
    - steroid responder
    - ocular hypertension
    - primary angle closure glaucoma without glaucoma damage
  - open angle glaucoma
    - low tension
    - pigmentary
    - capsular (with pseudoexfoliation of lens)
    - residual stage
- Primary angle-closure glaucoma; specify stage as
  - acute (attack) (crisis)
  - chronic

  - intermittent
  - residual
- Glaucoma secondary to eye trauma
  - specify underlying (causal) trauma and residual complications
- Glaucoma secondary to eye inflammation
  - specify underlying chronic inflammatory condition
- Glaucoma secondary to other eye disorder
  - specify underlying eye disorder
- Glaucoma secondary to drugs
  - specify drug, medication or substance, and intent (poisoning, adverse effect in therapeutic use, assault, underdosing)
- Other glaucoma
  - glaucoma with increased episcleral venous pressure
  - hypersecretion glaucoma
  - aqueous misdirection (malignant glaucoma)

When glaucoma is associated with an ocular disorder, adverse effects of drugs or medications, or sequel of previous trauma, relate the glaucoma to the causal or underlying condition or factor.

Document any associated or underlying chronic or systemic disease processes. If conditions are inter-related, document the cause-and-effect relationship.

Hearing Loss

Code Axes

Noise effects on inner ear	**H83.3**
Conductive and sensorineural hearing loss	**H9Ø.-**
Other and unspecified hearing loss	**H91.-**
Transient ischemic deafness	**H93.Ø1**

⇨ I-10 ALERT

ICD-10-CM classifies hearing loss in separate code categories based on the type or underlying cause of hearing loss; whether the hearing loss is caused by mechanical, sensory, vascular, neurological, or other causes such as noise-induced trauma.

Noise-induced (acoustic) hearing loss is classified to subcategory H83 Other diseases of inner ear. Category H9Ø Conductive and sensorineural hearing loss, includes auditory disorders of the external, middle, or inner ear of specific or mixed type. Category H91 Other and unspecified hearing loss, includes expanded subcategories, which include specific classifications for ototoxic hearing loss, sudden idiopathic hearing loss, and presbycusis. Subcategory H93.Ø Degenerative and vascular disorders of ear, includes classifications for transient ischemic deafness.

Note: Conditions classified to chapter 8 include laterality (right, left, bilateral) within the code structure. All conditions should specify the affected ear(s).

Description of Condition

Hearing loss

Clinical Tip

Acquired hearing loss (deafness) can be clinically categorized according to the type or underlying cause. The central nervous system, organs of the ear, and related structures are vulnerable to damage, disease, tumor and deterioration from multiple possible causes, and pathologies including genetic predisposition, drugs, trauma, infection, disease, and other inter-related or overlapping factors. Types of hearing loss include:

Conductive: mechanical external and middle ear malfunction

Sensory: cochlear or inner ear disorders

Neural: auditory nerve trauma, disease or other disorder

Sensorineural: damage to cochlea or inner ear pathways to the central nervous system

Combination (mixed): overlapping causal factors (e.g., conductive and sensorineural)

Otosclerosis: genetic-related bony overgrowth (hardening) of the stapes

Transient ischemic: circulatory compromise of the small cerebrovascular vessels that supply the cochlea in the inner ear

Presbycusis: normal, degenerative age-related hearing loss of high-frequency stimuli

Sudden idiopathic: abrupt onset of unilateral hearing loss without apparent cause with spontaneous recovery of hearing within two weeks.

Key Terms

Key terms found in the documentation may include:

Acoustic trauma of inner ear (noise-induced)

Central hearing loss

Congenital deafness

Deafness

High frequency/low frequency hearing loss
Neural hearing loss
Perceptive deafness
Presbyacusia

Clinical Findings

Physical Examination

History and review of systems may include:

- Gradual or acute hearing loss
- Ear pain
- Ear discharge
- Tinnitus
- Vertigo
- Exposure to an acute event (e.g., head trauma)
- Exposure to chronic loud noise
- External ear exam
  - obstruction
  - infection
- TM perforation or drainage
- Otitis media
- Neurologic examination

Diagnostic Procedures and Services

- Imaging
  - MRI or CT
- Other
  - audiologic tests

Therapeutic Procedures and Services

- Drainage of fluid from middle ear effusion
- Surgery for damaged TM or ossicles
- Hearing aid

Documentation Tip

Documentation must include the underlying cause or type of hearing loss to avoid reporting nonspecific diagnoses. The provider should qualify the loss as:

- Noise-induced
- Conductive
- Sensorineural (or mixed type; with conductive)
- Conductive (or mixed type; with sensorineural)
- Vascular (ischemic)
- Ototoxic

⇨ I-10 Alert

ICD-10-CM classifies hearing loss to separate categories, based on the underlying cause or pathology, for example:

H83	Other diseases of inner ear
H9Ø	Conductive and sensorineural hearing loss
H91	Other and unspecified hearing loss
H93.Ø	Degenerative and vascular disorders of ear includes classifications for transient ischemic deafness

Note: Conditions classified to chapter 8 include laterality (right, left, bilateral) within the code structure. All conditions should specify the affected ear(s).

Subcategory H83.3 Noise effects on inner ear, and H91.8 Other specified hearing loss, contain placeholders X to allow for future code expansion, without disturbing the code structure.

- Presbycusis (age related; degenerative)
- Idiopathic (sudden)
- Other (specify)

Documentation of laterality and status of hearing on contralateral side should be thorough and specific to avoid reporting unspecified codes.

Ototoxic hearing loss requires documentation of the causal drug or agent and intent (e.g., poisoning, overdose, adverse effect of drug in therapeutic use, underdosing, assault) to support complete, accurate reporting.

Ensure that all related conditions are coded appropriately, particularly if hearing loss is related to other underlying diseases or disorders (e.g., vascular disease, metabolic disturbances, congenital anomalies, infection).

Clinician Note

Specify the type of hearing loss. Differentiate between noise-induced, conductive, sensory, neural, ischemic, idiopathic and other. Document whether a combination of types or pathologies exist (e.g., sensorineural, mixed conductive and sensorineural).

Document the specific anatomic site affected. For example, for transient ischemic deafness, document whether the ischemia is related to inner ear or other cerebrovascular disease. Specify the site of ischemia and underlying pathology, if known.

Document the laterality of the affected site (left, right, bilateral), and the status of hearing on the contralateral side.

For example:

H9Ø.3 Sensorineural hearing loss, bilateral

H9Ø.42 Sensorineural hearing loss, unilateral, left ear, with unrestricted hearing on the contralateral side

Clinician Documentation Checklist

Clinician documentation should indicate the following:

Noise effects on inner ear

- Type
  - labyrinthitis
  - labyrinthine fistula
  - labyrinthine dysfunction
    - includes
      - labyrinthine hypersensitivity
      - labyrinthine hypofunction
      - labyrinthine loss of function
  - noise effects of inner ear
    - includes
      - acoustic trauma of inner ear

- ♦ noise-induced hearing loss of inner ear
  - other specified diseases of inner ear
  - unspecified disease of inner ear
- Identification of laterality of ear
  - right
  - left
  - bilateral

Conductive and sensorineural hearing loss

- Conductive hearing loss, bilateral
- Conductive hearing loss, unilateral with unrestricted hearing on contralateral side
  - identification of laterality of ear
    - — right
    - — left
- Unspecified conductive hearing loss
  - conductive deafness
- Sensorineural hearing loss, bilateral
- Sensorineural hearing loss, unilateral with unrestricted hearing on contralateral side
  - identification of laterality of ear
    - — right
    - — left
- Unspecified sensorineural hearing loss
  - includes
    - — central hearing loss
    - — congenital deafness
    - — neural hearing loss
    - — perceptive hearing loss
    - — sensorineural deafness
    - — sensory hearing loss
- Mixed conductive and sensorineural hearing loss, bilateral
- Mixed conductive and sensorineural hearing loss, unilateral with unrestricted hearing on contralateral side
  - identification of laterality of ear
    - — right
    - — left
- Unspecified mixed conductive and sensorineural hearing loss

Other and unspecified hearing loss

- Type
  - ototoxic hearing loss
    - — identification of the drug
    - —presbycusis

        - presbyacusia
    - sudden idiopathic hearing loss
        - sudden hearing loss
    - deaf nonspeaking
    - other specified hearing loss
    - unspecified hearing loss
        - high frequency
        - low frequency
        - deafness
        - complete deafness
        - partial deafness
- Identification of laterality of ear
    - right
    - left
    - bilateral

Heart Failure

Code Axes

Left ventricular failure	**I5Ø.1**
Systolic (congestive) heart failure	**I5Ø.2**
Diastolic (congestive) heart failure	**I5Ø.3**
Combined systolic (congestive) and diastolic (congestive) heart failure	**I5Ø.4**
Heart failure, unspecified	**I5Ø.9**
Postprocedural heart failure	**I97.13**
Heart failure due to hypertension	**I11.Ø**
Heart failure due to hypertension with chronic kidney disease (CKD)	**I13.Ø, I13.2**
Rheumatic heart failure	**IØ9.81**

Key Terms

Key terms found in the documentation may include:

- Biventricular (heart) failure
- Cardiac asthma
- Cardiac, heart or myocardial failure
- CHF
- Congestive heart disease
- Congestive heart failure
- Edema of lung with heart disease
- Edema of lung with heart failure
- Left heart failure
- Pulmonary edema with heart disease
- Pulmonary edema with heart failure
- Right ventricular failure (secondary to left heart failure)

⇨ I-10 ALERT

When documentation indicates that the patient has congestive heart failure (CHF), review for any hypertensive heart or hypertensive heart and kidney disease. Combination classifications (e.g., I11.Ø) may be required to fully describe the condition. This classification assumes a cause-and-effect relationship because the two conditions are linked by the term "with" in the index. Per 2017 guidelines, code these conditions as related even if provider documentation does not specifically link them, unless the provider clearly states the conditions are not related. ICD-10-CM codes contain the word "congestive" in their code titles, therefore, it is not necessary to assign a separate code for CHF.

Description of Condition

Systolic (congestive) heart failure (I5Ø.2-)

Systolic heart failure is characterized by impairment of myocardial contraction, resulting in inadequate emptying of the ventricle and associated ventricular dilation. Documentation that describes an "exacerbation" of congestive heart failure indicates an acute flare-up of the condition. If the patient also carries a chronic CHF diagnosis, classify the case to one of the "acute on chronic" CHF codes.

Diastolic (congestive) heart failure (I5Ø.3-)

Diastolic heart failure occurs in patients with CHF symptoms, yet with preserved left ventricular ejection fraction (> 0.50) in the absence of major valvular disease. Filling defect occurs as a result of impaired myocardial relaxation, resulting in increased diastolic pressure. Diastolic dysfunction accounts for 40 percent to 60 percent of patients with CHF.

Other forms of heart failure

When heart failure is documented as due to hypertension (I11.Ø), hypertension and CKD (I13.Ø, I13.2), rheumatic heart disease (I09.81), or is due to an obstetric (O75.4) or other procedure (I97.13-), the documentation should clearly indicate whether CHF is the precipitating factor. In these cases, a separate code should be assigned to appropriately classify the heart failure.

Clinical Findings

Physical Examination

History and review of systems may include:

- Myocardial infarction
- Hypertension
- Heart murmur
- Dyspnea
- Fatigue
- Reflecting low cardiac output
- Ankle swelling
- LV Failure
  - tachycardia
  - tachypnea
  - cyanosis
  - hypotension
  - LV systolic dysfunction
- RV failure
  - pitting edema of feet and ankles
  - enlarged liver
  - abdominal swelling
  - ascites
  - elevated jugular venous pressure

Diagnostic Procedures and Services

- Laboratory
  - CBC
  - creatinine
  - BUN
  - electrolytes

- albumin
- liver function
- Imaging
  - chest x-ray
  - echocardiogram
  - radionuclide imaging
  - cardiac MRI
- Other
  - ECG
  - coronary angiography
  - cardiac catheterization

Therapeutic Procedures and Services

- Treatment for the cause of heart failure
- Diet and lifestyle changes
- Medications
  - diuretics
  - nitrates
  - digitalis preparation
  - ACE inhibitors
  - vasodilators
  - beta blockers
  - angiotensin II receptor blockers (ARB)
  - aldosterone antagonists
- Device therapy, if applicable (i.e., pacemakers, ICD)
- Percutaneous intervention or surgery

Clinician Note

Code assignment for congestive heart failure is dependent upon both the type of failure (e.g., left systolic, diastolic, combined) as well as severity (e.g., acute chronic, acute on chronic). Documentation should be carefully reviewed for this type of information and, if not present, the physician should be queried. Code I5Ø.9 should only be reported if the type of heart failure can be further specified.

Clinician Documentation Checklist

Clinician documentation should indicate the following:

- Types
  - left ventricular
  - systolic
  - diastolic
  - combined systolic and diastolic
  - unspecified
- Severity

  - acute
  - chronic
  - acute on chronic
- Also document
  - associated hypertension
  - associated renal disease
  - congestive
  - neonatal

Postprocedural Heart Failure

- Postcardiotomy syndrome
- Postmastectomy lymphedema syndrome
- Postprocedural hypertension
- Type of surgery
  - following heart catheterization
  - following cardiac bypass
  - following cardiac surgery
  - following other circulatory surgery
  - following other surgery
- Timing
  - intraoperative
  - postoperative
- Other functional disturbances
  - cardiac insufficiency
  - cardiac arrest
  - heart failure
  - other functional disturbances
- Hemorrhage and/or hematoma
- Accidental puncture and laceration
- Cerebrovascular infarction

Hematuria in Glomerular Disease

Code Axes

Recurrent and persistent hematuria with minor glomerular abnormality	**NØ2.Ø**
Recurrent and persistent hematuria with focal and segmental glomerular lesions	**NØ2.1**
Recurrent and persistent hematuria with diffuse membranous glomerulonephritis	**NØ2.2**
Recurrent and persistent hematuria with diffuse mesangial proliferative glomerulonephritis	**NØ2.3**
Recurrent and persistent hematuria with diffuse endocapillary proliferative glomerulonephritis	**NØ2.4**
Recurrent and persistent hematuria with diffuse mesangiocapillary glomerulonephritis	**NØ2.5**
Recurrent and persistent hematuria with dense deposit disease	**NØ2.6**
Recurrent and persistent hematuria with diffuse crescentic glomerulonephritis	**NØ2.7**
Recurrent and persistent hematuria with other morphologic changes	**NØ2.8**
Recurrent and persistent hematuria with unspecified morphologic changes	**NØ2.9**

Clinical Tip

Glomerular disease affects the glomerulus, which is responsible for filtering toxins out of the blood and excreting them in the urine, while keeping red blood cells and proteins in the bloodstream. Hematuria (blood in the urine) may be a precursor to more serious renal disorders.

Note: The following definitions are related to the glomerular diseases discussed in this section:

Global: Affecting the whole of the glomerulus uniformly.

Segmental: Affecting one glomerular segment, leaving other segments unaffected.

Diffuse: Affecting all glomeruli in both kidneys.

Focal: Affecting a proportion of glomeruli, with others unaffected

⇨ I-10 Alert

Hematuria has been found to be a far more important symptom in the diagnosis and treatment of renal diseases than previously thought. When it is recurrent and persistent and diagnosed with several various glomerular diseases, combination codes are available in ICD-10-CM in category NØ2 to report the condition much more accurately than was possible in ICD-9-CM.

Description of Condition

Recurrent and persistent hematuria with minor glomerular abnormality (NØ2.Ø)

Clinical Tip

As the name implies, this form of glomerular disease is minor, but requires treatment to avoid further disease progression to nephrotic syndrome. The most common symptom is massive fluid accumulation, edema, and proteinuria. It affects the pediatric population at higher rates than that for adults and typically responds after three months of steroid treatment.

Key Terms

Key terms found in the documentation for recurrent and persistent hematuria with minor glomerular abnormality may include:

Minimal change disease

Minimal change lesion

Nil disease (lipoid nephrosis)

Nil lesions

Clinician Note

Documentation such as laboratory results should support the presence of blood in the urine.

Recurrent and persistent hematuria with focal and segmental glomerular lesions (NØ2.1)

Clinical Tip

This condition usually presents as nephrotic syndrome, especially in children, and is a cause of acute kidney failure in adults. Focal and segmental refer to the presentation of the kidney tissue on biopsy: focal—only some of the glomeruli are involved (as opposed to diffuse), and segmental refers to the fact that only part of each glomerulus is involved (as opposed to global).

Key Terms

Key terms found in the documentation for recurrent and persistent hematuria with focal and segmental glomerular lesions may include:

Focal glomerular sclerosis

Focal nodular glomerulosclerosis

Focal segmental glomerulosclerosis (FSGS)

Recurrent and persistent hematuria with focal and segmental hyalinosis

Recurrent and persistent hematuria with focal and segmental sclerosis

Recurrent and persistent hematuria with focal glomerulonephritis

Clinician Note

Documentation such as laboratory results should support the presence of blood in the urine.

Recurrent and persistent hematuria with diffuse membranous glomerulonephritis (NØ2.2)

Clinical Tip

This is a slowly progressive disease of the kidney affecting mostly patients between the ages of 30 and 50 years, characterized by inflammation of the basement membrane but not the mesangium (a structure in the glomerulus of the kidney, between the capillaries). It is the second most common cause of nephrotic syndrome in adults, with focal segmental glomerulosclerosis (FSGS) being the most common.

Key Terms

Key terms found in the documentation for recurrent and persistent hematuria with diffuse membranous glomerulonephritis may include:

Membranous glomerulopathy

Membranous nephritis

Membranous nephropathy

Clinician Note

Terms such as nephritic and nephrosis are often used when documenting glomerular diseases and require careful attention to the medical record documentation.

Recurrent and persistent hematuria with diffuse mesangial proliferative glomerulonephritis (NØ2.3)

Clinical Tip

This disease process is a form of glomerulonephritis associated primarily with the mesangium, a supportive structure in the glomerulus of the kidney, between the capillaries that assists with filtration. The condition also causes antibody deposits in the mesangium layer, which increases in size and number, giving the glomeruli a lumpy appearance. It usually causes nephrotic syndrome and may progress to chronic kidney failure.

Key Terms

Key terms found in the documentation for recurrent and persistent hematuria with diffuse mesangial proliferative glomerulonephritis may include:

Glomerulonephritis — mesangial proliferative

Mesangial proliferative GN

Clinician Note

Documentation such as laboratory results should support the presence of blood in the urine.

Recurrent and persistent hematuria with diffuse endocapillary proliferative glomerulonephritis (NØ2.4)

Clinical Tip

This condition is characterized by endocapillary hypercellularity, which is defined by the presence and proliferation of cells within the capillary lumina, affecting kidney function. Proliferating cells are mesangials, endothelials, and circulating inflammatory cells that have migrated to the capillary tuft. There is occlusion of capillary lumens due to cellular proliferation and endothelial cells edema. The lesion is usually diffuse, but, in some cases, it is segmental and focal.

Key Terms

Key terms found in the documentation for recurrent and persistent hematuria with diffuse endocapillary proliferative glomerulonephritis may include:

Diffuse proliferative endocapillary glomerulonephritis (EPGN)

Clinician Note

Documentation such as laboratory results should support the presence of blood in the urine.

Recurrent and persistent hematuria with diffuse mesangiocapillary glomerulonephritis (NØ2.5)

Clinical Tip

This condition is a chronic form of glomerulonephritis characterized by mesangial cell proliferation, irregular thickening of glomerular capillary walls, and thickening of the mesangial matrix and glomerular basement membrane.

Key Terms

Key terms found in the documentation for recurrent and persistent hematuria with diffuse mesangiocapillary glomerulonephritis may include:

Membranoproliferative glomerulonephritis

Clinician Note

Documentation such as laboratory results should support the presence of blood in the urine.

Recurrent and persistent hematuria with dense deposit disease (NØ2.6)

Clinical Tip

This is a type of glomerulonephritis caused by deposits in the kidney glomerular mesangium and basement membrane (GBM) thickening, which damages the glomeruli. The distinctive factor involves deposits at the intraglomerular mesangium.

Key Terms

Key terms found in the documentation for recurrent and persistent hematuria with dense deposit disease may include:

Membranoproliferative glomerulonephritis type II (MPGNII)

Clinician Note

Documentation such as laboratory results should support the presence of blood in the urine.

Recurrent and persistent hematuria with diffuse crescentic glomerulonephritis (NØ2.7)

Clinical Tip

This is an uncommon form of acute glomerulonephritis characterized by heavy proteinuria, microaneurysms, and hypertension. The primary distinguishing characteristic is crescent formation in the glomeruli; prognosis is related to the proportion of affected glomeruli. In true crescentic glomerulonephritis, crescents are present in 50 percent or more of the glomeruli. Crescents in 80 percent to 100 percent of the glomeruli have been described as rapidly progressive glomerulonephritis. This lesion usually progresses to renal insufficiency and/or failure in less than six months.

Key Terms

Key terms found in the documentation for recurrent and persistent hematuria with diffuse crescentic glomerulonephritis may include:

Extracapillary glomerulonephritis

Clinical Findings

Physical Examination

History and review of systems may include:

- Dark-colored urine
- Recent strep throat
- Fatigue
- Weight gain
- Vomiting
- Hypertension
- Edema
- Oliguria
- Fever
- Periorbital edema
- Respiratory crackles
- Elevated jugular venous pressure
- Abdominal pain
- Palpable kidneys
- Diagnostic Procedures and Services

- Laboratory
  - urinalysis
  - BUN
  - serum creatinine
  - CBC
  - serologic testing
  - urine culture
- Imaging
  - ultrasonography
  - CT scan
  - voiding cystourethrograms
  - radionuclide study

Clinician Note

Documentation such as laboratory results should support the presence of blood in the urine.

Clinician Documentation Checklist

Clinician documentation should indicate the following:

- Type of glomerular disease
  - global
  - segmental
  - diffuse
  - focal
  - mesangial/mesangium
  - endocapillary hypercellularity

Hemorrhoids and Perianal Venous Thrombosis

Code Axes

First degree hemorrhoids	**K64.Ø**
Second degree hemorrhoids	**K64.1**
Third degree hemorrhoids	**K64.2**
Fourth degree hemorrhoids	**K64.3**
Residual hemorrhoidal skin tags	**K64.4**
Perianal venous thrombosis	**K64.5**
Other and unspecified hemorrhoids	**K64.8, K64.9**

Clinical Tip

The definitions for the degrees of hemorrhoids are as follows:

First degree: No prolapse outside of the anal canal

Second degree: Prolapse with straining, but retract spontaneously

Third degree: Prolapse with straining and require manual replacement back inside the anal canal

Fourth degree: Prolapsed tissue that cannot be manually replaced

Key Terms

Key terms found in the documentation may include:

External hemorrhoids

External hemorrhoid with thrombosis

First degree internal hemorrhoid

Fourth degree internal hemorrhoid

Internal hemorrhoids

Perianal hematoma

Piles

Second degree internal hemorrhoid

Third degree internal hemorrhoid

Thrombosed hemorrhoids

Clinician Documentation Checklist

Clinician documentation should indicate the following:

- Piles
- Combined
- Hemorrhoid skin tag

⇨ I-10 ALERT

The classification axis for hemorrhoids is completely revised in ICD-10-CM. It has been moved from the circulatory chapter to the digestive system chapter. Instead of internal/external and bleeding/other complication axes, ICD-10-CM classifies these conditions according to degree, first through fourth.

CDI ALERT

Alert the medical staff to the need for documentation of the degree or stage of hemorrhoids and provide ICD-10-CM definitions, if necessary. Additionally, documentation often will indicate the location of the hemorrhoid using clock positioning.

CDI ALERT

Carefully examine the medical record documentation for indications of thrombosis. Thrombosis is a condition arising from the presence or formation of blood clots within a blood vessel that may cause vascular obstruction and insufficient oxygenation.

- Type
  - first-degree hemorrhoids
    - grade/stage I hemorrhoids
    - hemorrhoids (bleeding) without prolapse outside of anal canal
  - second-degree hemorrhoids
    - grade/stage II hemorrhoids
    - hemorrhoids (bleeding) that prolapse with straining, but retract spontaneously
  - third-degree hemorrhoids
    - grade/stage III hemorrhoids
    - hemorrhoids (bleeding) that prolapse with straining and require manual replacement into anal canal
  - fourth-degree hemorrhoids
    - grade/stage IV hemorrhoids
    - hemorrhoids (bleeding) with prolapsed tissue that cannot be manually replaced
  - residual hemorrhoids skin tags
    - external hemorrhoids
    - skin tags of anus
  - perianal venous thrombosis
    - external hemorrhoids with thrombosis
    - perianal hematoma
    - thrombosed hemorrhoids
  - other hemorrhoids:
    - internal hemorrhoids, without mention of degree
    - prolapsed hemorrhoids, degree not specified
  - unspecified hemorrhoids
    - hemorrhoids (bleeding)
    - hemorrhoids (bleeding) without mention of degree

Human Immunodeficiency Virus (HIV) Disease

Code Axes

Human immunodeficiency virus (HIV) disease **B2Ø**

Clinical Tip

Some conditions are considered opportunistic infections and are routinely associated with HIV disease; it is vitally important that these conditions be coded when documented.

Condition	ICD-10-CM Code
Tuberculosis, all types	A15–A19
Strep and other sepsis	A4Ø.9, A41.-
Herpesviral infections	A6Ø.Ø[Ø,1,4,9], A6Ø.1, A6Ø.9, BØØ.-
Candidal infections	B37.-
Cryptococcal infections	B45-
Pneumocystosis	B59
Kaposi's sarcoma	C46.-
Non-follicular lymphoma	C83.-
Mature T/NK-cell lymphoma	C84.-
Other specified and unspecified non-Hodgkin lymphoma	C85.-
Unspecified dementia	FØ3.-
Other and unspecified encephalopathy and disorder of brain	G93.4-, G93.9
Acute and subacute endocarditis	I33.-
Flu due to identified influenza A virus with pneumonia	JØ9.X1
Other and unspecified viral pneumonia	J12.8-, J12.9
Bacterial pneumonia, NEC	J15.-
Lobar and other pneumonia	J18.[1,8,9]

Note: The codes in the table above are not all-inclusive.

Key Terms

Key terms found in the documentation may include:

- Acquired immune deficiency syndrome (AIDS)
- AIDS related complex (ARC)
- HIV infection, symptomatic
- Primary HIV infection

Clinical Tip

According to the Centers for Disease Control and Prevention (CDC), in order to be diagnosed with AIDS, a person with HIV must have an AIDS-defining condition or have a baseline CD4 count less than 200 cells/mm.

⇨ I-10 ALERT

The guidelines for ICD-10-CM indicate that the code for HIV disease should only be assigned for confirmed cases, which may consist of a physician's diagnostic statement. Positive serology or culture is not specifically required in order to assign the HIV code. If the reason for the encounter is for treatment of an HIV related disease, the HIV code (B2Ø) should be assigned as the first-listed/principal diagnosis. Because of this guideline, it is essential that those staff members participating in the coding and/or documentation improvement efforts become knowledgeable about the disorders that are considered AIDS-defining conditions.

CDI ALERT

Carefully examine the medical record documentation. Terms such as "HIV positive," "known HIV," or "HIV test positive" refer to the patients' asymptomatic human immunodeficiency virus (HIV) status and do not refer to an HIV-related illness.

Ensure that the patient's HIV status is clearly documented. If a patient has inconclusive serologic evidence of an HIV infection, code R75 should be assigned. A patient that has tested positive for HIV, but as of yet has had no symptoms or AIDS-defining conditions, should be classified to code Z21. The documentation differentiating these three HIV status positions should be clear in the medical record.

Clinical Findings

Diagnostic Procedures and Services

- Laboratory
  - HIV antibody test
  - nucleic acid amplification assays
  - ELISA
  - Western blot
- Associated pathology
  - malignancies such as Kaposi's sarcoma, lymphoma and squamous cell carcinoma
  - fungal diseases such as candidiasis, cryptococcosis and penicilliosis
  - bacterial diseases such as tuberculosis, *Mycobacterium avium* complex, bacterial pneumonia, and septicemia
  - protozoal diseases such as *Pneumocystis carinii* pneumonia (PCP), toxoplasmosis, microsporidiosis, cryptosporidiosis, isosporiasis, and leishmaniasis
  - viral diseases such as those caused by cytomegalovirus, herpes simplex, and herpes zoster virus

Therapeutic Procedures and Services

- Therapy for opportunistic infections and malignancies: antibiotics for opportunistic infections and chemotherapy for malignancies
- Antiretroviral treatment: drugs that suppress the HIV infection. A combination of drugs is standard and using a single drug is discouraged.
- Hematopoietic stimulating factors: treatment of anemia
- Prophylaxis for opportunistic infections: prevention of certain infections before they develop. This should be offered to patients with CD4 counts below 200 cells/µl, weight loss, or oral candidiasis.
- Medications
- Antiretroviral treatment: nucleoside reverse transcriptase inhibitors (NRTI)
  - Combivir
  - Emtriva
  - Videx, Videx EC
  - Retrovir (AZT)
  - Epzicom
- Nonnucleoside reverse transcriptase inhibitors (NNRTI)
  - Viramune
  - Rescriptor
  - Sustiva

- Prophylaxis treatment
  - Trimethoprim-sulfamethoxazole
  - Dapsone
  - aerolized pentamidine
  - Clarithromycin
  - Rifabutin
- Hematopoietic stimulating factors
  - erythropoietin
- Treatment of opportunistic infections
  - Trimetrexate
  - Primaquine
  - Clindamycin
- Surgical procedures
  - placement of a vascular access device

Hypertension Complicating Childbirth, Pregnancy, and the Puerperium

CDI ALERT

Documentation must indicate if the hypertension is pre-existing or gestational as well as the following:

- Trimester
- Hypertensive heart disease when present
- Chronic kidney disease when present
- Pre-eclampsia if present

Code Axes

Pre-existing hypertension complicating pregnancy, childbirth and the puerperium	**O1Ø.Ø** **O1Ø.42** **O1Ø.43**
Pre-existing hypertension with pre-eclampsia	**O11.-**
Gestational (pregnancy-induced) hypertension without significant proteinuria	**O13.-**
Unspecified maternal hypertension	**O16.-**

CDI ALERT

In addition to identifying any conditions associated with the hypertension as shown in the Key Terms section, the documentation should also indicate whether the hypertension is essential, secondary, or unspecified. If unspecified, query the physician as to the type.

Description of Condition

The Pregnancy, Childbirth and the Puerperium chapter of the ICD-10-CM system contains codes which describe pregnancy complicated by hypertension.

I-10 ALERT

Category O1Ø Pre-existing hypertension complicating pregnancy, childbirth and the puerperium, includes codes for hypertensive heart and hypertensive chronic kidney disease. When assigning one of the O1Ø codes that includes hypertensive heart disease or hypertensive chronic kidney disease, it is necessary to add a secondary code from the appropriate hypertension category to specify the type of heart failure or chronic kidney disease.

Pre-existing hypertension complication pregnancy, childbirth and the puerperium (O1Ø.Ø1X–O1Ø.93)

Documentation should indicate pre-existing hypertension affecting the management of the pregnancy.

Key Terms

Key terms found in the documentation may include:

- Eclampsia complicated by pre-existing hypertension
- Pre-eclampsia complicated by pre-existing hypertension
- Pregnancy complicated by hypertension due to ______________
- Pregnancy complicated by hypertensive arteriosclerosis of kidney
- Pregnancy complicated by hypertensive cardiovascular disease
- Pregnancy complicated by hypertensive chronic kidney disease
- Pregnancy complicated by hypertensive chronic nephritis
- Pregnancy complicated by hypertensive chronic renal disease
- Pregnancy complicated by hypertensive heart disease
- Pregnancy complicated by hypertensive heart failure
- Pregnancy complicated by hypertensive interstitial nephritis
- Pregnancy complicated by hypertensive nephropathy
- Pregnancy complicated by hypertensive nephrosclerosis
- Pregnancy complicated by hypertensive renal disease
- Pregnancy complicated by secondary hypertension

Pre-existing hypertension with pre-eclampsia (O11.1–O11.9)

Pre-eclampsia is a complication of pregnancy manifesting in the development of borderline hypertension, protein in the urine, and unresponsive swelling between the 20th week of pregnancy and the end of the first week following birth in mild to moderate cases. Severe pre-eclampsia presents with hypertension (blood pressure greater than 150/100) associated with marked swelling, proteinuria, abdominal pain, and/or visual changes. Documentation must support that the patient had pre-existing hypertension or this code is not supported. ***Synonym(s):*** mild toxemia.

I-10 ALERT

When reporting a code from O11, an additional code from category O1Ø must be assigned to indicate the type of hypertension.

Key Terms

Key terms found in the documentation may include:

Essential hypertension (pre-eclampsia)

Hypertension with pre-eclampsia

Maternal hypertension superimposed with pre-eclampsia

Pre-existing hypertension (pre-eclampsia)

CDI ALERT

Documentation should indicate the type of hypertension present (essential, secondary) as well as any organ involvement (hypertensive heart disease, chronic kidney disease)

Gestational (pregnancy-induced) hypertension without significant proteinuria (O13.1–O13.9)

Gestational hypertension is a form of hypertension that forms during pregnancy. Gestational hypertension is diagnosed when blood pressure readings are higher than 140/90 mm Hg after 20 weeks of pregnancy with normal blood pressure.

Key Terms

Key terms found in the documentation may include:

Gestation hypertension

Gestational hypertension without proteinuria

Hypertension during pregnancy

Hypertension with pregnancy

CDI ALERT

When the physician documentation indicates that the patient has significant amounts of protein in the urine (proteinuria), query the physician to see if the patient may be pre-eclamptic.

Unspecified maternal hypertension (O16.1–O16.9)

Hypertension during pregnancy; documentation does not indicate if the hypertension is pre-existing or gestational.

CDI ALERT

Query the physician to determine if a more specific diagnosis is available.

Clinical Findings

Physical Examination

History and review of systems may include:

- Rapid weight gain
- Swelling of hands, face and feet that persists
- Decreased/no urine output
- Severe headaches
- Bloody urine
- Dizziness

- Excessive nausea and vomiting
- Visual disturbance
- Hypertension severity
- Reflex changes
- Abdominal pain

Diagnostic Procedures and Services

- Laboratory
  - urinalysis
  - urine dip
  - CBC
  - glucose levels
  - liver enzymes
  - creatinine clearance
  - serum creatinine
  - BUN
  - albumin
  - uric acid
  - TSH
- Other
  - fetal ultrasound transducer

Therapeutic Procedures and Services

- Home BP monitoring
- Patient education
- Bed rest
- Fetal monitoring
- Antihypertension medication if applicable

Clinician Documentation Checklist

Clinician documentation should indicate the following:

- At time of visit
  - antepartum (trimester #)
  - childbirth
  - puerperium
- Type
  - pre-existing
    - essential
    - secondary
      - etiology when known
    - hypertensive heart disease
      - type of heart disease
      - hypertensive chronic kidney disease

- stage of kidney disease
- hypertensive heart and chronic kidney disease
  - type of heart disease
  - stage of kidney disease
- unspecified
- with pre-eclampsia
  - type of heart disease
- gestational
  - without significant proteinuria
- unspecified maternal hypertension

Pre-existing Hypertension with Pre-eclampsia

- Trimester
- Gestational edema only
- Pre-eclampsia
  - Severity
    - mild
    - moderate
    - severe
  - HELLP syndrome, if present
  - with hypertension
    - gestational
    - pre-existing

Hypertensive Diseases

Code Axes

Essential (primary) hypertension	I1Ø
Hypertensive heart disease	I11
Hypertensive chronic kidney disease	I12
Hypertensive heart and chronic kidney disease	I13
Secondary hypertension	I15
Postoperative hypertension	I97.3

Description of Condition

Essential (primary) hypertension (I1Ø)

Elevated arterial blood pressure that occurs without an apparent organic cause. In the benign form, the blood pressure is mildly elevated. In the malignant form, the elevation is severe and may result in necrosis of the kidneys or retinas. Hemorrhage and death may occur, most often due to uremia or rupture of cerebral vessels.

I-10 ALERT

Hypertension no longer uses type as an axes of classification. Therefore, terms such as malignant, benign, or unspecified no longer require a different code assignment and are included in the essential (primary) hypertension category (I1Ø).

Key Terms

Key terms found in the documentation may include:

- Arterial hypertension
- Benign hypertension
- Controlled hypertension
- Essential hypertension
- HBP
- High blood pressure
- HTN
- Hypertension
- Malignant hypertension
- Primary hypertension
- Uncotrolled hypertension

Hypertensive heart disease (I11.Ø–I11.9)

A causal relationship is stated (due to hypertension) or implied (hypertensive).

The same heart conditions (I5Ø.-, I51.4–I51.9) with hypertension are also assigned a code from this category.

CDI ALERT

Documentation containing an elevated BP without mention of hypertension does not support a diagnosis of hypertension.

Key terms

Key terms found in the documentation may include:

- Hypertensive cardiovascular disease
- Hypertensive heart disease
- Hypertensive heart failure

Hypertensive chronic kidney disease (I12.Ø–I12.9)

Documentation indicates that both hypertension and a condition classifiable to category N18 Chronic kidney disease (CKD), are present. Since a cause-and-effect relationship is presumed, when documentation indicates both chronic kidney disease with hypertension this category is supported.

> ⇨ **I-10 ALERT**
>
> When documentation states the hypertension is due to kidney disease, the hypertension is considered secondary.

Key Terms

Key terms found in the documentation may include:

- Hypertension and arteriosclerosis of kidney
- Hypertension and chronic kidney disease
- Hypertension and chronic nephritis
- Hypertension and chronic renal disease
- Hypertension and interstitial nephritis
- Hypertension and nephrosclerosis
- Hypertensive chronic kidney disease
- Hypertensive nephropathy
- Hypertensive renal disease

>  **CDI ALERT**
>
> Documentation should also identify the stage of chronic kidney disease. This is reported separately.

Hypertensive heart and chronic kidney disease (I13.1–I13.9)

When both hypertensive kidney disease and hypertensive heart disease are stated in the diagnosis, the appropriate code from category I13 is supported. The ICD-10-CM system assumes a relationship between the hypertension and the chronic kidney disease, whether or not the condition is documented as related.

Key Terms

Key terms found in the documentation may include:

- Hypertensive chronic heart and kidney disease
- Hypertensive heart and renal disease
- Hypertensive heart disease and arteriosclerosis of kidney
- Hypertensive heart disease and chronic kidney disease
- Hypertensive heart disease and chronic nephritis
- Hypertensive heart disease and chronic renal disease
- Hypertensive heart disease and interstitial nephritis
- Hypertensive heart disease and nephrosclerosis
- Hypertensive nephropathy and hypertensive heart disease

> **CDI ALERT**
>
> When documentation indicates that heart failure is present, an additional code from category I5Ø to identify the type of heart failure is assigned.

Secondary Hypertension (I15.Ø-I15.9)

Secondary hypertension is hypertension that is due to an underlying condition.

Key Terms

Key terms found in the documentation may include:

Hypertension due to ____________

Renovascular hypertension

Secondary hypertension [condition causing the hypertension]

> **⇨ I-10 ALERT**
>
> Two codes are required: one to identify the underlying etiology and one from category I15 to identify the hypertension. Sequencing is determined by the reason for admission/encounter.

Postoperative hypertension (I97.3)

Documentation indicates that hypertension as the complication of a procedure is present.

Key Terms

Key terms found in the documentation may include:

Postprocedure hypertension

Clinical Findings

Physical Examination

Hypertension is typically asymptomatic until complications arise in other organ systems. History and review of symptoms may include:

- Dizziness
- Headache
- Epistaxis
- Flushed face
- Fatigue

Severe hypertension may cause major cardiovascular and renal symptoms including:

- Shortness of breath with minimal exertion
- Swollen ankles, legs, and feet
- Swelling in abdomen
- Pitting edema
- Jugular vein distention
- Confusion
- Blurry or double vision
- Bloody urine
- Decrease in urine output
- Exam
  - funduscopic exam
  - auscultation for bruits (neck and abdomen)
  - peripheral pulses

- complete cardiac, neurologic and respiratory exam

Diagnostic Procedures and Services

- Laboratory
  - urinalysis
  - albumin
  - creatinine
  - fasting plasma glucose
  - Na
  - TSH
  - lipid profile
- Imaging
  - chest x-ray
  - Doppler ultrasound
  - angiography
  - cardiac MRI
  - cardiac cath
  - echocardiogram
- Other
  - EKG
  - Holter monitor
  - stress test

Therapeutic Procedures and Services

- Low-salt diet
- Lifestyle changes
- Medication
  - diuretic
  - beta blocker
  - ACE inhibitor
  - Ca channel blockers
  - angiotensin II receptor blockers (ARB)
  - digoxin
  - aldosterone antagonists
  - direct vasodilators
- Smoking cessation
- Implantable cardioverter defibrillator (ICD)
- Left ventricular assist device

Clinician Documentation Checklist

Clinician documentation should indicate the following:

- Hypertension
- Heart disease
- Heart failure
  - diastolic
    - acute
    - chronic
  - systolic
    - acute
    - chronic
- Chronic kidney disease (CKD)
  - CKD stage

Hysterectomy

Code Axes

Hysterectomy procedures	**58150–58294**
Laparoscopic hysterectomy	**58541–58554**

Description of Procedure

A hysterectomy is the removal of the uterus. The tubes and/or ovaries may or may not be removed at the time of a hysterectomy procedure. There are three surgical approaches that can be used to perform a hysterectomy (abdominal incision or open, vaginal approach, or laparoscopic approach) and other services may be performed during the surgical encounter such as urethrocystopexy for urinary incontinence or lymph node sampling. It is also important to note that the size of the uterus may also affect code assignment.

OPEN APPROACH

Total abdominal hysterectomy (corpus and cervix), with or without removal of tube(s), with or without removal of ovary(s) (58150)

Total abdominal hysterectomy (corpus and cervix), with or without removal of tube(s), with or without removal of ovary(s); with colpourethrocystopexy (e.g., Marshall-Marchetti-Krantz, Burch) (58152)

Documentation will indicate a horizontal incision just within the pubic hairline. The physician removes the uterus including the cervix and may elect to remove one or both of the ovaries and one or both of the fallopian tubes (salpingo-oophorectomy). The supporting pedicles containing the tubes, ligaments, and arteries are clamped and cut free. The uterus and cervix are removed along with a narrow rim or cuff of vaginal lining. The vaginal defect may be left open for drainage.

At the time of a total hysterectomy, it may also be necessary to perform a colpourethrocystopexy for urinary incontinence. Documentation will indicate that the bladder neck is suspended by placing sutures through the tissue surrounding the urethra and into the back of the symphysis pubis, which is the midline junction of the pubic bones in the front (Marshall-Marchetti-Krantz or MMK), or sutures may be placed in the fascia on either side of the bladder and then through the Cooper's ligaments above. The sutures are then tied which elevates the vesical neck (the junction of the bladder and urethra) in the direction of the Cooper's ligament (Burch procedure). The sutures are pulled tight so that the tissues are tacked to the symphysis pubis and the urethra is moved forward.

CDI ALERT

When the documentation states that the uterus weighs more than 250 grams, see codes 58543–58544.

Supracervical abdominal hysterectomy (subtotal hysterectomy), with or without removal of tube(s), with or without removal of ovaries (58180)

Documentation for a supracervical abdominal hysterectomy will indicate the removal of the uterus above the cervix and may elect to remove one or both of the ovaries and one or both of the fallopian tubes (salpingo-oophorectomy) via a horizontal incision just within the pubic hairline. It is important to note that the uteri cervix is not removed during this service.

LAPAROSCOPIC APPROACH

Laparoscopy, surgical, supracervical hysterectomy, for uterus greater than 250 g (58543)

Laparoscopy, surgical, supracervical hysterectomy, for uterus greater than 250 g; with removal of tube(s) and ovary(s) (58544)

Key terms in the documentation for these procedures will indicate that the patient is placed in the dorsal lithotomy position, that a speculum is placed in the vagina so that the clinician may grasp the cervix with an instrument to manipulate the uterus during the surgery, and that trocars are inserted periumbilically in the right and left lower quadrants of the abdomen. Documentation will also indicate that the uterus is morcellized and removed using endoscopic tools. In 58544, one or both ovaries and/or one or both fallopian tubes are removed in similar fashion. Once the excisions are complete, the abdominal cavity is deflated and instruments and trocars removed. The fascia and skin are closed with sutures.

Vaginal hysterectomy, with total or partial vaginectomy (58275)

Vaginal hysterectomy, with total or partial vaginectomy; with repair of enterocele (58280)

Vaginal hysterectomy, radical (Schauta type operation) (58285)

Schauta procedure

The Schauta procedure is the surgical removal through a vaginal approach of the uterus, cervix, upper vagina, and parametrium. This procedure does not permit pelvic lymph node dissection but is useful in certain patients, such as in obese patients. Other parts such as the lymph nodes, ovaries, and fallopian tubes are also usually removed if clinically indicated. It is usually performed for early malignancy of the cervix but can also be performed on patients who have severe uterine prolapse or prolapse accompanied by stress incontinence and for patients with pelvic relaxation, history of myomata, and irregular uterine bleeding.

Vaginal hysterectomy for uterus greater than 250 g (58290–58294)

Vaginal Hysterectomy

A vaginal hysterectomy is the removal of the uterus through the vagina. During a vaginal hysterectomy, the surgeon detaches the uterus from the ovaries, fallopian tubes, and upper vagina, as well as from the blood vessels and connective tissue that support it. The uterus is then removed through the vagina. This service can be done either open (by incision) or laparoscopically.

When reviewing the clinical documentation for vaginal hysterectomies it is important to determine:

- Size of the uterus
- If the procedure was open or laparoscopic
- If the ovaries and/or tubes were removed
- Any additional services performed at the time of the procedure (such as urethrocystopexy or vaginectomy)

Below are some key items to look for in documentation for specific procedures.

- Codes 58260–58264 are used to report an open vaginal hysterectomy of a uterus 250 grams or less. Correct code assignment is determined based on whether the ovaries and/or fallopian tubes were removed or not and what additional services were performed during the same operative session.
- Codes 58275 and 58280 are used to report a vaginal hysterectomy with a total or partial vaginectomy. Report 58280 when documentation indicates that an enterocele was also performed.
- When the uterine weight is over 250 grams, codes 58290–58294 are reported. As with codes 58260–58270, appropriate code selection is dependent upon what, if any, other procedures are performed during the surgical encounter.

Clinician Documentation Checklist

Clinician documentation should indicate the following:

- Medical condition being treated
- Surgical approach
  - abdominal or open
  - vaginal
  - laparoscopic
- Weight of uterus (g)
- Vaginectomy performed
  - total
  - partial
  - radical

- Other procedures performed
  - removal of tubes
  - removal of ovary(s)
  - removal of bladder
  - urethral transplantations
  - resection of rectum
  - resection of colon
  - colostomy
  - repair of enterocele
  - lymph node sampling (biopsy)

Influenza

Code Axes

Influenza due to identified novel influenza A virus with pneumonia **JØ9.X1**

Influenza due to identified novel influenza A virus with other respiratory manifestations **JØ9.X2**

Influenza due to identified novel influenza A virus with gastrointestinal manifestations **JØ9.X3**

Influenza due to identified novel influenza A virus with other manifestations **JØ9.X9**

Influenza due to other identified influenza virus with unspecified type of pneumonia **J1Ø.ØØ**

Influenza due to other identified influenza virus with the same other identified influenza virus pneumonia **J1Ø.Ø1**

Influenza due to other identified influenza virus with other specified pneumonia **J1Ø.Ø8**

Influenza due to other identified influenza virus with other respiratory manifestations **J1Ø.1**

Influenza due to other identified influenza virus with gastrointestinal manifestations **J1Ø.2**

Influenza due to other identified influenza virus with other manifestations **J1Ø.8**

Subcategories represent conditions with encephalopathy, myocarditis, otitis media, and other manifestations.

Influenza due to unidentified influenza virus with pneumonia **J11.Ø**

Subcategories identify whether the pneumonia is unspecified or specified.

Influenza due to unidentified influenza virus with other respiratory manifestations **J11.1**

Influenza due to unidentified influenza virus with gastrointestinal manifestations **J11.2**

Influenza due to unidentified influenza virus with other manifestations **J11.8**

Subcategories represent conditions with encephalopathy, myocarditis, otitis media, and other manifestations.

⇨ I-10 ALERT

Codes in these categories representing specific forms of influenza should only be assigned if the specific disease process (e.g., novel influenza A virus) is documented as confirmed. The specific codes in these categories should not be assigned if the corresponding documentation contains terminology such as "possible," "suspected," or "probable." In those instances, assign the appropriate code(s) for the presenting symptoms.

Description of Condition

Influenza (all types) with pneumonia (JØ9.X1, J1Ø.Ø[Ø,1,8], J11.Ø[Ø,8])

Clinical Tip
Influenza due to novel virus A is most commonly isolated from birds, whether domestic poultry or wild birds, which act as asymptomatic carriers of influenza A virus. The category also includes influenza designated as that due to swine or other animals. The course of the disease largely depends on the manifestations, which can range from pneumonia or other respiratory conditions, to encephalopathy or myocarditis.

 **CDI ALERT**

Ensure that the medical record indicates the causal agent or virus, if possible. If the condition is due to influenza A virus, treatment typically involves oseltamivir or zanamivir.

Key Terms
Key terms found in the documentation for novel influenza A virus may include:

Avian flu

Avian influenza

Bird flu

Bird influenza

H5N1

Influenza A/H5N1

Influenza of other animal origin, not bird or swine

Swine influenza (viruses that normally cause infections in pigs)

Clinician Note
Documentation must indicate the presence of pneumonia to support code assignment. When documentation does not specifically indicate pneumonia, see Influenza (all types) with other respiratory manifestations.

Influenza (all types) with other respiratory manifestations (JØ9.X2, J1Ø.1, J11.1)

Clinical Tip
Patients with influenza may demonstrate respiratory conditions other than pneumonia, which may include laryngitis, pharyngitis, or other upper respiratory symptoms. Ensure that any associated pleural effusion and/or sinusitis is documented and coded separately.

Key Terms
Key terms found in the documentation for influenza-related respiratory manifestations may include:

Influenzal laryngitis

Influenzal pharyngitis

Influenzal upper respiratory symptoms

Clinical Tip

Chest pain, cough, fever, hiccups, rapid breathing, or shortness of breath are symptoms of pleural effusion; however, unless specifically indicated by the physician the code for pleural effusion should not be reported.

Influenza (all types) with other manifestations (JØ9.X9, J1Ø.8-, J11.8-)

Key Terms

Key terms found in the documentation for influenza-related manifestations may include:

Influenzal encephalopathy

Influenzal myocarditis

Influenzal otitis media

> **CDI ALERT**
>
> Conditions such as encephalopathy, myocarditis, and other serious clinical conditions are very rare when associated with the influenzal virus. Ensure that documentation clearly links the conditions before assigning the condition to this classification.

Clinical Findings

Physical Examination

History and review of symptoms include fever, cough, sudden onset of chills, headache sometimes with photophobia, and general aches and pains. In mild cases symptoms may resemble a common cold. Respiratory symptoms may start as a scratchy sore throat and nonproductive cough and progress to a persistent, productive cough.

Diagnostic Procedures and Services

- Reverse transcriptase assays
- Rapid diagnostic testing
- Pulse oximetry
- Imaging
  - chest x-ray

Therapeutic Procedures and Services

- Treat symptoms
- Rest
- Hydration
- Medications
  - antiviral drugs

Clinician Documentation Checklist

Clinician documentation should indicate the following:

- Influenza due to
  - novel influenza a virus (certain identified virus)
    - avian influenza
    - bird influenza
    - influenza a/h5n1

        - influenza of other animal origin, not bird or swine
        - swine influenza virus
    - other identified influenza virus
        - identification of the virus
    - unidentified influenza virus
- Influenza with
    - pneumonia
        - identify for
            - associated lung abscess
            - type of pneumonia
                - same as other identified influenza virus
                - other specified
                - unspecified
    - other respiratory manifestations
        - laryngitis
        - pharyngitis
        - upper respiratory symptoms
        - identify for associated
            - pleural effusion
            - sinusitis
    - gastrointestinal manifestations
        - gastroenteritis
    - other manifestations
        - encephalopathy
        - myocarditis
        - otitis media
            - identify for associated perforated tympanic membrane
        - other
            - identify the manifestations

Injections and Infusions (Non-chemotherapy)

Code Axes

Hydration, therapeutic, prophylactic, and diagnostic injections and infusions (nonchemotherapy) **96360–96379**

Key Terms

Key terms found in the documentation may include:

IM Inj

Inf

Inj

Intradermal Inj

IV Inf

SQ Inj

CDI ALERT

Documentation should state why the patient required these services to support the medical necessity.

Clinician Documentation Checklist

Clinician documentation should indicate the following:

- The site of the injection or infusion
- The route of administration
  - subcutaneous
  - intramuscular
  - intravenous
  - intradermal
- The substance administered
  - fluids
  - medication
  - sequential
  - combined
  - the number of units

In the instance of infusions the documentation should also include:

- If the IV therapy was the main service
- The amount of time
- Technique (i.e., push or drip)
- If for hydration

CDI ALERT

The volume of hydration therapy and the doses of nonchemotherapy drugs administered should be clearly documented.

CDI ALERT

The stop and start time of infusion therapy should be documented in order to support code assignment.

Intracranial Injury

Code Axes

Concussion	**SØ6.ØX**
Traumatic cerebral edema	**SØ6.1X**
Diffuse traumatic brain injury	**SØ6.2X**
Focal traumatic brain injury, unspecified	**SØ6.3Ø**
Contusion and laceration of cerebrum (right, left, unspecified)	**SØ6.3[1,2,3]**
Traumatic hemorrhage of cerebrum (right, left, unspecified)	**SØ6.3[4,5,6]**
Contusion, laceration, and hemorrhage of cerebellum	**SØ6.37**
Contusion, laceration, and hemorrhage of brainstem	**SØ6.38**
Epidural hemorrhage	**SØ6.4X**
Traumatic subdural hemorrhage	**SØ6.5X**
Traumatic subarachnoid hemorrhage	**SØ6.6X**
Injury of [right, left] internal carotid artery, intracranial portion, NEC	**SØ6.8[1,2]**
Other specified and unspecified intracranial injury	**SØ6.89, SØ6.9X**

Classification Note

All of the code subcategories listed above are also differentiated along two additional code axes: one related to duration of loss of consciousness and one related to type of encounter. The additional character choices are as follows:

Sixth character: Loss of consciousness:

Ø without loss of consciousness

1 with loss of consciousness of 30 minutes or less

2 with loss of consciousness of 31 minutes to 59 minutes

3 with loss of consciousness of 1 hour to 5 hours 59 minutes

4 with loss of consciousness of 6 hours to 24 hours

5 with loss of consciousness greater than 24 hours with return to pre-existing conscious level

6 with loss of consciousness greater than 24 hours without return to pre-existing conscious level with patient surviving

7 with loss of consciousness of any duration with death due to brain injury prior to regaining consciousness

8 with loss of consciousness of any duration with death due to other cause prior to regaining consciousness

9 with loss of consciousness of unspecified duration

Seventh character: Type of encounter:

A initial encounter

D subsequent encounter

S sequela

Concussion (SØ6.ØX-)

Clinical Tip

A concussion is the most common and mildest form of traumatic brain injury (TBI) with a variety of symptoms, including somatic (e.g., headache), cognitive (e.g., feeling dazed), and emotional (e.g., increased irritability). In addition, some patients experience physical signs, such as loss of consciousness or amnesia, cognitive impairment, such as slowed reaction times, or sleep disturbances. Patients with a personal history of concussion are at higher risk for another, particularly if the new injury occurs before symptoms from the initial injury have resolved. Symptoms typically resolve within seven to 10 days, with no serious long-term effects. Varying definitions exist, but it is thought that a concussion is a functional state, meaning that symptoms are caused primarily by temporary biochemical changes in neurons, taking place at their cell membranes and synapses.

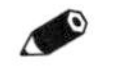 **CDI ALERT**

If a concussion is documented along with a more specific intracranial injury, the case should be classified to that specific intracranial injury.

Key Terms

Key terms found in the documentation for concussion may include:

Commotio cerebri

Mild brain injury

Mild head injury (MHI)

Minor head trauma

Mild traumatic brain injury (MTBI)

Traumatic cerebral edema (SØ6.1X-)

Clinical Tip

Cerebral edema following a traumatic event can lead to an expansion of brain volume and has a crucial impact on morbidity and mortality as it increases intracranial pressure, impairs cerebral perfusion and oxygenation, and contributes to additional ischemic injuries. It has been determined that the formation of cerebral edema is one of the major factors leading to the high mortality and morbidity in a traumatic brain injury (TBI) patient. Recently, significant progress has been made toward identifying factors that contribute to edema formation after TBI, most notably both vasogenic and cytotoxic cerebral edema that causes the blood brain barrier (BBB) to remain open. Managing BBB permeability has increasingly become a promising approach to managing brain edema and associated swelling.

 **CDI ALERT**

Ensure that any connection between cerebral swelling or edema and the patient's personal history of trauma are documented clearly in the medical record.

Key Terms
Key terms found in the documentation for traumatic cerebral edema may include:

Diffuse traumatic cerebral edema

Focal traumatic cerebral edema

Diffuse traumatic brain injury (SØ6.2X-)

Clinical Tip
Diffuse traumatic brain injury occurs over a widespread area of the brain as opposed to focal brain injury, which is confined to one specific area. It is common for both focal and diffuse damage to occur as the result of the same event; many traumatic brain injuries have aspects of both focal and diffuse injury. Diffuse injuries are most often found in acceleration/deceleration injuries in which the head does not necessarily hit anything, but brain tissue is damaged because tissue types with varying densities accelerate at different rates. This also includes brain injury due to hypoxia, meningitis, or damage to blood vessels. Diffuse injuries may be difficult to detect and define because often, much of the damage is microscopic.

Key Terms
Key terms found in the documentation for diffuse traumatic brain injury may include:

Acceleration/deceleration brain injury

Diffuse axonal brain injury

Unspecified focal traumatic brain injury (SØ6.3Ø-)

Clinical Tip
Focal brain injury occurs in a specific location and it is common for both focal and diffuse damage to occur as the result of the same event; many traumatic brain injuries have aspects of both focal and diffuse injury. Focal injuries are most commonly associated with an injury in which the head strikes or is struck by an object and is usually associated with brain tissue damage visible to the naked eye. The manifestations associated with this type of injury generally relate to the area that has been damaged.

Key Terms
Key terms found in the documentation for focal traumatic brain injury may include:

Focal neurological deficit brain injury

Contusion and laceration of cerebrum (right, left, unspecified) (SØ6.3[1,2,3]-)

Clinical Tip

A cerebral laceration is a type of traumatic brain injury that involves the tissue of the brain being mechanically cut or torn, while a cerebral contusion does not involve the tears. Lacerations are very common in penetrating and perforating head trauma injuries and in many cases accompany skull fractures. They are particularly common in the inferior frontal lobes and the poles of the temporal lobes. Both conditions are considered more serious than concussions and can cause bleeding or swelling in the brain. Intracranial pressure is monitored and surgical treatment may be required.

Traumatic hemorrhage of cerebrum (right, left, unspecified) (SØ6.3[4,5,6]-)

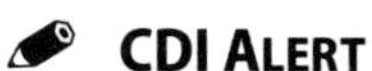

CDI ALERT

Ensure that any signs of either contusion and/or laceration are documented clearly in the medical record, with differentiation of each.

Clinical Tip

Three criteria that are typically used to classify cerebral hemorrhages are: location (i.e., subarachnoid, extradural, subdural), kind of vessel involved (i.e., arterial, venous, capillary), and origin (i.e., traumatic, degenerative). Each kind of cerebral hemorrhage has distinctive clinical characteristics. The hemorrhage may lead to displacement or destruction of brain tissue and in some cases an extensive hemorrhage can be fatal.

Key Terms

Key terms found in the documentation for traumatic hemorrhage of cerebrum may include:

Traumatic cerebral hematoma

Traumatic intracerebral hemorrhage

Contusion, laceration, and hemorrhage of cerebellum (SØ6.37-)

CDI ALERT

Ensure that any signs of either contusion and/or laceration are documented clearly in the medical record, with differentiation of each.

Clinical Tip

The cerebellum is located at the base of the skull and controls coordination, balance, and equilibrium. Hemorrhaging into this area causes dizziness, loss of coordination, and/or vomiting. In most cases, a patient who is awake and has a Glasgow coma scale score of 14 or greater with a small hemorrhage, without hydrocephalus, may be a candidate for conservative supportive care with close monitoring. Ventriculostomy may be indicated in patients with hemorrhage and hydrocephalus, but is controversial.

Contusion, laceration, and hemorrhage of brainstem (SØ6.38-)

Clinical Tip

Traumatic brainstem hemorrhage after blunt head injury is an uncommon event, although the most frequent site of hemorrhage is the midline rostral brainstem. The prognosis of these patients is poor because of its critical location. Traumatic brainstem hemorrhage typically results in coma, decerebrate posturing, and autonomic nervous system dysfunction.

Epidural hemorrhage (SØ6.4X-)

Clinical Tip

An epidural or extradural hematoma is a type of traumatic brain injury (TBI) in which a buildup of blood occurs between the dura mater, the tough outer membrane of the central nervous system) and the skull. The condition can be life threatening because the buildup of blood may increase pressure in the intracranial space, compress delicate brain tissue, and cause brain shift. There may be a lucid period of time after the injury and a time lag before symptoms appear, which may rapidly progress to coma. This typically occurs at six to eight hours post injury.

Traumatic subdural hemorrhage (SØ6.5X-)

CDI ALERT

Ensure that documentation of the timing between injury and symptoms is clearly defined in the medical record, particularly if the patient has a history of both acute and chronic subdural hematoma.

Clinical Tip

A subdural hematoma is a collection of blood in the space between the outer layer (dura) and middle layers of the covering of the brain (the meninges). The time between the injury and the appearance of symptoms can vary from less than 48 hours to several weeks or more. Symptoms appearing in less than 48 hours are due to an acute subdural hematoma. This type of bleeding is often fatal and results from tearing of the venous sinus. If more than two weeks have passed before symptoms appear, the condition is called a chronic subdural hematoma resulting from tearing of the smaller vein.

Key Terms

Key terms found in the documentation for traumatic subdural hemorrhage may include:

Extradural hemorrhage

Clinician Note

Coordination of benefits is often required for payment from third-party payers; therefore, the documentation should indicate how the injury occurred (e.g., auto accident, fall from ladder at work, fall when riding a bike).

Traumatic subarachnoid hemorrhage (SØ6.6X-)

Clinical Tip

Traumatic subarachnoid hemorrhage refers to bleeding into the subarachnoid space that is found between the middle (arachnoid) and the innermost (pia mater) membranes that cover the brain. The condition occurs as the result of severe blunt head trauma. In this condition the brain may be subject to severe twisting and torsion that can shear blood vessels between the arachnoid and pia mater resulting in subarachnoid hemorrhage. Swelling of brain tissue with an increase in pressure in the brain may result. A blood clot and increased intracranial pressure can obstruct the flow of cerebrospinal fluid resulting in hydrocephalus.

Clinician Note
Coordination of benefits is often required for payment from third-party payers; therefore, the documentation should indicate how the injury occurred (e.g., auto accident, fall from ladder at work, fall when riding a bike).

Injury of [right, left] internal carotid artery, intracranial portion, NEC (SØ6.8[1,2]-)

Clinical Tip
Carotid artery injury is relatively rare and is reported to occur in approximately 1 percent of individuals who experience severe blunt head trauma. Arterial dissections in the head and neck usually are associated with deceleration and shear injuries and treatment of carotid and vertebral arterial dissections remains somewhat controversial. The most conservative approach includes medical management, with ongoing debate as to whether anticoagulation with heparin and/or antiplatelet therapy is more effective. Stents have been used to treat patients who have contraindications to anticoagulation or antiplatelet therapy.

CDI ALERT

Ensure that documentation clearly indicates the site of the injury, particularly the portion of the carotid artery involved.

Clinician Note
Coordination of benefits is often required for payment from third-party payers; therefore, the documentation should indicate how the injury occurred (e.g., auto accident, fall from ladder at work, fall when riding a bike).

Clinical Findings

Physical Examination

History and review of symptoms may include:

- Rapid trauma assessment
- Glasgow coma scale (GCS)
- Neurological examination
- Common symptoms
  - fatigue
  - headache
  - memory loss
  - sleep disturbance
  - irritability
  - vision problems (blurred, loss of, sensitivity to light, diplopia)
  - depression
  - poor concentration
  - seizures
  - confusion
  - nausea
  - loss of smell
  - lack of concentration

  - slurred speech
  - difficulty conversing
  - tinnitus
  - sensitivity to sound
  - impaired hearing
  - papilledema

Diagnostic Procedures and Services

- Laboratory
  - blood test
  - toxicology
- Imaging
  - CT
  - MRI
  - PET scan
- Other
  - EEG
  - sensor to monitor intracranial pressure (ICP)

Therapeutic Procedures and Services

- Monitor pupillary reaction, BP, pulse frequently
- Discharge home if TBI is mild
- Patients with moderate TBI are observed in the hospital
- Patients with severe TBI are admitted to a critical care unit
- Surgery
- Antiseizure medication
- Mechanical ventilation
- Barbiturates to lower ICP
- Oxygen therapy
- Corticosteroids

Intraoperative and Postprocedural Complications and Disorders of Ear and Mastoid Process

Code Axes

Recurrent cholesteatoma of postmastoidectomy cavity	H95.Ø
Chronic inflammation of postmastoidectomy cavity	H95.11
Granulation of postmastoidectomy cavity	H95.12
Mucosal cyst of postmastoidectomy cavity	H95.13
Intraoperative hemorrhage and hematoma of ear and mastoid process complicating a procedure	H95.2
Accidental puncture and laceration of ear and mastoid process during a procedure	H95.3
Postprocedural hemorrhage of ear and mastoid process following a procedure	H95.4
Postprocedural hematoma of ear and mastoid process following a procedure	H95.5
Postprocedural stenosis of external ear canal	H95.81

Description of Condition

Intraoperative and postprocedural complications and disorders of the ear and mastoid process

Clinical Tip

Surgical intervention on the external, middle, or inner ear entails certain operative and postoperative risks. Similar to other surgery, these risks include intraoperative or postoperative (delayed) hemorrhage, intraoperative puncture or laceration and infection. However, certain procedures (e.g., mastoidectomy) carry risk for certain delayed complications which may require further care and treatment. Such specific complications include:

Cholesteatoma (recurrent): Abnormal growth of keratinous squamous epithelial cells forming a mass within the middle ear extending to the external meatus.

Granulation: Accumulation of fibrous, collagen-rich connective tissue that provides a barrier against infectious microorganisms to facilitate healing.

Mucosal cyst: Mucous-lined cyst cavity following removal of mastoid bone.

⇨ I-10 ALERT

ICD-10-CM classifies postoperative complications to (typically) the end of the body system classification chapter, where possible. Chapter 8 contains multiple specific intraoperative and postoperative complication codes.

Note: Conditions classified to chapter 8 include laterality (right, left, bilateral) within the code structure. All conditions should specify the affected ear(s).

CDI ALERT

Documentation must include the specific nature of the complication to avoid reporting nonspecific diagnoses. The documentation should qualify the disorder as:

- Intraoperative (complication during surgery requiring care, correction)
- Postoperative (complication developing after surgery for which the patient seeks care)
- Documentation should state whether the procedure that resulted in a complication was:
- Performed on the ear or mastoid process
- Other (non-ear/mastoid process) procedure
- Documentation should specify the nature of the complication as:
- Recurrent cholesteatoma
- Chronic inflammation
- Granulation of postmastoidectomy cavity
- Mucosal cyst of postmastoidectomy cavity
- Hemorrhage or hematoma
- Accidental puncture or laceration
- Stenosis
- Other (provider must document specifics)
- A separate or additional code may be reported, if necessary, to specify the nature of the complication.

Documentation of laterality (i.e., right, left, bilateral) should be present to avoid reporting unspecified codes.

Stenosis of ear canal: Narrowing of ear canal due to trauma, scar tissue, surgery, osteoma (bony overgrowth).

Key Terms

Key terms found in the documentation may include:

Cholesteatoma (middle ear postmastoidectomy cavity):

- Cholesterosis
- Keratosis

Granulation:

- Granuloma
- Proud flesh

Clinical Findings

Physical Examination

History and review of systems may include:

- Hearing loss
- Vertigo
- Balance issues
- Facial nerve paralysis
- Tinnitus
- Altered taste
- Chronic drainage
- Fistula
- Dural injury

Diagnostic Procedures and Services

- Long-term monitoring
- MRI

Therapeutic Procedures and Services

- Second surgery

Clinician Note

Specify the nature of the complication. Document a link or otherwise clearly associate the complicating condition/manifestation to the causal procedure. Specify the causal/precipitating procedure.

Document whether complications exist in combination with other systemic disease or auditory disorder. Specify any contributory history of trauma, infection or other related condition or status (e.g., deafness).

Document the laterality of the affected site (left, right, bilateral).

Clinician Documentation Checklist

Clinician documentation should indicate the following:

- Type
  - recurrent cholesteatoma of postmastoidectomy cavity
  - other disorders of ear and mastoid process following mastoidectomy
    - subtype
      - chronic inflammation of postmastoidectomy cavity
      - granulation of postmastoidectomy cavity
      - mucosal cyst of postmastoidectomy cavity
      - other disorders following mastoidectomy
  - intraoperative hemorrhage and hematoma of ear and mastoid process complicating a procedure
    - identify the procedure as
      - procedure on ear and mastoid process
      - other procedure
  - accidental puncture and laceration of ear and mastoid process during a procedure
    - identify the procedure as
      - procedure on ear and mastoid process
      - other procedure
  - postprocedural hemorrhage and hematoma of ear and mastoid process following a procedure
    - identify the procedure as
      - procedure on ear and mastoid process
      - other procedure
  - other intraoperative and postprocedural complications and disorders of ear and mastoid process
    - postprocedural stenosis of external ear canal
    - other intraoperative complications and disorders of ear and mastoid process
      - specify the disorder
    - other postprocedural complications and disorders of ear and mastoid process
      - specify the disorder
- Identification of laterality of ear
  - right
  - left
  - bilateral

Intraoperative and Postprocedural Complications and Disorders of Genitourinary System

Code Axes

Postprocedural (acute) (chronic) kidney failure	**N99.Ø**
Postprocedural urethral stricture	**N99.1-**
Postprocedural adhesions of vagina	**N99.2**
Prolapse of vaginal vault after hysterectomy	**N99.3**
Postprocedural pelvic peritoneal adhesions	**N99.4**
Complications of stoma of urinary tract	**N99.5-**

Note: Official coding guideline I.B.16 indicates: Code assignment is based on the provider's documentation of the relationship between the condition and the care or procedure, unless otherwise instructed by the classification. The guideline extends to any complications of care, regardless of the chapter in which the code is located. It is important to note that not all conditions that occur during or following medical care or surgery are classified as complications. There must be a cause-and-effect relationship between the care provided and the condition, and an indication in the documentation that it is a complication. Query the provider for clarification, if the complication is not clearly documented.

⇨ I-10 Alert

Like other chapters within ICD-10-CM related to specific body systems, the genitourinary chapter contains a section at the end that contains many common postoperative and postprocedural complications. Unlike ICD-9-CM, where many of these complications were found within one chapter and were more general in nature, the complication categories within the specific chapters of ICD-10-CM provide much more detail and are tailored to the types of complications typically encountered for that type of disease process.

Description of Condition

Postprocedural (acute) (chronic) kidney failure (N99.Ø)

Clinical Tip

Postoperative acute renal failure (ARF) is a serious complication resulting in a prolonged acute care stay and high mortality. An increase in the intra-abdominal pressure above 20 mm Hg is associated with an increase in the incidence of postop ARF and the only proven management strategies for prevention are adequate volume expansion and avoidance of hypovolemia.

⇨ I-10 Alert

If either acute or chronic postoperative or postprocedural kidney failure is documented, assign an additional code to identify the specific type of kidney disease/failure.

Key Terms

Key terms found in the documentation for postprocedural (acute) (chronic) kidney failure may include:

- Post-op acute renal failure
- Post-op chronic renal failure

Clinician Note

Ensure that all related conditions are coded, particularly those related to underlying kidney disease.

Postprocedural urethral stricture (N99.1-)

Clinical Tip

Urethral stricture is an abnormal narrowing of the urethra that occurs in male patients more often than in females, due to the longer urethral structure. The condition is the most common late complication of transurethral prostatectomy (TURP), but patient predisposing factors include previous trauma or infection or presence of a long-term urinary catheter.

Key Terms

Key terms found in the documentation for postprocedural urethral stricture may include:

Postcatheterization urethral stricture

Clinician Note

Ensure that all related conditions are coded, particularly those related to underlying urinary system disease.

Postprocedural adhesions of vagina (N99.2)

Clinical Tip

Adhesions form when there is damage to the visceral or parietal peritoneum and the basement membrane of the mesothelial layer is exposed to the surroundings. Adhesion formation at the vaginal cuff and pelvic sidewall frequently involves bowel, omentum, and adnexa.

Clinician Note

Ensure that all related conditions are coded, particularly those related to underlying female genital system disease.

Prolapse of vaginal vault after hysterectomy (N99.3)

Clinical Tip

Vaginal vault prolapse involves a descent of the vaginal cuff below a point that is 2 cm less than the total vaginal length above the plane of the hymen. It occurs when the upper vagina bulges into or outside the vagina. The condition is a common complication following vaginal hysterectomy and pre-existing pelvic floor defect prior to hysterectomy is the single most important risk factor for vault prolapse.

Clinician Note

Ensure that all related conditions are coded, particularly those related to underlying female genital system disease.

Postprocedural pelvic peritoneal adhesions (N99.4)

Clinical Tip

Peritoneal adhesions are a consequence of peritoneal irritation by surgical trauma and may be considered as the pathological part of healing following any peritoneal injury, particularly due to abdominal surgery. Postoperative

⇨ I-10 ALERT

Because the condition occurs much more frequently in the male population, there are four codes related to male postprocedural urethral stricture, differentiated by type:

Meatal: Occurring at the opening of the urethra at the external meatus

Membranous: Occurs in up to 6 percent of patients who undergo transurethral resection of the prostate (TURP). The scar tissue is caused by the trauma of using too large a resectoscope/catheter or from overly aggressive distal prostate resection.

Anterior: The bulbar and penile urethra, fossa navicularis, and meatus together represent the anterior urethra

Unspecified: Strictural process that is not specified as any of the remaining types above.

CDI ALERT

Review medical record documentation for any indication of urinary incontinence and, if present, report separately.

⇨ I-10 ALERT

Ensure proper code selection: code N73.6 is assigned when the pelvic peritoneal adhesions are not specified as postprocedural and code N73.6 is assigned when the adhesions are specified as being postinfective.

peritoneal adhesions are a major cause of morbidity resulting in multiple complications, many of which can manifest several years after the initial surgical procedure. They may cause pelvic or abdominal pain, small bowel obstruction, and infertility.

Clinician Note
Ensure that all related conditions are coded, particularly those related to underlying female genital system disease.

Complications of stoma of urinary tract (N99.5-)

Clinical Tip
For patients with long-term suprapubic catheters (cystostomies), postprocedural complications, particularly related to urinary tract infections, are not uncommon. Duration of catheterization is the leading risk factor for the development of urinary tract infections. Macroscopic hematuria and blockage of catheter are frequent complications as well.

Clinician Note
Ensure that all related conditions are coded, particularly those related to underlying urinary system disease.

Clinician Documentation Checklist

Clinician documentation should indicate the following:

- Postprocedural (acute) (chronic) kidney failure
  - identify type of kidney disease
- Postprocedural urethral stricture
  - includes postcatheterization urethral stricture
  - identify
    - postprocedural urethral stricture, male
      - postprocedural urethral stricture, meatal
      - postprocedural bulbous urethral stricture
      - postprocedural membranous urethral stricture
      - postprocedural anterior urethral stricture
      - postprocedural fossa navicularis urethral stricture
      - unspecified postprocedural urethral stricture
    - postprocedural urethral stricture, female
- Postprocedural adhesions of vagina
- Prolapse of vaginal vault after hysterectomy
- Postprocedural pelvic peritoneal adhesions
- Complications of stoma of urinary tract
  - identify
    - complication of cystostomy
      - cystostomy hemorrhage
      - cystostomy infection

- cystostomy malfunction
- other cystostomy complications
- complication of other external stoma of urinary tract
  - hemorrhage of incontinent external stoma of urinary tract
  - infection of incontinent external stoma of urinary tract
  - malfunction of incontinent external stoma of urinary tract
  - herniation of incontinent stoma of urinary tract
  - stenosis of incontinent stoma of urinary tract
  - other complication of incontinent external stoma of urinary tract
- complication of other stoma of urinary tract
  - hemorrhage of continent stoma of urinary tract
  - infection of continent stoma of urinary tract
  - malfunction of continent stoma of urinary tract
  - herniation of continent stoma of urinary tract
  - stenosis of continent stoma of urinary tract
  - other complication of continent stoma of urinary tract

Malignant Neoplasm of Breast

Note: Each of the subcategories listed below for malignant neoplasm of breast are subdivided based on the following components: sex (female versus male), and laterality (right, left, unspecified).

I-10 ALERT

The number of specific codes for malignant neoplasm of breast has increased from 11 in ICD-9-CM to 54 in ICD-10-CM. These codes include sex and laterality indicators and also more specific and all-inclusive body sites. An additional code should be assigned for estrogen receptor status, if available. In addition, there are 12 codes related to carcinoma in situ of breast, still considered to be a malignancy, but the tumor cells are noninvasive and have not spread to any surrounding tissue at the time of diagnosis.

Code Axes

Malignant neoplasm of nipple and areola	**C5Ø.Ø--**
Malignant neoplasm of central portion of breast	**C5Ø.1--**
Malignant neoplasm of upper-inner quadrant of breast	**C5Ø.2--**
Malignant neoplasm of lower-inner quadrant of breast	**C5Ø.3--**
Malignant neoplasm of upper-outer quadrant of breast	**C5Ø.4--**
Malignant neoplasm of lower-outer quadrant of breast	**C5Ø.5--**
Malignant neoplasm of axillary tail of breast	**C5Ø.6--**
Malignant neoplasm of overlapping sites of breast	**C5Ø.8--**
Malignant neoplasm of unspecified site of breast	**C5Ø.9--**
Lobular carcinoma in situ of breast	**DØ5.Ø--**
Intraductal carcinoma in situ of breast	**DØ5.1--**
Other specified type of carcinoma in situ of breast	**DØ5.8--**
Unspecified type of carcinoma in situ of breast	**DØ5.9--**

CDI ALERT

- Documentation of risk factors should be included in the current record.
- Family history of breast history
- Estrogen receptor status
- Genetic susceptibility to malignant neoplasm of breast (BRCA1, BRCA2)
- Personal history of breast cancer
- Personal history of postmenopausal hormone replacement status
- Personal history of radiation therapy
- Postmenopausal status
- Obesity

Key Terms

Key terms found in the documentation for malignant neoplasm of the breast may include:

Colloid carcinoma of breast
Infiltrating lobular carcinoma of the breast
Inflammatory breast cancer (IBC)
Invasive cribriform carcinoma of the breast
Invasive ductal carcinoma (IDC) of breast
Invasive lobular carcinoma of the breast
Invasive papillary carcinoma of the breast
Malignant phyllodes tumors of the breast
Medullary carcinoma of breast
Mucinous carcinoma of breast
Paget's disease of the breast
Paget's disease of the nipple
Triple negative breast cancer
Tubular carcinoma of breast

Key Terms

Key terms found in the documentation for carcinoma in situ of the breast may include:

Ductal carcinoma in situ (DCIS)

Lobular carcinoma in situ (LCIS)

Clinical Findings

The most common symptom of breast cancer is a mass or lump in the breast, while early stage breast cancer may be asymptomatic and discovered during a routine screening exam.

Physical Examination

History and review of systems may include:

- Breast/nipple pain
- Scaling or thickening of breast skin
- Swelling of the breast
- Irritation or dimpling
- Retracted nipple
- Enlarged lymph nodes

Diagnostic Procedures and Services

- Imaging
  - mammogram
  - ultrasound
  - MRI
  - ductogram
  - biopsy

Therapeutic Procedures and Services

- Surgery
- Radiation therapy
- Hormone therapy
- Chemotherapy
- Targeted therapy for certain types

Clincian Note

Prior authorization of treatment is often dependent upon the type of carcinoma, therefore, careful attention to the medical record documentation including pathology reports is crucial.

The provider is responsible for confirming the findings of pathology and radiology reports within their documentation for inpatient records.

The provider should document admissions for screening mammogram or routine mammogram, including risk factors for the patient. If the patient is having a mammogram due to symptoms, report the symptoms as the reason for the encounter.

Clinician Documentation Checklist

Clinician documentation should indicate the following:

- Includes
  - Connective tissue of breast
  - Paget's disease of breast
  - Paget's disease of nipple
- Identification of
  - estrogen receptor status
    - positive
    - negative
  - laterality
    - right
    - left
  - gender
    - male
    - female
  - site
    - nipple and areola
    - central portion
    - quadrant
      - upper-inner
      - lower-inner
      - upper-outer
      - lower-outer
    - axillary tail
    - overlapping sites of breast
    - unspecified

Carcinoma in situ of breast, other and unspecified sites

- Carcinoma in situ of breast
  - type
    - lobular
    - intraductal
    - other
    - unspecified
- Identification of the laterality of breast
  - right
  - left

Malignant Neoplasm of Liver and Intrahepatic Bile Ducts

Code Axes

Liver cell carcinoma	**C22.Ø**
Intrahepatic bile duct carcinoma	**C22.1**
Hepatoblastoma	**C22.2**
Angiosarcoma of liver	**C22.3**
Other sarcomas of liver	**C22.4**
Other specified carcinomas of liver	**C22.7**
Malignant neoplasm of liver, primary, unspecified as to type	**C22.8**
Malignant neoplasm of liver, not specified as primary or secondary	**C22.9**

⇨ I-10 ALERT

There are currently eight ICD-10-CM codes available to report malignant neoplasms of the liver and intrahepatic bile ducts, as opposed to only three in ICD-9-CM.

Description of Condition

Liver cell carcinoma (C22.Ø)

Clinical Tip

Liver cell carcinoma is a primary tumor and is the most common type of malignancy involving the liver. There are two main causes: one is due to a viral hepatitis B or C infection, and the other is due to hepatic cirrhosis, most commonly caused by alcoholism. The tumor involves the hepatocyte cells, which comprise approximately 80 percent of the liver. Prognosis is typically poor with this type of malignancy.

Cholangiocarcinoma with hepatocellular carcinoma, combined, is found in code C22.Ø. Liver cholangiocarcinoma is found in code C22.1.

CDI ALERT

Physicians will be required to document specific forms of liver malignancies under ICD-10-CM. Ensure that they are aware of the eight different classifications available (i.e., hepatocellular, intrahepatic, angiosarcoma, etc.).

Key Terms

Key terms found in the documentation for liver cell carcinoma may include:

HCC

Hepatocellular carcinoma

Hepatoma

Malignant hepatoma

Primary liver carcinoma

Primary liver cell carcinoma

Clinician Note
Because there appears to be a direct correlation to the increased incidence of HCC and alcohol abuse, alcohol dependence, hepatitis B and hepatitis C these conditions should be documented when present and reported separately using the appropriate code.

CDI Alert

Manifestations of cancer that are not integral to the cancer (i.e., not one of the clinical indicators for the cancer) should be documented and reported when they meet criteria as an additional diagnosis:

- Anemia in neoplastic disease
- Ascites
- Coagulation defect due to liver disease
- Encephalopathy due to hepatic failure
- Hemorrhage/bleeding (of site)
- Peritonitis

Intrahepatic bile duct carcinoma (C22.1)

Clinical Tip
A malignancy that invades bile ducts within the liver is called an intrahepatic bile duct carcinoma; only about 10 percent of all bile duct carcinomas are intrahepatic. Prognosis depends on location of the tumor and the extent of spread, or stage.

Key Terms
Key terms found in the documentation for intrahepatic bile duct carcinoma may include:

- Adenocarcinoma of intrahepatic bile duct
- Cholangiocarcinoma
- Intracholangiocarcinoma

I-10 Alert

In ICD-9-CM, both hepatocellular (liver cell) carcinomas and hepatoblastomas were indexed and classified to the same code (155.Ø). In ICD-10-CM, they each have a separate subclassification: C22.Ø for liver cell carcinoma and C22.2 for hepatoblastoma. This should be kept in mind when using mapping processes and reviewing longitudinal clinical data.

Hepatoblastoma (C22.2)

Clinical Tip
Hepatoblastoma is a rare liver malignancy that typically affects infants and small children, usually no more than three years of age. The tumor originates from immature liver precursor cells, most often involving the right liver lobe. Several genetic conditions can increase a patient's risk for developing hepatoblastoma, including Beckwith-Wiedemann syndrome, hemihypertrophy, and familial adenomatous polyposis.

Angiosarcoma of liver (C22.3)

Clinical Tip
A liver angiosarcoma is a tumor that arises from the endothelial cells that line the walls of the blood vessels. The portal vein or central and sublobular veins are often involved. The causes of angiosarcoma include toxic exposure to thorium dioxide (Thorotrast), vinyl chloride, and arsenic, which may have occurred 30 or more years previously.

Key Terms
Key terms found in the documentation for angiosarcoma of liver may include:

- Hemangioendothelioma
- Hepatic angiosarcoma
- Kupffer cell sarcoma

Other sarcomas of liver (C22.4)

Clinical Tip

Besides angiosarcoma of the liver (classified above), there are several other forms of liver sarcomas, which include those listed below. Symptoms, treatment, and prognosis depend upon the stage and progression of the tumor at the time of diagnosis.

Key Terms

Key terms found in the documentation for other sarcomas of liver may include:

Epithelioid hemangioendothelioma

Fibrosarcoma

Leiomyosarcoma

Malignant fibrous histiocytoma

Malignant histiocytoma

Primary hepatic sarcoma

Undifferentiated embryonal sarcoma of the liver

Undifferentiated liver sarcoma

Malignant neoplasm of liver, primary, unspecified as to type (C22.8) and Malignant neoplasm of liver, not specified as primary or secondary (C22.9)

Clinical Tip

Secondary liver carcinoma (C78.7) has metastasized from another primary cancer, such as that of the colon, breast, pancreas, stomach, or lung. It occurs much more frequently than primary liver carcinoma. Primary liver cancer (hepatocellular carcinoma) tends to occur in livers damaged by alcoholic cirrhosis, birth defects, or chronic infection with diseases such as hepatitis B and C, or hemochromatosis.

⇨ I-10 ALERT

Codes C22.8 and C22.9 represent residual subcategories for liver tumors that are not well defined. If the malignancy is documented as primary but no type is specified, code C22.8 should be reported. If no indication of primary or secondary tumor is documented, code C22.9 must be reported, although it is preferable that the attending physician be queried as to specific type.

Clinical Findings

Physical Examination

History and review of symptoms may include:

- Weight loss
- Enlarged liver
- Abdominal pain
- Loss of appetite
- Abdominal swelling
- Jaundice (yellowing of skin/eyes)
- Fever
- Nausea and vomiting

Diagnostic Procedures and Services

- Laboratory
  - alpha-fetoprotein levels
  - liver function
  - prothrombin time
  - BUN
  - CBC
  - viral hepatitis
  - blood chemistry (calcium, glucose)
  - cholesterol
- Imaging
  - ultrasound
  - MRI
  - CT scan
  - angiogram
  - bone scan
  - biopsy

Therapeutic Procedures and Services

- Surgery
- Radiation
- Chemotherapy
- Tumor ablation
- Targeted therapy
- Embolization

Clinician Note

Careful review of the medical record documentation is required to prevent incorrect classification. When documentation indicates terms such as extrahepatic or hepatic duct, the condition is more than likely classified elsewhere.

Clinician Documentation Checklist

Clinician documentation should indicate the following:

- Malignant neoplasm of liver and intrahepatic bile ducts
  - identification of
    - alcohol abuse and dependence
    - hepatitis b
    - hepatitis c
  - type
    - liver cell carcinoma
      - hepatocellular carcinoma
      - hepatoma

- intrahepatic bile duct carcinoma
- cholangiocarcinoma

— hepatoblastoma

— angiosarcoma of liver

- Kupffer cell sarcoma

— other sarcoma of liver

— other specified carcinomas of liver

— malignant neoplasm of liver, primary, unspecified as to type

— malignant neoplasm of liver, not specified to primary or secondary

- Malignant neoplasm of gallbladder
- Malignant neoplasm of other and unspecified parts of biliary tract
  - identification of the site

— extrahepatic bile duct

- common bile duct
- cystic duct
- hepatic duct
- biliary duct or passage

— ampulla of vater

— overlapping sites of biliary tract

- malignant neoplasm involving both intrahepatic and extrahepatic bile ducts
- primary malignant neoplasm of two or more contiguous sites of biliary tract

— unspecified

Malignant Neoplasm of Unspecified Site

Code Axes

Secondary malignant neoplasm of unspecified site	**C79.9**
Disseminated malignant neoplasm, unspecified	**C8Ø.Ø**
Malignant (primary) neoplasm, unspecified	**C8Ø.1**
Carcinoma in situ, unspecified	**DØ9.9**

Description of Condition

Secondary malignant neoplasm of unspecified site (C79.9)

Clinical Tip
This condition may be documented as metastatic cancer or metastatic disease, with no further specification. The diagnosis refers to the site to which the primary tumor has spread. In most cases, the site of metastasis should be known, particularly if treatment has been provided. The most common sites of cancer metastasis are the lungs, bones, and liver. Metastatic cancer cells have the same attributes and are similar, if not identical, to the cancer cells of the primary tumor, regardless of differing body sites. If a primary site is not found, clinicians know by the cell type that the tumor is metastatic.

Key Terms
Key terms found in the documentation for secondary malignant neoplasm of unspecified site may include:

Metastatic cancer

Metastatic disease

Clinician Note
Ensure that all related conditions are coded, particularly neoplasms of other site or pathological fracture.

Disseminated malignant neoplasm, unspecified (C8Ø.Ø)

Clinical Tip
A disseminated malignant neoplasm is defined as one that has widely metastasized and has spread throughout the body. Besides local invasion, whereby the tumor infiltrates and destroys tissues surrounding the original site, there are other ways that a tumor can metastasize:

- Lymphangitic system or lymph nodes
- Hematogenous: through the blood vessels
- Direct seeding, such as spread to the peritoneum from other abdominal sources

⇨ I-10 ALERT

Providing precise classifications for malignancies without specification of site has always presented challenges, particularly in the ICD-9-CM system, where both primary and secondary malignant neoplasm of unspecified sites were classified to the same code (199.1). ICD-10-CM provides four separate codes for classification of these neoplasms.

CDI ALERT

ICD-10-CM often requires more specificity regarding the anatomical location of the malignancy and if it does not, the physician should be queried and the documentation updated accordingly. Clinicians should be educated that when documenting a malignant condition, the specific site should be indicated as to whether the malignancy is primary or secondary, and if secondary, the primary site should be indicated.

Key Terms

Key terms found in the documentation for disseminated malignant neoplasm may include:

- Carcinomatosis
- Generalized cancer, unspecified site
- Generalized malignancy, unspecified site

Clinician Note

Ensure that all related conditions are coded, particularly neoplasms of other sites or pathological fracture.

> ⇨ **I-10 ALERT**
>
> Official Coding Guideline I.C.2.j indicates that: Code C80.0 Disseminated malignant neoplasm, unspecified, is for use only in those cases where the patient has advanced metastatic disease and no known primary or secondary sites are specified. It should not be used in place of assigning codes for the primary site and all known secondary sites.

Malignant (primary) neoplasm, unspecified (C80.1)

Clinical Tip

If a patient is diagnosed with metastatic neoplasm and the primary site cannot be determined due to cancer cells too small to be detected or to regression of the disease, the patient is said to have a cancer of unknown primary origin (CUPO).

> ⇨ **I-10 ALERT**
>
> Official Coding Guideline I.C.2.k indicates that: Code C80.1 Malignant (primary) neoplasm, unspecified, equates to Cancer, unspecified. This code should only be used when no determination can be made as to the primary site of a malignancy.

Key Terms

Key terms found in the documentation for malignant (primary) neoplasm, unspecified may include:

- Cancer NOS
- Cancer unspecified site (primary)
- Carcinoma unspecified site (primary)
- Malignancy unspecified site (primary)

Clinician Note

Ensure that all related conditions are coded, particularly neoplasms of other sites or pathological fracture.

Carcinoma in situ, unspecified (D09.9)

> ⇨ **I-10 ALERT**
>
> In most cases, the site of the carcinoma in-situ is known and a code from category range D00–D09 should be assigned.

Clinical Tip

Carcinoma in-situ (CIS) cells do not penetrate the tissue barriers around them and are not considered invasive. Although CIS cells are growing in the characteristic disorganized way that identifies the tumor as a cancer, they do not have the ability to metastasize or have not gained access to the blood or lymph stream to spread to other parts of the body. Although not immediately life threatening, CIS cases should be treated (typically via surgical removal) because they can transform into invasive malignant tumors if left untreated.

 **CDI ALERT**

For an encounter in which both the primary site and a metastatic site(s) are initially diagnosed and (equally) treated during the admission, apply the OCG on Selection of Principal Diagnosis for two or more diagnoses that equally meet the definition of principal diagnosis.

Key Terms

Key terms found in the documentation for carcinoma in situ, unspecified may include:

Bowen's disease

Erythroplasia

Grade III intraepithelial neoplasia

Queyrat's erythroplasia

Clinician Note

Review the clinical documentation to ensure that all related conditions are coded, particularly neoplasms of other sites or pathological fracture.

Clinical Tip

Pulmonary lymphangitic spread refers to the small lymph vessels within the lungs and does not mean lymph node metastasis. When documented, it would be reported as metastasis to the lung (C78.Ø-).

Clinician Documentation Checklist

Clinician documentation should indicate the following:

- Carcinoma in situ of breast
  - Type
    - unspecified
- Carcinoma in situ of other and unspecified sites
  - identification of the site
    - urinary organs
      - unspecified
    - other
    - unspecified

Malnutrition

Code Axes

Kwashiorkor	E4Ø
Nutritional marasmus	E41
Marasmic kwashiorkor	E42
Unspecified severe protein-calorie nutrition	E43
Moderate protein-calorie malnutrition	E44.Ø
Mild protein-calorie malnutrition	E44.1
Retarded development following protein-calorie malnutrition	E45
Unspecified protein-calorie malnutrition	E46

Description of Condition

Malnutrition, also known as protein-energy undernutrition and protein-calorie malnutrition, is an energy (calorie) deficit due to a chronic deficiency of nutrients. There are ranges of severity and several causes, including but not limited to, an unbalanced diet, GI disorders, AIDS, malignancy, anorexia, depression, and systemic infection. Malnutrition may result from complications of these other diseases because these illnesses impair the body's ability to absorb or use nutrients.

 **CDI ALERT**

Body mass index (BMI) may be reported based on documentation by nurses, dietitians, etc., who are not the patient's provider. However, a diagnosis of malnutrition must be based on clinician documentation.

Kwashiorkor (E4Ø)

A form of severe malnutrition that may develop from a diet low in protein and high in carbohydrates, the characteristics of this type of malnutrition include nutritional edema, distended abdomen, hepatomegaly, and dyspigmentation of skin and hair. This form of severe malnutrition is very rarely seen in the U.S. except among the elderly and children who may be victims of abuse or neglect.

Nutritional Marasmus (E41)

Nutritional marasmus is a form of severe malnutrition that is caused by a lack of total nutrition in the diet and is characterized by energy deficiency, peeling skin, and hair discoloration. Marasmus is more common in the U.S. than Kwashiorkor but usually only affects very young children.

Marasmic kwashiorkor (E42)

This form of malnutrition is considered an intermediate form of severe protein-calorie malnutrition with signs of both kwashiorkor and marasmus.

Unspecified severe protein-calorie nutrition (E43)

Key Terms

Key terms found in the documentation may include:

- BMI <16
- Cachexia
- Dehydration
- Diminished functional status
- Feeding tube
- Hepatomegaly
- IV nutrition
- Normocytic anemia
- Nutritional edema
- Periorbital edema
- Protein-calorie malnutrition
- Severe malnutrition
- Severe muscle mass loss
- Starvation edema
- Subcutaneous fat loss
- Undernutrition

Moderate protein-calorie malnutrition (E44.Ø)

The moderate form of malnutrition involves more intense symptoms and intracellular changes.

Mild protein-calorie malnutrition (E44.1)

Mild malnutrition may have little if any symptoms.

Unspecified protein-calorie malnutrition (E46)

Conditions are caused by not getting enough calories or the right amount of key nutrients, such as vitamins and minerals that are needed for health. Malnutrition may occur when there is a lack of nutrients in the diet or when the body cannot absorb nutrients from food.

Clinical Tip

Malnutrition or protein-energy undernutrition can be primary or secondary. Primary malnutrition results from a diet with insufficient nutrient intake. Secondary malnutrition is more common in the U.S. and occurs as a result of other disease/disorders (e.g., GI disorders, malignancy, AIDS, alcoholism, anorexia nervosa), or drugs that interfere with nutrient use.

Providers must assess the following six characteristics in the context of an acute illness or injury, a chronic illness, or social or environmental circumstances to determine if malnutrition is present and whether it is severe or nonsevere (moderate): Insufficient energy intake, weight loss, loss of muscle mass, loss of subcutaneous fat, localized/generalized fluid accumulation (edema), and diminished functional status (hand grip strength).

Key Terms

Key terms found in the documentation may include:

BMI <16-18.9

Dehydration

Diminished functional status

Fluid accumulation

Malnutrition

Mild malnutrition

Moderate malnutrition

Muscle mass loss

Subcutaneous fat loss

Weight loss

Clinical Findings

This disease occurs in stages over a period of time, starting with low levels of nutrients within the blood and tissues that progress to changes in the intracellular function and structure. Once these changes are severe, signs and symptoms appear. Signs and symptoms of protein calorie malnutrition vary greatly and affect multiple body parts and organ systems.

Physical Examination

History and review of symptoms may include:

- Weight loss
- Fluid accumulation (edema)
- Muscle mass loss (severity based on degree of malnutrition)
- Insufficient energy intake
- Loss of subcutaneous fat
- Diminished functional status (hand grip strength)
- BMI <19
- Apathy
- Weakness
- Dizziness
- Lethargy
- Cachexia
- Swollen/bleeding gums
- Tooth decay
- Pale conjunctiva
- Periorbital edema
- Developmental delay
- Loss of knee reflexes

- Impaired cognition
- Bradycardia
- Tachycardia
- Hypotension
- Impaired wound healing
- Brittle/thin hair
- Dry/thin/inelastic skin
- Pallor
- Skin hypopigmentation
- Anemia
- Dehydration
- Enlarged liver
- Renal impairment
- Decreased respiratory rate

Diagnostic Procedures and Services

- Laboratory
  - CBC
  - serum albumin
  - serum electrolytes
  - total lymphocyte count
  - CD4+ T lymphocytes
  - transferrin
  - response to skin antigens
  - BUN
  - glucose
- Imaging
  - decreased bone mineralization
- Other
  - swallow function study

Clinician Note

Protein calorie malnutrition is classified by the extent of progression, from mild to severe. Mild malnutrition has little, if any symptoms and may be described as grade 1. Moderate malnutrition involves additional intracellular changes along with more symptoms and may be described as grade 2. In severe malnutrition the patient clearly exhibits several symptoms and may be described as grade 3.

Severe malnutrition is further subdivided by type such as kwashiorkor and marasmus. Kwashiorkor is a lack of protein in the diet and is characterized by more severe manifestations such as edema, distended abdomen, ulcerating dermatoses, and hepatomegaly. Kwashiorkor is also very rare in the U.S. and should not be routinely reported. Marasmus is more common in the U.S., usually only affects very young children and is characterized by energy deficiency, hair discoloration, growth retardation, and peeling skin.

Clinician Documentation Checklist

Clinician documentation should indicate the following:

- History including dietary intake relevant to the encounter
- Procedures performed (CT, MRI, laboratory, cardiovascular, swallow testing, etc.)

Clinical guidelines have been established to appropriately code mild to severe malnutrition. At least two of the following six conditions should be present and documented before assigning an ICD-10-CM code for malnutrition/undernutrition.

- Insufficient energy (calorie) intake
- Weight loss
- Loss of muscle mass
- Loss of subcutaneous fat
- Localized/generalized fluid accumulation that may mask weight loss (edema)
- Diminished functional status (measured by hand grip strength)

In order to report severe malnutrition such as marasmus or kwashiorkor, more severe symptoms outlined in the physical examination section must be present and documented in addition to those bulleted above.

In addition, the following clinical values commonly used to confirm if protein calorie malnutrition is present and the severity of malnutrition should be documented when indicated:

Measurement	Normal	Mild Malnutrition	Moderate Malnutrition	Severe Malnutrition
% Normal body weight	90–110%	85–90%	75–85%	<75%
Body mass index (BMI)	19–24	18–18.9	16–17.9	<16
Serum albumin (g/dL)	3.5–5.0	3.1–3.4	2.4–3.0	<2.4
Serum transferrin (mg/dL)	220–400	201–219	150–200	<150
Total Lymphocyte count (per µL)	2000–3500	1501–1999	800–1500	<800

⇨ I-10 ALERT

When "emaciated" or "emaciation" is documented in the medical record but no indication of whether or not the patient is suffering from malnutrition is documented, assign code E41 Nutritional marasmus. This is a change from ICD-9-CM coding for "emaciated" without any documentation of malnutrition. In ICD-9-CM, the code for nutritional marasmus was not assigned when malnutrition was not documented, instead a code for cachexia was reported.

Migraine

Code Axes

Migraine without aura	**G43.Ø**
Migraine with aura	**G43.1**
Hemiplegic migraine	**G43.4**
Persistent migraine aura without cerebral infarction	**G43.5**
Persistent migraine aura with cerebral infarction	**G43.6**
Chronic migraine without aura	**G43.7**
Cyclical vomiting	**G43.A**
Ophthalmoplegic migraine	**G43.B**
Periodic headache syndromes in child or adult	**G43.C**
Abdominal migraine	**G43.D**
Other migraine	**G43.8**
Migraine, unspecified	**G43.9**

CDI ALERT

Migraine as adverse effect of medication: documentation must link the nature of the adverse effect as the type of migraine and state the drug or classification, when known.

Clinical Tip

Migraine is defined as a moderate to severe headache that is intermittent, lasts four to 72 hours, and is throbbing in quality. Some patients experience nausea and become sensitive to lights and noise, in association with the headache. Migraine mechanisms are believed to involve chemical substances such as serotonin, increased stickiness of blood platelets, alterations in cerebral blood flow, and increased irritability of the nerve cells in the brain.

The following definitions should be used for all subclassifications related to migraine:

Intractable migraine: Sustained and severe migraine headaches, along with their manifestations, that are not adequately controlled by standard outpatient treatments. Other terms may include: pharmacoresistant, pharmacologically resistant, treatment resistant, medically refractory, or poorly controlled.

Status migrainosus: A debilitating migraine headache lasting more than 72 hours.

Migraine with aura: A less common type of migraine that includes symptoms or feelings that occur immediately preceding a migraine headache. The symptoms are also called a prodrome, which may last for five to 20 minutes, or may continue with the headache. Some of the most common prodromes include the following:

- Blind spots or scotomas
- Weakness

- Hallucinations
- Blindness in half of the visual field in one or both eyes (hemianopsia)
- Seeing zigzag patterns (fortification)
- Seeing flashing lights (scintilla)
- Feeling prickling skin (paresthesia)

Description of Condition

Migraine without and with aura (G43.Ø-, G43.1-)

Clinical Tip
Migraine is defined as a moderate to severe headache that it is intermittent, lasts four to 72 hours, and is throbbing in quality. Some patients experience nausea and become sensitive to lights and noise, in association with the headache. Migraine mechanisms are believed to involve chemical substances such as serotonin, increased stickiness of blood platelets, alterations in cerebral blood flow and increased irritability of the nerve cells in the brain. A migraine with aura is a less common type of migraine that includes symptoms or feelings that occur immediately preceding a migraine headache. The symptoms are also called a prodrome, which may last for five to 20 minutes, or may continue with the headache.

Key Terms
Key terms found in the documentation may include:

Basilar migraine

Classical migraine

Common migraine

Migraine equivalents

Migraine preceded or accompanied by transient focal neurological phenomena

Migraine triggered seizures

Migraine with acute-onset aura

Migraine with aura without headache (migraine equivalents)

Migraine with prolonged aura

Migraine with typical aura

Retinal migraine

Without aura

Clinician Note
Ensure that all related conditions are coded appropriately, particularly if seizure activity is documented.

CDI ALERT

Ensure that not only are conditions related to intractability and status migrainosus clearly documented, but if any associated seizure activity is present, it should be documented and classified separately.

Hemiplegic migraine (G43.4-)

> **CDI ALERT**
>
> If hemiplegia or a related condition is documented on a record with a migraine, ensure that the physician links the conditions before assigning codes from this subcategory.

Clinical Tip

Hemiplegic migraine is a rare, neurological disease that is characterized by a migraine with aura accompanied by motor weakness. The patient may experience visual disturbances, sensory loss, weakness to paralysis on one side of the body, confusion, speech difficulty, impaired consciousness, coma, or memory loss. Familial hemiplegic migraine (FHM) is a variation of hemiplegic migraine where at least one first-degree or second-degree relative also has hemiplegic migraine.

Key Terms

Key terms found in the documentation may include:

Familial migraine

Sporadic migraine

> **I-10 ALERT**
>
> If a patient has a persistent migraine aura with a cerebral infarction, a separate code should be assigned to classify the type of cerebral infarction (I63.-).

Clinician Note

Ensure that all related conditions are coded appropriately, particularly if seizure activity is documented.

Persistent migraine aura without and with cerebral infarction (G43.5-, G43.6-)

> **CDI ALERT**
>
> If a cerebral infarction or a related condition is documented on a record with a migraine, ensure that the physician links the conditions before assigning codes from this subcategory.

Clinical Tip

Persistent migraine aura without infarction (PAWOI) is a relatively rare condition that can cause neurological symptoms such as loss of vision, visual snow, increased afterimages, or tinnitus. The condition is typically diagnosed when there are aura symptoms lasting more than a week without evidence of cerebral infarction. A 2006 study published in the Journal of the American Medical Association indicated that active migraines with aura in women were associated with an increased risk of vascular disease, including cerebral infarction, although the overall occurrence of a stroke during or immediately following a migraine attack is fortunately a rare event.

Clinician Note

Telephone transmission of electroencephalograms (EEG) is considered medically necessary for the diagnosis of certain types of migraines. For this reason, careful attention to the medical record documentation is crucial to correct code assignment and, therefore, substantiating the medical necessity of the procedure.

> **I-10 ALERT**
>
> Codes in subcategory G43.7- Chronic migraine without aura, are differentiated from codes in subcategory G43.Ø- Migraine without aura, by the frequency of the migraines, as defined above.

Chronic migraine without aura (G43.7-)

Clinical Tip

A chronic migraine is defined as a headache that occurs 15 or more days a month with headache lasting four hours or longer for at least three consecutive months in patients with current or prior diagnosis of migraine.

Key Terms
Key terms found in the documentation may include:

Chronic migraine without aura, without refractory migraine
Chronic migraine without aura, with refractory migraine
Transformed migraine

Clinician Note
Ensure that all related conditions are coded appropriately, particularly if seizure activity is documented.

Cyclical vomiting (G43.A-)

Clinical Tip
Cyclical vomiting syndrome is a condition whose symptoms are recurring attacks of intense nausea, vomiting, and sometimes abdominal pain in the setting of migraine headaches. There are three criteria used to diagnose the condition:

- A history of three or more periods of acute, intense nausea with unrelenting vomiting and sometimes pain lasting hours to days; in some cases several months duration has been reported.
- Intervening symptom-free intervals, which can last weeks to months.
- Diagnostic workup that excludes metabolic, gastrointestinal, or central nervous system structural or biochemical disease.

Clinician Note
Ensure that all related conditions are coded appropriately, particularly if seizure activity is documented.

⇨ I-10 ALERT

The codes in subcategory G43.A- include those related to the presence of intractability. Ensure that this is clearly documented in the medical record.

Ophthalmoplegic migraine (G43.B-)

Clinical Tip
An ophthalmoplegic migraine is a very rare eye disorder that is also classified as a cranial neuralgia. Symptoms include headaches and a weakening of muscles around the eye, oculomotor nerve palsy. In some cases, these headaches commonly precede episodes of partial paralysis of one or more ocular nerve (most commonly the third cranial nerve), drooping of the eyelid, double vision, and dilation of pupils. Onset is typically in infancy or early childhood. The exact etiology is unknown.

Key Terms
Key terms found in the documentation may include:

Acephalgic migraine
Basilar migraine
Ocular migraine
Ophthalmic migraine
Silent migraine

⇨ I-10 ALERT

The codes in subcategory G43.B- include those related to the presence of intractability. Ensure that this is clearly documented in the medical record.

Clinician Note
Ensure that all related conditions are coded appropriately, particularly if seizure activity is documented.

⇨ I-10 ALERT

The codes in subcategory G43.C- include those related to the presence of intractability. Ensure that this is clearly documented in the medical record.

Periodic headache syndromes in child or adult (G43.C-)

Clinical Tip
The childhood periodic syndromes include cyclical vomiting syndrome (CVS), abdominal migraine (AM), and benign paroxysmal vertigo of childhood (BPVC) as migraine precursors. It is also widely believed that periodic syndrome is a common childhood precursor of adult migraine.

Clinician Note
Ensure that all related conditions are coded appropriately, particularly if seizure activity is documented.

⇨ I-10 ALERT

The codes in subcategory G43.D- include those related to the presence of intractability. Ensure that this is clearly documented in the medical record.

Abdominal migraine (G43.D-)

Clinical Tip
A variant of classical migraine headaches, abdominal migraines involve abdominal pain, usually near the midline or navel. Children with abdominal migraines typically develop migraine headaches as they age. Diagnosis of the condition requires ruling out other causes of the pain, particularly of GI origin.

Clinician Note
Ensure that all related conditions are coded appropriately, particularly if seizure activity is documented.

⇨ I-10 ALERT

The codes in subcategory G43.8- include those related to the presence of intractability. Ensure that this is clearly documented in the medical record.

Menstrual migraine (G43.82-, G43.83-)

Clinical Tip
There are two subsets of menstrual migraines. The first, menstrually related migraine without aura, must have an onset during the perimenstrual time period (two days before to three days after the onset of menstruation) and this relationship must be confirmed in two to three of menstrual cycles, regardless of whether attacks occur at other times of the menstrual cycle. Symptoms of the second type, pure menstrual migraine without aura, are similar to the above criteria except that migraine headaches are strictly limited to the perimenstrual time period and do not occur at other times of the month. Estrogen and serotonin levels and interactions are thought to be the underlying cause of the condition.

Key Terms

Key terms found in the documentation may include:

Menstrual headache

Menstrually related migraine

Premenstrual headache

Premenstrual migraine

Pure menstrual migraine

Clinical Findings

Recurrent moderate to severe headaches are most commonly caused by a migraine. There are many possible triggers for migraines including: head trauma, neck pain, fluctuating estrogen levels, skipping meals, weather changes, stress, sleep deprivation, specific foods, etc. Migraine pain may be unilateral or bilateral and may last from four hours to several days.

Physical Examination

History and review of systems may include:

- Moderate to severe headache
- Nausea
- Sensitivity to light and certain sounds
- Fifteen or more days with a headache per month
- Vertigo
- Imbalance
- Speech disturbance
- Visual disturbance
- Sensory disturbance
- Focal weakness
- Complete neurological examination

Diagnostic Procedures and Services

- Laboratory
  - blood tests
- Imaging
  - MRI or CT

Therapeutic Procedures and Services

- Medication
  - pain relievers (NSAIDs, ibuprofen, acetaminophen, etc.)
  - antiemetics
  - triptans
  - ergots
  - glucocorticoids
  - opioids

- IV fluids
- preventive medication
  - beta blockers
  - calcium channel blockers
  - antidepressants
  - naproxen
  - antiseizure medication
  - onabotulinumtoxinA

Clinician Note
Ensure that all related conditions are coded appropriately, particularly if seizure activity is documented.

Clinician Documentation Checklist

Clinician documentation should indicate the following:

- Drug, if responsible
- Type
  - migraine without aura
    - common migraine
  - migraine with aura
    - identify any associated seizure
    - includes
      - basilar migraine
      - classical migraine
      - migraine equivalents
      - migraine preceded or accompanied by transient focal neurological phenomena
      - migraine triggered seizures
      - migraine with acute-onset aura
      - migraine with aura without headache
      - migraine with prolonged aura
      - migraine with typical aura
      - retinal migraine
  - hemiplegic migraine
    - includes
      - familial migraine
      - sporadic migraine
  - Persistent migraine aura without cerebral infarction
  - Persistent migraine aura with cerebral infarction
    - document type of cerebral infarction

- Chronic migraine without aura
  - includes
    - transformed migraine
- cyclical vomiting
- ophthalmoplegic migraine
- periodic headache syndromes in adult or child
- abdominal migraine
- other migraine
  - other specified migraine
  - menstrual migraine
    - identify associated premenstrual tension syndrome
    - includes
      - menstrual headache
      - menstrual migraine
      - menstrually related migraine
      - premenstrual headache
      - premenstrual migraine
      - pure menstrual migraine
- unspecified migraine

- Document each type of migraine as:
  - not intractable
  - intractable
    - includes
      - pharmacoresistant (pharmacologically resistant)
      - treatment resistant
      - refractory (medically)
      - poorly controlled
  - with status epilepticus
  - without status epilepticus

Nerve Blocks

Code Axes

Introduction/injection of anesthetic agent (nerve block), diagnostic or therapeutic **64400–64530**

Description of Procedure

These services are for the injection of an anesthetic agent or other substance and are most frequently used for the treatment of chronic pain. These codes are not used to report anesthesia services.

Introduction/injection of anesthetic agent (nerve block), diagnostic or therapeutic, somatic nerves (64400–64489)

Key Terms

Key terms found in the documentation may include:

Block

Inj

Injection

TAP block

Clinical Tip

Somatic nerves are a part of the peripheral nervous system and are associated with the voluntary control of body movements through the skeletal muscles.

Documentation for nerve blocks of the somatic nerves should include:

- The specific nerve(s) injected
- The substance administered
- The strength and amount of the substance

Documentation should also include the reason for the nerve block and the response of prior treatment if any.

Introduction/injection of anesthetic agent (nerve block), diagnostic or therapeutic, paravertebral spinal nerves (64490–64495)

Facet joint injections should be reported using the appropriate codes from range 64490–64495. Correct code selection is dependent upon:

- Level of the spine injected
- Number of levels reported
- Whether the service was performed unilaterally or bilaterally

Single level: A single level injection occurs when the physician administers one or more substances to a level using one or more needles. A physician may insert a needle and attach a small tube through which the first substance is administered via a syringe. The physician may then change out the syringe and administer a second substance. However, only one needle puncture is performed.

In another method, the physician inserts the needle, administers a substance, and then removes the needle and makes a second puncture with a new needle and syringe to administer an additional substance. Despite the fact that there are two puncture sites, only a single level is being treated.

Multiple levels: When the physician documentation clearly indicates that multiple levels of the spine were injected, add-on codes 64491–64492 and 64494–64495, respectively, are reported.

Bilateral injections: Modifier 50 should be appended when the documentation states that injections were made on the same level but on different sides. Add-on codes 64491–64492 or 64494–64495 are not appropriate when the documentation indicates that the injections were performed bilaterally.

Anesthetic/steroids: Examine the documentation for the name and dosage of the anesthetic agent and/or steroid agent administered. List the appropriate HCPCS Level II code separately.

Clinician Note

Documentation must indicate if the procedure was performed unilaterally or bilaterally. This supports the use of modifier 50 when documentation indicates that the injection was performed bilaterally.

Clinical Tip

Medicare considers facet joint blocks to be reasonable and necessary for chronic pain (persistent pain for three (3) months or greater) suspected to originate from the facet joint. Facet joint block is one of the methods used to document/confirm suspicions of posterior element biomechanical pain of the spine. Hallmarks of posterior element biomechanical pain are as follows:

- The pain does not have a strong radicular component
- There is no associated neurological deficit and the pain is aggravated by hyperextension, rotation, or lateral bending of the spine, depending on the orientation of the facet joint at that level
- A paravertebral facet joint represents the articulation of the posterior elements of one vertebra with its neighboring vertebrae; it is further noted that there are two (2) facet joints at each level, left and right

During a paravertebral facet joint block procedure, a needle is placed in the facet joint or along the medial branches that innervate the joints under fluoroscopic guidance and a local anesthetic and/or steroid is injected. After the injection(s) has been performed, the patient is asked to indulge in the activities that usually aggravate his/her pain and to record his/her impressions of the effect of the procedure. Temporary or prolonged abolition of the pain suggests that the facet joints are the source of the symptoms and appropriate treatment may be prescribed in the future. Some patients have long-lasting relief with local anesthetic and steroid; others require a denervation procedure for more permanent relief. Before proceeding to a denervation treatment, the patient should experience at least a 50 percent reduction in symptoms for the duration of the local anesthetic effect.

Diagnostic or therapeutic injections/nerve blocks may be required for the management of chronic pain. It may take multiple nerve blocks targeting different anatomic structures to establish the etiology of the chronic pain in a given patient. It is standard medical practice to use the modality most likely to establish the diagnosis or treat the presumptive diagnosis. If the first set of procedures fails to produce the desired effect or to rule out the diagnosis, the provider should proceed to the next logical test or treatment indicated. For the purpose of this paravertebral facet joint block, an anatomic region is defined per the CPT manual as cervical/thoracic (64490, 64491, 64492) or lumbar/sacral (64493, 64494, 64495).

Introduction/injection of anesthetic agent (nerve block), diagnostic or therapeutic, autonomic nerves (64505–64530)

The autonomic nervous system is a part of the peripheral nervous system and controls visceral functions, which occur below the level of consciousness. It can be further subdivided into the parasympathetic nervous system and the sympathetic nervous system.

Key Terms

Key terms found in the documentation may include:

ANS

PSNS

SNS

Documentation Tip

Documentation for nerve blocks of the autonomic nerves should include:

- The specific nerve(s) injected
- The substance administered
- The strength and amount of the substance

Documentation should also include the reason for the nerve block and the response of prior treatment if any.

Clinician Documentation Checklist

Clinician documentation should indicate the following:

- Medical condition being treated
- Reason for the nerve block
- Patient response to prior pain treatment
- Nerves injected
- Substance administered
  - strength administered
  - amount administered

- Facet joint injections
- Anatomic region
  - cervical/thoracic
  - lumbar/sacral
  - number of levels reported
    - single level
    - second level
    - third or additional levels
  - bilateral injections
  - anesthetic/steroids
- Contrast used
  - fluoroscopy
  - CT

Nicotine Dependence (Cigarettes, Chewing Tobacco, Other Tobacco Product)

Code Axes

Description	Code
Nicotine dependence, unspecified, uncomplicated	**F17.200**
Nicotine dependence, unspecified, in remission	**F17.201**
Nicotine dependence unspecified, withdrawal	**F17.203**
Nicotine dependence, unspecified, with other nicotine-induced disorders	**F17.208**
Nicotine dependence, unspecified, with unspecified nicotine-induced disorders	**F17.209**
Nicotine dependence, cigarettes, uncomplicated	**F17.210**
Nicotine dependence, cigarettes, in remission	**F17.211**
Nicotine dependence, cigarettes, with withdrawal	**F17.213**
Nicotine dependence, cigarettes, with other nicotine-induced disorders	**F17.218**
Nicotine dependence, cigarettes, with unspecified nicotine-induced disorders	**F17.219**
Nicotine dependence, chewing tobacco, uncomplicated	**F17.220**
Nicotine dependence, chewing tobacco, in remission	**F17.221**
Nicotine dependence, chewing tobacco, with withdrawal	**F17.223**
Nicotine dependence, chewing tobacco, with other nicotine-induced disorders	**F17.228**
Nicotine dependence, chewing tobacco, with unspecified nicotine-induced disorders	**F17.229**
Nicotine dependence, other tobacco product, uncomplicated	**F17.290**
Nicotine dependence, other tobacco product, in remission	**F17.291**
Nicotine dependence, other tobacco product, with withdrawal	**F17.293**
Nicotine dependence, other tobacco product, with other nicotine-induced disorders	**F17.298**
Nicotine dependence, other tobacco product, with unspecified nicotine-induced disorders	**F17.299**

Description of Condition

Nicotine dependence (F17)

Nicotine dependence, the most common chemical dependence, is a chronic disorder characterized by use of high quantities of or frequent use of nicotine products in which the individual becomes physically and mentally dependent upon to function. Long-term consequences are physical, psychological, and behavioral. Some of the physical consequences of nicotine use are emphysema, heart disease, stroke, and cancer. Criterion denoting dependence is increased tolerance and continued use despite impairment of health and social life. Cessation results in withdrawal symptoms. Nicotine dependence without negative consequences documented (e.g., uncomplicated) is reported with subcategory F17.2Ø0.

Key Terms

Key terms found in the documentation may include:

Smoker (current usage)

Smoker under treatment for tobacco dependence

Tobacco dependence

Clinical Findings

Physical Examination

History and review of systems may include some of the following criteria over the past 12 months:

- Increased heart rate
- Elevated BP
- Weight loss
- Respiratory bronchitis
- Larger amounts of tobacco used
- Constant need or unsuccessful attempts to stop or cutback
- Strong craving to use tobacco
- Considerable time spent on activities needed to obtain tobacco
- Tobacco use that conflicts with work or school performance
- Continued use despite tobacco causing persistent social and interpersonal issues
- Smoking in situations that may be hazardous (e.g., in bed)
- Continued use despite persistent physical and psychological problems related to tobacco
- Use of tobacco to avoid or relieve withdrawal symptoms

Withdrawal symptoms may include:

- Nervousness
- Weight gain
- Headache

- Decreased heart rate
- Irritability
- Difficulty concentrating
- Insomnia

Therapeutic Procedures and Services

- Smoking cessation counseling
  - individual or group counseling
- Nicotine replacement therapy
- Hypnosis
- Medication
  - antidepressant
  - bupropion
  - varenicline
  - nortriptyline
  - clonidine

Clinician Note

Documentation of smoking status should indicate the frequency and amount used and identifies the type of nicotine product. If dependency is not indicated, report as tobacco use. Note in the medical record when smoking cessation counseling was provided (Z71.6). A periodic update of smoking status should be performed. The providers' clinical judgment is required for the documentation of "in remission."

Clinician Documentation Checklist

Clinician documentation should indicate the following:

- Exposure to environmental tobacco smoke
- History of tobacco use
- Occupational exposure to environmental tobacco smoke
- Tobacco dependence (e.g., current regular cigarette smoker)
- Tobacco use (e.g., unknown usage of cigarettes)

Obstetrical Package

When documenting obstetrical care, it is important to understand the global obstetrical care package. The concept is similar to the global surgical package. The global obstetrical package includes all the services normally provided during an uncomplicated pregnancy including the antepartum (during pregnancy), delivery, and postpartum (puerperium). The following definitions apply:

Antepartum care: This includes the initial prenatal history and physical examination as well as the history and physical examination (including weight, blood pressure, fetal heart tone, and routine chemical urinalysis) performed during the monthly visits up to 28 weeks gestation; biweekly visits up to 36 weeks gestation, and weekly visits until the time of delivery.

Delivery: The delivery portion of the global obstetrical package includes admission to the hospital or birthing center including the admission history and physical examination, the management of uncomplicated labor and either vaginal or cesarean delivery. Vaginal delivery includes episiotomy and forceps. Also included is any postdelivery management such as discharge services.

Postpartum care: This includes all routine services required up to six weeks postdelivery.

Any services provided outside of those listed above should be documented and reported separately. For example, if a patient has a pregnancy complicated by hyperemesis and therefore needs additional evaluation and management services during the first trimester, these additional E/M services are reported using the appropriate code from the Evaluation and Management section of the CPT manual.

Vaginal delivery, antepartum and postpartum care (59400–59430)

The provider uses these codes to report routine obstetrical care including all antepartum, delivery, and postpartum care or a portion of the global surgical package. Codes from this section should not be used to report the vaginal delivery when the patient has had a previous cesarean delivery (vaginal birth after cesarean or VBAC). In those instances, a code from the 59610–59622 range is used. Correct code assignment is dependent upon the services rendered. For example, if only the vaginal delivery and postpartum care are provided, code 59410 would be reported. However, if the provider managed the entire pregnancy, delivery, and postpartum care, code 59400 is reported.

Also within this section are codes used to report antepartum care only (59425–59426). Correct code selection is dependent upon the number of visits provided. Likewise, code 59430 is used to report only postpartum care.

External cephalic version (59412) is performed by manipulating the fetus from the outside of the abdominal wall, turning the fetus from a breech position to a cephalic position. The clinician places both hands on the patient's abdomen and locates each pole of the fetus by palpation. The fetus is shifted so that the breech or rear end of the fetus is moved upward and the head downward. The physician may elect to use tocolytic drug therapy to suppress uterine contractions during the manipulation. This code may be used for manipulation prior to or during delivery. It may be reported in addition to any of the delivery codes. This includes the cesarean delivery as the physician may attempt to perform the external cephalic version but is unable to manipulate the fetus to a normal cephalic presentation and, therefore, must deliver the infant by cesarean delivery.

Cesarean delivery (59510–59525)

Codes within this range are used to report all or a portion of the global obstetrical package when the delivery is by cesarean section. As with the vaginal delivery codes, correct code selection is dependent upon what portions of the global obstetrical package are provided.

Also within this section is code 59525. This code is used to report a subtotal or total hysterectomy that is performed at the same surgical encounter as the cesarean delivery. Note that this is an add-on code and is listed in addition to the cesarean delivery code.

For those patients who have had a previous cesarean delivery, are expecting to deliver vaginally but require a cesarean delivery, a code from the 59620–59622 range is reported. Again, correct code assignment is dependent upon the level of care provided.

Delivery after previous cesarean (59610–59622)

As mentioned above, there are times when a patient has had a previous cesarean birth and presents with the expectation of delivering vaginally (VBAC). Because previous cesarean delivery can complicate the vaginal delivery and may require a cesarean delivery, separate codes have been developed to report these services.

Codes 59610–59614 are used to report a vaginal delivery after previous cesarean delivery. Correct code selection is dependent upon how much of the global obstetrical package was provided.

Codes 59618–59622 are reported when a vaginal delivery was attempted but delivery had to be by cesarean section after a previous cesarean delivery.

Clinician Documentation Checklist

Clinician documentation should indicate the following:

- Antepartum care
  - prenatal history
  - physical exam
  - weight
  - blood pressure
  - fetal heart tone
  - urinalysis
- Delivery
  - management of labor

  - vaginal delivery w no prior Cesarean
  - cesarean
    - classical
    - low
  - delivery after previous cesarean
- Postpartum
  - weight
  - blood pressure
  - urinalysis

Other Specified Disorders of Kidney and Ureter

Code Axes

Hypertrophy of kidney	**N28.81**
Megaloureter	**N28.82**
Nephroptosis	**N28.83**
Pyelitis cystica	**N28.84**
Pyeloureteritis cystica	**N28.85**
Ureteritis cystica	**N28.86**
Other specified disorders of kidney and ureter	**N28.89**

Description of Condition

Hypertrophy of kidney (N28.81)

Clinical Tip
Kidney hypertrophy is a general increase in the size of the kidney due to an increase in cell volume, but not due to tumor formation, or to an increase in the number of cells. If the other kidney has been surgically removed, compensatory kidney hypertrophy is a result and the remaining kidney takes on the work previously performed by both kidneys.

Key Terms
Key terms found in the documentation for hypertrophy of kidney may include:

Compensatory kidney hypertrophy

Clinician Note
Ensure that all related conditions are coded, particularly those related to underlying kidney function.

CDI ALERT

Ensure that documentation is complete for these conditions and that they are not classified inappropriately as unspecified disorders of kidney and ureter.

CDI ALERT

Although the term hypertrophy is often used to indicate enlargement, documentation stating enlarged kidney should not be assumed to mean hypertrophy of kidney. There are many other conditions that may cause enlargement of the kidney such as polycystic kidney disease or hydronephrosis. Query the physician to determine the exact nature of the condition.

Megaloureter (N28.82)

Clinical Tip
Megaloureter is a descriptive term that represents a ureter that is dilated out of proportion to the remainder of the urinary tract. The condition may be congenital or acquired, in some cases caused by infection or obstruction. It is normally surgically repaired, because retrograde flow of urine can result.

Key Terms
Key terms found in the documentation for megaloureter may include:

Idiopathic megaureter

Megaureter

Nonreflux megaureter

Obstructed ureter

Reflux megaureter

Clinician Note
Ensure that all related conditions are coded, particularly those related to underlying ureter obstruction or malfunction.

Nephroptosis (N28.83)

Clinical Tip
Nephroptosis is a condition in which the kidney descends more than two vertebral bodies (or > 5 cm) during a position change from supine to upright. The condition affects generally more female than male patients and is often asymptomatic but can be treated with nephropexy, a surgical procedure that secures the floating kidney to the retroperitoneum. It is thought to be due to a deficiency in the supporting perirenal fascia.

Key Terms
Key terms found in the documentation for nephroptosis may include:

Floating kidney

Renal ptosis

Clinician Note
Ensure that all related conditions are coded, particularly those related to underlying kidney disorder.

Pyelitis cystica (N28.84)

Clinical Tip
This condition consists of small subepithelial cysts which elevate the mucous membrane of the renal pelvis and appear as round radiolucent areas on urographic studies. It is related to chronic irritation of the urinary collecting system and recurring urinary tract infections, most frequently due to a stone or infection.

Key Terms
Key terms found in the documentation for pyelitis cystica may include:

Ureteritis cystica

Pyeloureteritis cystica (N28.85)

Clinical Tip
This condition is similar to pyelitis cystica (above) but the cysts extend into the ureter as well. It is related to chronic irritation of the urinary collecting system and recurring urinary tract infections, most frequently due to a stone or infection.

Clinician Note
Intravenous pyelography and/or retrograde urography are the gold standard for diagnosis and support code assignment. Findings reveal small and multiple filling defects of the ureter and pelvis. Ureteroscopy can provide pathological confirmation of the benign diagnosis. Differential diagnosis to ureteritis cystica includes tumors of the ureters and pelvis, nonopaque calculi, blood clots and iatrogenically induced air-bubbles.

Ureteritis cystica (N28.86)

CDI ALERT

Carefully examine the clinical documentation as ureteritis cystica (UC) can mimic other conditions such as transitional cell carcinoma, blood clots, air bubbles, radiolucent stones, fibroepithelial polyps, and sloughed renal papillae. Do not report ureteritis cystica unless confirmed by the clinician's documentation.

Clinical Tip
This condition is similar to pyelitis cystica (above) but the cysts involve only the ureter. It is related to chronic irritation of the urinary collecting system and recurring urinary tract infections, most frequently due to a stone or infection.

Clinician Note
Intravenous pyelography and/or retrograde urography are the gold standard for diagnosis and support code assignment. Findings reveal small and multiple filling defects of the ureter and pelvis. Ureteroscopy can provide pathological confirmation of the benign diagnosis. Differential diagnosis to ureteritis cystica includes tumors of the ureters and pelvis, nonopaque calculi, blood clots and iatrogenically induced air-bubbles.

Clinician Documentation Checklist

Clinician documentation should indicate the following:

- Other disorders of kidney and ureter
  - type
    - cyst of kidney, acquired
      - cyst (multiple) (solitary) of kidney, acquired
    - other specified disorders of kidney and ureter
      - hypertrophy of kidney
      - megaloureter
      - nephroptosis
      - pyelitis cystica
      - pyeloureteritis cystica
      - ureteritis cystica
      - other disorders of kidney and ureter
      - unspecified disorder of kidney and ureter

- nephropathy
- renal disease (acute)
- renal insufficiency (acute)

- Other disorders of kidney and ureter in diseases
  - identify underlying disease, such as
    - amyloidosis
    - nephrocalcinosis
    - schistosomiasis

⇨ I-10 ALERT

Very few and very general ICD-9-CM codes for signs and symptoms involving cognitive functioning have been replaced by more specific ICD-10-CM codes. These conditions may not represent fully diagnosed conditions, but do provide more detailed codes during work-up and can classify symptoms whose work-up do not progress to a clearly identifiable condition.

Other Symptoms and Signs Involving Cognitive Functions and Awareness

Code Axes

Age-related cognitive decline	**R41.81**
Altered mental status, unspecified	**R41.82**
Borderline intellectual functioning	**R41.83**
Attention and concentration deficit	**R41.840**
Cognitive communication deficit	**R41.841**
Visuospatial deficit	**R41.842**
Psychomotor deficit	**R41.843**
Frontal lobe and executive function deficit	**R41.844**
Other and unspecified symptoms and signs involving cognitive functions and awareness	**R41.89, R41.9**

Clinician Note
Many payers, including Medicare, have quality measures in place to determine that quality and cost effective care is provided to the patient. It is imperative that the results of cognitive screening and any associated conditions be documented in the medical record.

Description of Condition

Age-related cognitive decline (R41.81)

Clinical Tip
Normal aging is associated with a decline in abilities related to numeric/arithmetic and processing speed, memory, reasoning, verbal ability, and visuoperceptual skills. Patients for whom response and skills are worse than expected for the current age are difficult to clearly diagnose. Research is currently being conducted to determine where normal aging stops and pathology begins.

Key Terms
Key terms found in the documentation for age-related cognitive decline may include:

Senility

Clinician Note
Many payers will not provide coverage of psychotherapy services for age-related cognitive decline unless the medical record documentation can indicate that an improvement in the patients status is expected.

Altered mental status, unspecified (R41.82)

Clinical Tip

Altered mental status is a very general term that refers to general changes in brain function, such as confusion, amnesia (memory loss), loss of alertness, loss of orientation (not cognizant of self, time, or place), defects in judgment or thought, poor regulation of emotions, and disruptions in perception, psychomotor skills, and behavior. Other medical conditions and trauma must be ruled out before a full neurological work-up is performed.

Key Terms

Key terms found in the documentation for altered mental status, unspecified may include:

Change in mental status

Clinician Note

Many payers will not provide coverage of psychotherapy services for altered mental status unless the medical record documentation can indicate that an improvement in the patients status is expected.

Borderline intellectual functioning (R41.83)

Clinical Tip

This condition is broadly defined as a person with an IQ stated to be between 71 and 84. The designation is meant to differentiate these patients from those in the "intellectual disabilities" categories. Research has shown that borderline intellectual functioning is developmental, can be present in both children and adults, and can be a factor associated with relatively poor outcomes in psychiatric disorders.

 **CDI ALERT**

If the specific IQ score is not documented, clarify whether a patient would be classified in the intellectual disabilities category or more appropriately in the borderline intellectual functioning category.

Attention and concentration deficit (R41.840)

Clinical Tip

A variety of environmental factors can negatively affect attention and concentration. Some of these include caffeine, some antidepressant medications, sleep disorders, heavy metal poisoning, and traumatic brain injury, just to name a few. Problems with attention and concentration may also be due to deficiencies in magnesium, thyroid, B-12, or iron levels. Patients undergoing work up for attention or concentration problems should not be classified with ADHD.

Clinician Note

Ensure that all other related diagnoses are coded appropriately, particularly that for underlying neurological disorders.

⇨ **I-10 ALERT**

This particular code, being in the symptoms and signs chapter of ICD-10-CM, is not intended to be assigned for patients who have been diagnosed with one of the attention-deficit hyperactivity disorders (ADHD) (refer to category F90). The code is intended to be reported either when a patient suffers from these symptoms temporarily or as the initial symptom code when being worked up for ADHD.

Cognitive communication deficit (R41.841)

Clinical Tip
This condition involves the breakdown of applied communication skills. Cognitive-communication assessment refers to appraisal of thought processes, including attention, orientation, organization/sequencing, recall and problem solving, insight, processing speed, and pragmatics.

Clinician Note
Ensure that all other related diagnoses are coded appropriately, particularly that for underlying neurological disorders.

Visuospatial deficit (R41.842)

Clinical Tip
The condition involves an inability or deterioration in the ability to comprehend and conceptualize visual representations and spatial relationships in learning and performing a task. The two components of visual processing are: locating an object in space (where?) and determining the identity of an object (what?).

Clinician Note
Ensure that all other related diagnoses are coded appropriately, particularly that for underlying neurological disorders.

Psychomotor deficit (R41.843)

Clinical Tip
This condition involves relating the psychologic processes associated with muscular movement to the production of voluntary movements. Examples include decreased rate of speech, decreased energy, decreased libido and anhedonia (an absence of pleasure from the performance of acts that would ordinarily be pleasurable).

Clinician Note
Ensure that all other related diagnoses are coded appropriately, particularly that for underlying neurological disorders.

Coverage may be provided for occupational therapy and/or activities of daily living for this condition when documentation also indicates that the patient's status is likely to improve.

Frontal lobe and executive function deficit (R41.844)

Clinical Tip
Executive function describes a set of cognitive abilities that control and regulate other abilities and behaviors and are necessary for goal-directed behavior. They include the ability to initiate and stop actions, to monitor and change behavior as needed, and to plan future behavior when faced with novel tasks and situations. Patients with this deficit are unable or hindered in

their ability to anticipate outcomes and adapt to changing situations. The ability to form concepts and think abstractly is often affected.

Clinician Note

Ensure that all other related diagnoses are coded appropriately, particularly that for underlying neurological disorders.

Pacemakers and Implantable Defibrillators

Code Axes

Pacemaker or implantable defibrillators	**33202–33273**

Description of Procedure

A pacemaker may be either permanent or temporary. A permanent pacemaker is used to maintain cardiac stability and a normal sinus rhythm. A temporary pacemaker is used to treat transient bradycardia that may be due to conditions such as acute myocardial infarction or drug toxicity and may be followed by the insertion of a permanent pacemaker.

An implantable cardio-defibrillator monitors heart rhythms and if a potentially dangerous rhythm is sensed it delivers a shock to restore normal rhythm.

Both systems have two major components, an operating system and electrodes. Either of these components may need to be removed and replaced at some point.

Documentation should provide the following information:

What type of system?

Is the device permanent or temporary?

How many leads are placed?

Are any components being removed without replacement?

Are components being replaced and if so which components?

Is the system being converted to a biventricular system (additional lead being placed)?

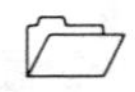

CPT Alert

Note that the insertion of a temporary pacemaker is considered an integral part of critical care and is not reported separately.

Key Terms

Dual lead pacemaker

Dual lead defibrillator

Leadless pacemaker

Multiple lead defibrillator

Permanent pacemaker

Temporary pacemaker

Clinical Tip

There is a new, experimental technology called a leadless cardiac pacemaker. This system includes a pulse generator with built-in battery and electrode for implantation in a cardiac chamber via transcatheter approach. Documentation will indicate that the physician made a small puncture in the groin and using a transcatheter placed the pacemaker into the heart. There will be no documentation indicating a lead placement. Services related to the leadless pacemaker are reported with the appropriate code from 0387T–0391T.

Clinician Documentation Checklist

Clinician documentation should indicate the following:

- Approach
  - open
  - endoscopic
  - transvenous
  - atrial
  - ventricular
- Purpose of the procedure
  - insertion
  - replacement
  - revision
  - repair
- Type of system inserted
  - single chamber
  - dual chamber
- Device expected length of service
  - permanent
  - temporary
- How many leads are placed
- Identification of
  - components being removed without replacement
  - components being replaced
- System conversion to biventricular system

Preventive Services — Prostate Cancer Screening

Code Axes

Prostate cancer screening; digital rectal examination	**G0102**
Prostate cancer screening; prostate specific antigen test (PSA)	**G0103**

Description of Procedure

For Medicare and many other third-party payers, coverage of prostate cancer screening tests includes the following procedures furnished to an individual for the early detection of prostate cancer:

- Screening digital rectal examination
- Screening prostate specific antigen blood test

⇨ I-10 ALERT

When reporting prostate cancer screening, digital rectal examinations, and screening prostate-specific antigen (PSA) blood tests, diagnosis code Z12.5 Encounter for screening for malignant neoplasm of prostate, must be used to indicate the screening nature of the service.

Prostate cancer screening; digital rectal examination (G0102)

Screening digital rectal examinations are covered at a frequency of once every 12 months for men who have attained age 50 (at least 11 months have passed following the month in which the last Medicare-covered screening digital rectal examination was performed). Documentation will indicate that the health care provider performed an examination of an individual's prostate for nodules or other abnormalities of the prostate.

Key Terms

DRE

Clinician Note

The size and any abnormalities should be noted in the medical record as well as any changes from previous examinations.

Prostate cancer screening; prostate specific antigen test (PSA) (G0103)

Screening prostate specific antigen (PSA) tests are performed to detect the marker for adenocarcinoma of prostate. PSA is a reliable immunocytochemical marker for primary and metastatic adenocarcinoma of prostate. Documentation supporting this service will include a laboratory result.

Prostatectomy

Code Axes

Prostatectomy **55801–55866**

Description of Procedure

Excision of the prostate, other than by transurethral methods, is reported with the appropriate code from range 55801–55845, 55866. Documentation should be carefully reviewed to determine:

- The approach
  - perineal
  - retropubic
  - laparoscopic
- The extent
  - total
  - subtotal
- The method
  - one stage
  - two stage
- If lymphadenectomy was performed

Prostatectomy, perineal, subtotal (including control of postoperative bleeding, vasectomy, meatotomy, urethral calibration and/or dilation, and internal urethrotomy) (55801)

Documentation supporting a subtotal perineal radical prostatectomy will indicate that the prostate was removed through an incision made in the perineum. The bladder outlet is revised; however, the seminal vesicles remain intact.

Key Terms

Key terms found in the documentation may include:

Subtotal radical prostatectomy

 **CDI ALERT**

Terms such as biopsy, lymphadenectomy, perineal, retropubic, radical, subtotal or nerve sparing provide the guidance needed to ensure correct code assignment.

Prostatectomy, perineal, radical (55810)

Documentation for this service will indicate that the seminal vesicles and vas deferens are also removed. When documentation indicates that local lymph nodes were removed for analysis, code 55812 is supported. When a separate incision is made and all lymph nodes are removed from the back wall of the pelvis, code 55815 is supported.

Prostatectomy (including control of postoperative bleeding, vasectomy, meatotomy, urethral calibration and/or dilation, and internal urethrotomy); suprapubic, subtotal, stages 1 or 2 (55821)

Prostatectomy (including control of postoperative bleeding, vasectomy, meatotomy, urethral calibration and/or dilation, and internal urethrotomy); retropubic, subtotal (55831)

Prostatectomy retropubic radical, with or without nerve sparing (55840)

When documentation indicates that an incision was made in the lower abdomen just above the pubic area, a suprapubic approach is performed. However, when the documentation indicates that the incision was made in the lower abdomen and the physician approached the prostate by going behind the pubic bone, a retropubic prostatectomy was performed. Note that if the seminal vesicles are not removed, a subtotal prostatectomy was performed. Documentation supporting a retropubic radical prostatectomy states that the seminal glands and vas deferens were also removed.

Clinician Documentation Checklist

Clinician documentation should indicate the following:

- Medical condition being treated
- Approach
  - perineal
  - retropubic
  - laparoscopic
- Extent
  - total
  - subtotal
- Method
  - one stage
  - two stages
- Other services
  - radiation application
  - lymph node biopsy

Respiratory Distress of Newborn

Code Axes

Respiratory distress syndrome of newborn	**P22.Ø**
Transient tachypnea of newborn	**P22.1**
Other respiratory distress of newborn	**P22.8**
Respiratory distress of newborn, unspecified	**P22.9**

Description of Condition

Respiratory distress syndrome of newborn (P22.Ø)

Respiratory distress syndrome (RDS) is a breathing disorder that affects newborns. RDS rarely occurs in full-term infants. Respiratory distress syndrome is the most common disorder of the premature infant, generally less than 34 weeks gestation. The incidence and severity increase with decreasing gestational age. RDS is more common in premature infants because their lungs are unable to produce enough surfactant.

Key Terms

Key terms found in the documentation may include:

Cardiorespiratory distress syndrome of newborn

Hyaline membrane disease

Idiopathic respiratory distress syndrome [IRDS or RDS] of newborn

Pulmonary hypoperfusion syndrome

Respiratory distress syndrome, type I

 **CDI ALERT**

Documentation should include prematurity or documentation of other deficiency of surfactant, progressively more severe respiratory distress after birth, as well as findings of cyanosis, grunting, nasal flaring, intercostal and subcostal retractions and tachypnea. Chest x-rays frequently have a ground-glass appearance. Oxygen requirements progressively increase over the first few hours after birth. There may also be documentation of apnea and refractory hypoxemia and acidosis.

Treatments include endotracheal intubation, positive pressure ventilation, continuous positive airway pressure (CPAP), supplementary oxygen, and surfactant placement via ET tube.

Clinical Findings

RDS is caused by pulmonary surfactant deficiency in the lungs and risk increases with the degree of prematurity.

Physical Examination

The following symptoms will occur immediately or within a few hours of delivery.

- Nasal flaring
- Rapid and labored breathing
- Grunting respirations
- Use of accessory muscles
- Cyanosis
- Apnea
- Lethargy
- Decreased breath sounds

- Diagnostic Procedures and Services
- Laboratory
  - arterial blood gas
  - blood cultures
  - tracheal aspirate cultures
  - cerebrospinal fluid culture
- Imaging
  - chest x-ray
- Other
  - transcutaneous CO_2 monitor

Therapeutic Procedures and Services

- Surfactant therapy
- Mechanical ventilation
- Supplementary oxygen

Transient tachypnea of newborn (P22.1)

Transient tachypnea of the newborn (TTN) is the most common respiratory disorder of the mature newborn and is self-limited, due to the inability to absorb fetal lung fluid. Infants with transient tachypnea of newborn present within the first few hours of life with tachypnea, increased oxygen requirement, and ABGs negative for carbon dioxide retention.

Treatment is generally close observation and symptomatic care with low flow supplemental oxygen.

Key Terms

Key terms found in the documentation may include:

Idiopathic tachypnea of newborn

Respiratory distress syndrome, type II

Wet lung syndrome

Other respiratory distress of newborn (P22.8)

Documentation Tip

Codes are not assigned for respiratory distress syndrome (RDS type I) or transitory tachypnea of newborn (RDS type II) unless the provider specifically documents these conditions. Code P22.8 would be assigned if the provider has documented a specific type of respiratory distress syndrome in the newborn that is not coded elsewhere.

Respiratory distress of newborn, unspecified (P22.9)

Documentation Tip

If the provider indicates "respiratory distress of newborn" without further documentation code P22.9 is assigned.

Clinician Documentation Checklist

Clinician documentation should indicate the following:

- Conditions acquired in utero, during birth, or during the first 28 days after birth
- Type of disorder
  - metabolic acidemia
    - before onset of labor
    - during labor
    - at birth
- Respiratory distress
  - respiratory distress syndrome of newborn
    - cardiorespiratory distress syndrome
    - hyaline membrane disease
    - pulmonary hypoperfusion syndrome
  - transient tachypnea
    - idiopathic tachypnea
    - respiratory distress type II
    - wet lung syndrome
- Congenital pneumonia
  - specify the organism
  - pneumonia due to
    - viral agent
    - *Chlamydia*
    - *Staphylococcus*
    - *Streptococcus*
    - *Escherichia coli*
    - pseudomonas
    - bacterial agent
- Neonatal aspiration
  - specify with or without respiratory symptoms
  - specify any pulmonary hypertension
  - due to
    - meconium
    - amniotic fluid and mucus
    - blood
    - milk and food
- Interstitial emphysema
  - interstitial
  - pneumothorax
  - pneumomediastinum
  - pneumopericardium

- Pulmonary hemorrhage
  - tracheobronchial hemorrhage
  - massive pulmonary hemorrhage
- Chronic respiratory disease
  - Wilson-Mikity syndrome
  - bronchopulmonary dysplasia
  - congenital pulmonary fibrosis
  - ventilator lung
- Other respiratory perinatal conditions
  - primary atelectasis
    - primary failure to expand terminal respiratory units
    - pulmonary hypoplasia associated with short gestation
    - pulmonary immaturity
  - atelectasis
  - resorption atelectasis without respiratory distress syndrome
  - cyanotic attacks
  - primary sleep apnea
  - apnea of prematurity
  - obstructive apnea of newborn
  - respiratory failure
  - respiratory arrest
  - respiratory depression
  - laryngeal stridor
  - sniffles
  - snuffles

Respiratory Failure

Code Axes

Note: All four subcategories of respiratory failure contain fifth characters that represent the following code classification axes: unspecified whether with hypoxia or hypercapnia; with hypoxia: defined as a condition in which the body is deprived of an adequate oxygen supply, regardless of whether the body has an adequate perfusion by blood; with hypercapnia: defined as an increased level of carbon dioxide in the blood, usually exhaled during regular breathing.

Acute respiratory failure	**J96.Ø**
Chronic respiratory failure	**J96.1**
Acute and chronic respiratory failure	**J96.2**
Respiratory failure, unspecified	**J96.9**
Acute respiratory distress syndrome	**J8Ø**
Postprocedural respiratory failure	**J95.82**

I-10 Alert

Although the major subcategories of respiratory failure remain the same between ICD-9-CM and ICD-10-CM, the secondary classification axes, involving the presence of hypoxia or hypercapnia are new. Understanding these conditions is essential for appropriate classification.

Description of Condition

Acute respiratory failure (J96.Ø-)

Clinical Tip

Acute respiratory failure may be life-threatening and involve the most abnormal arterial blood gas measurements, but the two types (hypoxic and hypercapnic) are very different. Hypoxemic is the most common form and can be associated with most lung diseases, representing a lower than normal arterial oxygen level. Hypercapnic respiratory failure, with a high level of carbon dioxide ($PaCO_2$) is most often associated with drug overdoses, severe airway disorders, or neuromuscular diseases. Acute RF develops within minutes or hours.

CDI Alert

Ensure that the documentation is adequate and can differentiate between acute respiratory failure and acute respiratory distress syndrome, which is classified to category J8Ø.

Clinician Note

Note that a documentation of respiratory insufficiency does not support the assignment of an acute respiratory failure code.

Chronic respiratory failure (J96.1-)

Chronic or long-term respiratory failure is most often caused by various types of chronic obstructive pulmonary diseases (COPD), neuromuscular diseases (e.g., myasthenia gravis), cystic fibrosis, and even morbid obesity. Chronic RF develops over days or longer, worsens over time, and triggers should be identified, which are most commonly related to a superimposed infection. Although chronic in presentation, this condition is sufficiently severe and may cause major complications, such as organ failure or dysfunction, acute myocardial infarction (AMI), respiratory arrest, or shock.

 **CDI ALERT**

If chronic respiratory failure is documented, ensure that there is no superimposed acute component as well. Acute on chronic respiratory failure is a common condition in this patient group.

Acute and chronic respiratory failure (J96.2-)

Acute and rapid deterioration of a patient with chronic respiratory failure is known as acute on chronic respiratory failure. These are typically COPD patients or those with neuromuscular disease or chest wall disorders. Patients with this condition may require long-term mechanical ventilation.

⇨ **I-10 ALERT**

For ICD-10-CM the word "adult" was changed to "acute" in the "respiratory distress syndrome" terminology. It is now understood that the disease process can occur in either an adult or a pediatric patient. However, be aware that a separate classification category exists for respiratory distress syndrome of the newborn (P22.Ø).

Acute respiratory distress syndrome (ARDS) (J8Ø)

Acute respiratory distress syndrome is considered the most acute form of acute lung injury (ALI) (nontraumatic). The syndrome is defined by the ratio of the partial pressure of oxygen in the patient's arterial blood (PaO_2) to the fraction of oxygen in the inspired air (FIO_2). In ARDS, the PaO_2/FIO_2 ratio is less than 200, and in ALI, it is less than 300. Patients with ARDS typically have pulmonary edema, as the alveolar space fills with fluid. Many patients also develop pulmonary hypertension, which usually resolves as the syndrome resolves.

Key Terms

Key terms found in the documentation may include:

Adult hyaline membrane disease

⇨ **I-10 ALERT**

Codes in subcategory J95.82 are differentiated by severity; code J95.821 represents acute postprocedural respiratory failure and code J95.822 represents the acute and chronic form of the condition.

Postprocedural respiratory failure (J95.82-)

Postoperative respiratory failure is the need for ventilation for more than 48 hours after surgery or reintubation with mechanical ventilation post extubation. Comorbid conditions that are risk factors are obstructive sleep apnea, COPD, CHF, advanced age, ASA class ≥ 2 and pulmonary hypertension. Patients who have had surgery of the aortic, thoracic, and upper abdomen areas have higher odds of developing postoperative respiratory failure.

Clinician Note

Differentiate between *expected* respiratory requirements postsurgery and a condition or complication requiring additional ventilation time or reintubation. Identify the causative condition when known (aspiration, exacerbation of COPD, pneumonia, etc.).

 **CDI ALERT**

The documentation for postprocedural respiratory failure must clearly make the cause-and-effect relationship between the condition and the fact that it was a result of the procedure or surgery in order to assign a code from this subcategory.

Clinical Findings

Conditions or diseases that may lead to respiratory failure are disorders that affect the nerves, muscles, tissues, or bones that support breathing or have a direct effect on the lungs. Examples include: muscular dystrophy, spinal cord injuries, chest injury that damages the tissues and ribs around the lungs, scoliosis, COPD, pneumonia, and ARDS.

Physical Examination

History and review of systems may include:

- Shortness of breath
- A feeling of the inability to breath in enough air
- Rapid breathing
- Abnormal lung sounds (crackling)

- Arrhythmia
- Asterixis
- Cyanosis
- Dyspnea
- Confusion
- Severe sleepiness
- Cor pulmonale—may be present with chronic respiratory failure
- Hypotension
- Gastric distention
- Diarrhea

Diagnostic Procedures and Services

- Laboratory
  - arterial blood gas
  - CBC
  - chemistry panel
  - serum creatinine
  - TSH—in chronic respiratory failure
- Imaging
  - chest x-ray
- Other
  - pulse oximetry
  - EKG
  - PFT—in evaluation of chronic respiratory failure

Therapeutic Procedures and Services

Treatment will depend on severity, if the condition is acute or chronic and the underlying cause.

- Oxygen therapy
- Mechanical ventilation
- Tracheostomy
- IV fluids
- CPAP—useful with chronic respiratory failure
- Medications may be given to treat the underlying cause

Clinician Documentation Checklist

Clinician documentation should indicate the following:

- Respiratory failure
  - with hypoxia
  - with hypercapnia
  - unspecified whether with hypoxia or hypercapnia
- Type
  - acute

- chronic
- acute and chronic
  - acute on chronic respiratory failure
- unspecified

Respiratory Diseases Affecting Interstitium

- Acute respiratory distress syndrome
  - in adult or child
  - adult hyaline membrane disease
- Pulmonary edema
  - identify
    - exposure to environmental tobacco smoke
    - history of tobacco use
    - occupational exposure to environmental tobacco smoke
    - tobacco dependence
    - tobacco use
  - type
    - acute
      - acute edema of lung
    - chronic
      - pulmonary congestion (chronic) (passive)
      - pulmonary edema
- Pulmonary eosinophilia
  - includes
    - allergic pneumonia
    - eosinophilic asthma
    - eosinophilic pneumonia
    - Loffler's pneumonia
    - tropical (pulmonary) eosinophilia

Intraoperative and Postprocedural Complications, Disorders of Respiratory System

- Procedure that was performed
- Specific part of respiratory tract that was involved
- Complications that occurred were
  - during procedure (intraoperative)
  - after procedure (postprocedural)
- Type of complications
  - tracheostomy complications
    - hemorrhage from tracheostomy stroma
    - infection of tracheostomy stroma
      - identify type of infection such as:
        - cellulitis

- sepsis
- malfunction of tracheostomy stroma
  - tracheal stenosis due to tracheostomy
  - obstruction of tracheostomy airway
  - mechanical complication
- tracheoesophageal fistula following tracheostomy
- other
- unspecified

- acute pulmonary insufficiency following
  - thoracic surgery
  - nonthoracic surgery
- chronic pulmonary insufficiency following
  - surgery
- chemical pneumonitis due to anesthesia
  - identify
    - Mendelson's syndrome
    - postprocedural aspiration pneumonia
    - the drug, if responsible
- postprocedural subglottic stenosis
- intraoperative hemorrhage and hematoma of respiratory system organ complicating a procedure
  - respiratory system procedure
  - other procedure
- postprocedural hematoma or hemorrhage of respiratory organ following a procedure
  - respiratory system procedure
  - other procedure
- accidental puncture and laceration during a procedure
  - respiratory system procedure
  - other procedure
- postprocedural pneumothorax
- postprocedural airleak
- postprocedural respiratory failure
  - acute
  - acute and chronic
- transfusion-related acute lung injury
- complication of respirator (ventilator)
  - mechanical complication
  - ventilator associated pneumonia
    - identification of the causal organism
  - other

- other complications and disorders
  - intraoperative
  - postprocedural
    - identification of disorders such as
      - aspiration pneumonia
      - bacterial or viral pneumonia

Rhythm and Conduction Disorders

Code Axes

Atrioventricular and left bundle-branch block	**I44.Ø–I44.7**
Other and unspecified conduction disorders	**I45.Ø–I45.9**
Atrial fibrillation and flutter	**I48.Ø–I48.9-**
Other cardiac arrhythmias	**I49.Ø–I49.9**

Clinical Tip

Mobitz I and Mobitz II AV blocks are both classified as second degree AV blocks, and are based on electrocardiographic (ECG) patterns, not on location. Even though slightly different, the conditions were classified to two different codes in ICD-9-CM, but in ICD-10-CM, both are classified to code I44.1.

Key Terms

Key terms found in the documentation for conduction disorders may include:

Accelerated atrioventricular conduction
Accessory atrioventricular conduction
A-fib
Anomalous atrioventricular excitation
Atrial fibrillation
Atrial flutter
Atrioventricular (AV) block, type I and II
Atrioventricular (AV) dissociation
Bifascicular block
Complete heart block Mobitz block, type I and II
Fascicular block
Interference dissociation
Isorhythmic dissociation
Left bundle branch block (LBBB)
Left bundle-branch hemiblock
Lown-Ganong-Levine syndrome
Nonparoxysmal AV nodal tachycardia
Pre-excitation atrioventricular conduction
Right bundle branch block (RBBB)
Sick sinus syndrome (SSS)
Sinoatrial block
Sinoauricular block
Stokes-Adams syndrome

⇨ I-10 ALERT

ICD-10-CM codes for cardiac arrhythmia conditions are much more specific than those for ICD-9-CM. For example, unlike ICD-9-CM, which contained single codes for atrial and ventricular fibrillation and flutter, ICD-10-CM provides code options for paroxysmal, persistent, chronic, typical, and atypical forms of atrial fibrillation and flutter.

Third degree AV block

Trifascicular block

Ventricular fibrillation

Ventricular flutter

Wenckebach's block

Wolff-Parkinson-White (WPW) syndrome

Clinical Tip

Atrial fibrillation may be classified into one of three categories:

Paroxysmal: These episodes end spontaneously within seven days and most episodes last less than 24 hours

Persistent: These episodes last more than seven days and may require electrical or pharmacologic intervention

Permanent (chronic): This atrial fibrillation has lasted more than one year, regardless of whether cardioversion has been attempted and has failed or has never been attempted

Atrial flutter is classified into two categories, Type I and Type II:

Type I: Typical (common) atrial flutter has an atrial rate of 240 to 340 beats/minute

Type II: Atypical atrial flutter follows a significantly different re-entry pathway than Type I and is faster; usually 340 to 440 beats/minute

Ensure that documentation is consistent when involving the different types of atrial fibrillation and flutter.

Clinical Findings

Bundle branch and fascicular blocks are generally asymptomatic and are diagnosed by ECG. Atrioventricular (AV) blocks may be asymptomatic or exhibit mild to severe symptoms including bradycardia, fatigue, light-headedness, presyncope, syncope, or heart failure. AV blocks are diagnosed by ECG and may be treated with medication or often require a pacemaker.

Atrial fibrillation affects nearly 2.3 million adults in the U.S. and is the most common type of irregular heartbeat.

Physical Examination

A-fib may be asymptomatic or the patient history or current symptoms may include one or more of the following:

- Irregularly irregular pulse
- Rapid and irregular heartbeat
- Weakness
- Light-headedness
- Dyspnea
- Fatigue
- Fluttering in the chest

- Vague chest discomfort/pain
- Palpitations
- Shortness of breath
- Swollen feet or legs

Diagnostic Procedures and Services

- Laboratory
  - TFTs
- Imaging
  - chest x-ray
  - echocardiography
- Other
  - ECG
  - Holter monitor

Therapeutic Procedures and Services

- Medications
  - blood clot prevention
    - antiplatelets
    - anticoagulants
  - heart rate/rhythm control
    - antiarrhythmic drugs
    - beta blockers
    - calcium channel blockers
    - digitalis
- Procedures
  - electrical cardioversion
  - ablation
  - pacemaker

Clinician Note

Many of the conduction disorders support the medical necessity of pacemaker insertion, cardioverter-defibrillator insertion, and intracardiac electrophysiologic procedures. Physician documentation should be examined to determine if there are other underlying conditions which should be reported separately.

Clinician Documentation Checklist

Clinician documentation should indicate the following:

- Heart blocks
  - atrioventricular block
    - first degree
    - second degree (Mobitz type I and II, Wenckebach)
    - third degree (complete NOS)

    - other
    - unspecified
  - left anterior fascicular block
  - left posterior fascicular block
  - other (left bundle branch hemiblock NOS)
  - unspecified (other fascicular block)
- Other conduction disorders
  - right fascicular block
  - other and unspecified right bundle branch block
  - bifascicular block
  - trifascicular block
  - nonspecific intraventricular block
  - other specified heart block (sinoatrial block, sinoauricular block)
  - pre-excitation syndrome
  - accelerated atrioventricular conduction
  - accessory atrioventricular conduction
  - anomalous atrioventricular excitation
  - Lown-Ganong-Levine syndrome
  - pre-excitation atrioventricular conduction
  - Wolff-Parkinson-White syndrome
  - other
    - long qt syndrome
    - other specified conduction disorder
    - AV dissociation
    - interference dissociation
  - unspecified
- Cardiac arrest
  - due to underlying cardiac condition
  - due to other underlying condition
  - cause unspecified

Cardiac Arrhythmias

- Tachycardia
  - re-entry ventricular
  - supraventricular
  - atrioventricular
  - atrioventricular re-entrant (nodal)
  - junctional
  - ventricular
  - unspecified (paroxysmal)
- Atrial fibrillation and flutter
  - paroxysmal

- persistent
- chronic
- typical
- atypical
- unspecified

- Other cardiac arrhythmias
  - ventricular fibrillation
  - ventricular flutter
  - atrial premature depolarization
  - junctional premature depolarization
  - ventricular premature depolarization
  - premature beats NOS
  - other premature depolarization
  - sick sinus syndrome
  - other specified cardiac arrhythmias
  - unspecified cardiac arrhythmias

Sepsis (Systemic, Generalized, Complication)

Code Axes

The majority of the ICD-10-CM sepsis codes are in categories A4Ø and A41:

Streptococcal sepsis	**A4Ø.Ø–A4Ø.9**
Sepsis due to Staphylococcus aureus	**A41.Ø1–A41.4**
Sepsis due to other Gram-negative organisms	**A41.5Ø–A41.59**
Other and unspecified sepsis	**A41.81, A41.89**

Description of Condition

Clinical Tip

Sepsis is a life-threatening systemic infection of the bloodstream, most typically originating in the urinary tract, lungs, GI systems, or via a surgical wound or infected implanted device. Symptoms may progress to shock or organ failure, and the condition may be fatal.

Bacteremia is an abnormal finding on blood culture that indicates bacteria in the blood and does not represent an infectious state. Bacteremia elicits an immune response which can exhibit as fever. If bacteremia is stated but clinical evidence supports the presence of sepsis, a systemic infection with features of a more severe immune response, query the provider for clarification.

Documentation Tip

Physician documentation must demonstrate the severity of the illness through the history and physical, progress notes, review and comment on all consults, and review and comment on ancillary test results indicating either the improvement or worsening of the patient status.

Streptococcal sepsis (A4Ø), including codes for sepsis due to strep, group A (A4Ø.Ø), group B (A4Ø.1), strep pneumoniae (A4Ø.3), and other and unspecified strep (A4Ø.8, A4Ø.9)

ICD-10-CM contains multiple codes in this category, including those for group A, group B, strep pneumoniae, and other and unspecified forms of the disease. Group B is most commonly responsible for infections in the pediatric population and also in pregnant patients.

CDI ALERT

Negative or inclusive blood cultures do not preclude a diagnosis of sepsis. The presence of one or more risk factors, the appropriate clinical presentation, and specific treatment in conjunction with physician confirmation validates the diagnosis.

Documentation Tip

The diagnosis of sepsis cannot be made based solely on laboratory or blood work findings. The physician must document the systemic infection.

Key Terms

Key terms found in the documentation may include:

Bloodstream infection (although necessary to differentiate from bacteremia)

Septicemia

Septic intoxication

Septic syndrome

Severe sepsis

Severe sepsis with organ failure

Toxemia

Urosepsis (antiquated term; necessary to differentiate from UTI)

Sepsis due to Staphylococcus aureus, including codes and for methicillin susceptible Staphylococcus aureus (MSSA) (A41.Ø1), for methicillin resistant Staphylococcus aureus (MRSA) (A41.Ø2)

ICD-10-CM diagnosis codes representing staph sepsis conditions mirror those in ICD-9-CM, with specific codes for MRSA and MSSA.

Key Terms

Key terms found in the documentation may include:

Bloodstream infection (although necessary to differentiate from bacteremia)

MRSA sepsis

MSSA sepsis

Septicemia

Septic intoxication

Septic syndrome

Severe sepsis

Toxemia

Urosepsis (antiquated term; necessary to differentiate from UTI)

Sepsis due to Hemophilus influenzae is (A41.3) and sepsis due to anaerobes is (A41.4) which would include Clostridium and Bacteroides.

ICD-10-CM diagnosis codes representing Gram-negative *Haemophilus influenzae* and anaerobic sepsis mirror those in ICD-9-CM. While the code for *Haemophilus influenzae* is specific, code A41.4 includes any (gram positive or negative) anaerobic organism, classified as such but for which there is no assigned index entry (unlike actinomycosis which is A42.7).

 **CDI ALERT**

In some cases skin bacteria contaminates the blood sample, which is another reason physician correlation and clarification of diagnosis is essential before code assignment.

Sepsis due to other Gram-negative organisms (A41.5-), including specific codes for sepsis due to Escherichia coli (A41.51), Pseudomonas(A41.52), Serratia (A41.53), and other and unspecified Gram-negative sepsis (A41.59, A41.5Ø)

ICD-10-CM diagnosis codes representing Gram-negative sepsis conditions mirror those in ICD-9-CM, with specific codes for sepsis due to E. coli, Pseudomonas, Serratia, and infections due to other Gram-negative organisms such as *Acinetobacter baumanni, Klebsiella pneumoniae.* Gram-negative sepsis is an increasingly common disorder and, with problems due to multiple drug resistance, the symptoms can lead to such serious complications as shock, adult respiratory distress syndrome, and disseminated intravascular coagulation.

CDI ALERT

Colonization is the presence of an organism without current disease; it should be documented when confirmed or suspected as it has potential risks for both patient and care-givers; colonization is reported as "carrier" from category Z22.

Key Terms

Key terms found in the documentation may include:

Bloodstream infection (although necessary to differentiate from bacteremia)

Septicemia

Septic intoxication

Severe sepsis

Toxemia

Urosepsis (antiquated term; necessary to differentiate from UTI)

Other specified sepsis (A41.89), includes sepsis due to Enterococcus (Strep group D) (A41.81).

Enterococcus faecalis and *Enterococcus faecium* are the most common of these pathogens. *Enterococcus* species are important nosocomial pathogens because of their resistance to antibiotics; *E. faecium* represents most vancomycin-resistant *Enterococcus* (VRE).

CDI ALERT

When the documentation indicates that the patient has severe sepsis, sepsis with acute organ dysfunction, sepsis with multiple organ dysfunction, or systemic inflammatory response syndrome (SIRS) due to infectious process with acute organ dysfunction, the appropriate code from R65.2- should also be assigned.

Viral sepsis (A41 and B97)

Viral sepsis, other than disseminated herpesviral disease, will require two codes. Sepsis will be identified by A41.89 when the organism is specified, or A41.9 when unspecified, in addition to a code from category B97 to identify the viral organism or a code to identify the localized infection.

Candidal sepsis (B37.7)

Candidiasis is a yeast fungal (mycosis) infection. Disseminated or invasive candidiasis is considered sepsis, also known as candidemia. Fungemia NOS (B49) is a fungal sepsis due to an unspecified mycosis. Treatment is by antifungals, such as fluconazole and amphotericin.

ICD-10-CM sepsis codes in chapter 1 but not in categories A4Ø or A41 are found in the following table.

Code	Description
A42.7	Actinomycotic sepsis
A22.7	Anthrax sepsis
B37.7	Candidal sepsis
A26.7	Erysipelothrix sepsis
A28.2	Extraintestinal yersiniosis (sepsis)
A54.86	Gonococcal sepsis
BØØ.7	Disseminated herpesviral disease (sepsis)
A32.7	Listerial sepsis
A24.1	Acute and fulminating melioidosis (sepsis)
A39.2–A39.4	Acute, chronic, or unspecified meningococcemia (sepsis)
AØ2.1	Salmonella sepsis
A2Ø.7	Septicemic plague
A21.7	Generalized tularemia (sepsis)

ICD-10-CM sepsis codes related to the pregnant patient are found in the following table.

Code	Description
OØ3.37	Sepsis following incomplete spontaneous abortion
OØ3.87	Sepsis following complete or unspecified spontaneous abortion
OØ4.87	Sepsis following (induced) termination of pregnancy
OØ7.37	Sepsis following failed attempted termination of pregnancy
OØ8.82	Sepsis following ectopic and molar pregnancy
O75.3	Other infection during labor (sepsis)
O85	Puerperal sepsis

ICD-10-CM sepsis codes in chapter 19 and represent postprocedural complications are found in the following table.

Code	Description
J95.Ø2	Infection of tracheostomy stoma
T8Ø.211	Bloodstream infection due to central venous catheter
T8Ø.22- T8Ø.29-	Acute infection following transfusion, infusion, or injection of blood and blood products; infection following other infusion, transfusion and therapeutic injection
T81.4-	Infection following a procedure (sepsis)
T82.6- T82.7-	Infection and inflammatory reaction due to cardiac valve prosthesis; infection and inflammatory reaction due to other cardiac and vascular devices, implants and grafts
T83.5- T83.6-	Infection and inflammatory reaction due to indwelling urinary catheter; infection and inflammatory reaction due to prosthetic device, implant and graft in urinary system; infection and inflammatory reaction due to prosthetic device, implant and graft in urinary tract

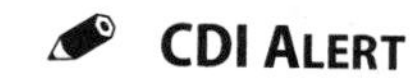

CDI ALERT

Vasopressors, such as norepinephrine, dopamine and epinephrine are used to reverse hypoperfusion, increase cardiac output and facilitate oxygen delivery in severe sepsis or septic shock that fails fluid resuscitation or as an adjunct to fluid resuscitation. A central catheter line is needed for delivery. The procedure of introduction of vasopressor in central vein would be reported.

Code	Description
T84.5- T84.6- T84.7-	Infection and inflammatory reaction due to internal joint prosthesis; infection and inflammatory reaction due to internal fixation device; infection and inflammatory reaction due to other internal orthopedic prosthetic devices, implants and grafts
T85.7-	Infection and inflammatory reaction due to other internal prosthetic devices, implants and grafts (peritoneal dialysis catheter; insulin pump; other)
T86.-	Transplanted organ infection
T88.Ø-	Infection following immunization (sepsis)

Clinician Note

Physician documentation must provide the cause and effect relationship between the procedure and the postprocedural sepsis.

Clinical Findings

Sepsis is a systemic response to bacterial infection in which chemicals released in the bloodstream to fight the infection cause an inflammatory state throughout the body.

Physical Examination

History and review of symptoms may include:

- Fever
- Tachycardia
- Rapid respiratory rate
- Mental status change
- Difficulty breathing
- Chills
- Major decrease in urine output
- Diaphoresis
- Decreased BP
- Organ dysfunction

Diagnostic Procedures and Services

- Laboratory
  - blood culture
  - electrolyte panel
  - urinalysis
  - procalcitonin levels
  - arterial blood gas
  - CBC
  - liver and renal function
- Imaging
  - chest x-ray
  - CT

- MRI
- ultrasound

- Other
  - pulse oximetry

Therapeutic Procedures and Services

- IV antibiotics
- Oxygen therapy
- Therapy to support any organ dysfunction
- Infection control
  - Surgery

Clinician Documentation Checklist

Clinician documentation should indicate the following:

Streptococcal

- Group a
- Group b
- Pneumonia
  - pneumococcal

Other sepsis

- *Staphylococcus aureus*
  - methicillin susceptible
  - methicillin resistant
  - *Haemophilus influenzae*
  - anaerobes
  - coagulase negative staphylococcus sepsis
- Gram-negative organisms
  - *Escherichia coli*
  - *Pseudomonas*
  - *Serratia*
- Other specified sepsis
  - *Enterococcus*

Shoulder Disorders

I-10 ALERT

There are several more specific ICD-10-CM codes available for shoulder lesions; the other classification axis that provides additional codes is that related to laterality. These codes specify that the condition is nontraumatic.

CDI ALERT

Ensure that laterality (right, left) is specified in the documentation for any of the musculoskeletal disorders that occur on paired body sites.

Code Axes

Adhesive capsulitis of shoulder	**M75.Ø**
Rotator cuff tear or rupture, not specified as traumatic	**M75.1**
Tendinitis (bicipital or calcific)	**M75.2, M75.3**
Impingement syndrome of shoulder	**M75.4**
Bursitis of shoulder	**M75.5**
Other and unspecified shoulder lesions	**M75.8, M75.9**

Description of Condition

Adhesive capsulitis of shoulder (M75.Ø-)

Clinical Tip

Adhesive capsulitis is a very common shoulder disorder and is caused by shoulder joint capsule inflammation. Symptoms include pain, stiffness, and loss of motion.

Key Terms

Key terms found in the documentation for adhesive capsulitis may include:

Frozen shoulder

Periarthritis of shoulder

Clinician Note

Ensure that all related conditions are coded appropriately.

Rotator cuff tear or rupture, not specified as traumatic (M75.1-)

Clinical Tip

Rotator cuff tears affect the shoulder tendons and most commonly involve the supraspinatus tendon. Many rotator cuff tears are chronic in nature and occur due to age degeneration. The tears can be classified as incomplete (partial thickness) or complete (full thickness), the latter involving through-and-through tears.

Key Terms

Key terms found in the documentation for rotator cuff tear may include:

Rotator cuff syndrome

Supraspinatus syndrome

Supraspinatus tear or rupture, not specified as traumatic

Clinical Findings

Physical Examination

History and review of systems may include:

- Shoulder pain-mild to severe
- Increased pain with abduction or flexion
- Decreased range of motion
- Shoulder weakness
- Palpation
- Neck
- Assessment of:
  - supraspinatus
  - infraspinatus
  - teres minor
  - subscapularis
- Neer test
- Hawkins test
- Apley scratch test

Diagnostic Procedures and Services

- Imaging
  - MRI
  - x-rays
  - ultrasound

Therapeutic Procedures and Services

- NSAID
- Strengthening exercises
- Surgery

Clinician Note

Ensure that all related conditions are coded appropriately and that if the tear is traumatic, category S46.Ø1- is referenced.

Tendinitis (bicipital or calcific) (M75.2-, M75.3-)

Clinical Tip

Calcific tendinitis is a condition that causes small 1 to 2 cm calcium deposits in the tendinous areas of the shoulder's rotator cuff. It may also be documented as calcified bursa of the shoulder. Bicipital tendinitis is an inflammation of the long head of biceps tendon, which can be due to instability of the tendon, bone spurs on the biceps tendon, or as a result of a previous injury.

Clinician Note
Ensure that all related conditions are coded appropriately and that if the tendinitis is due to a traumatic injury, that a code from the injuries chapter is referenced.

⇨ I-10 ALERT

ICD-10-CM includes a specific subcategory for impingement syndrome of the shoulder. This condition was previously classified to code 726.2 Other affections of shoulder region, NEC, in ICD-9-CM.

Impingement syndrome of shoulder (M75.4-)

Clinical Tip
When the tendons of the rotator cuff muscles become irritated and inflamed as they pass through the subacromial space, an impingement syndrome may result. There are many potential causes, including subacromial bone spurs, osteoarthritic spurs on the acromioclavicular (AC) joint, and variations in the shape of the acromion. Documentation may include information related to the three stages of impingement syndrome:

Stage I: Hemorrhage and edema are present, with palpable tenderness over the greater tuberosity at supraspinatus insertion

Stage II: Fibrosis and thickening of supraspinatus, biceps, and subacromial bursa due to chronic inflammation or repeated episodes of impingement

Stage III: Prolonged history of refractory tendinitis, significant tendon degeneration, and associated rotator cuff tears, biceps ruptures, and bone changes.

Key Terms
Key terms found in the documentation for shoulder impingement syndrome may include:

Painful arc syndrome

Supraspinatus syndrome

Swimmer's shoulder

Thrower's shoulder

Clinician Note
Ensure that all related conditions are coded appropriately and that if the impingement is due to a traumatic injury, that a code from the injuries chapter is referenced.

Bursitis of shoulder (M75.5-)

Clinical Tip
There are several bursae in the shoulder region: the subacromial, the subdeltoid, the subcoracoid, and the subscapular and their main function is to facilitate the gliding of soft tissue structures over bony surfaces. Any of the above bursae can become irritated, inflamed, and painful as a result of overuse of or trauma to the shoulder region, but the subacromial bursa is most commonly the culprit in this condition.

Clinician Note

Ensure that all related conditions are coded appropriately and that if bursitis is due to a traumatic injury, that a code from the injuries chapter is referenced.

Clinician Documentation Checklist

Clinician documentation should indicate the following:

- Type
  - due to use, overuse, pressure
  - gonococcal
  - infective
  - rheumatoid
  - syphilitic
  - other specified
    - adhesive
    - idiopathic
    - gouty
- Anatomic site

Skin Lesions — Removal of

Code Axes

Paring or cutting	**11055–11057**
Removal of skin tags	**11200–11201**
Shaving of epidermal or dermal lesions	**11300–11313**
Excision—benign lesions	**11400–11471**
Excision—malignant lesions	**11600–11646**

Description of Procedure

There are many methods that may be utilized to treat skin lesions and often the method employed is determined by the type of lesion being treated. There are a number of components that should be recorded in the documentation regardless of the methodology used:

- Anatomical location
- Preoperative diagnosis
- Postoperative diagnosis
- Size of the lesion
- Number of lesions
- Methodology used
- Type of closure is required
- Any complications

Paring or cutting of benign hyperkeratotic lesion (e.g., corn or callus) (11055–11057)

Documentation will indicate that the provider removed tissue by cutting away the edge or surface of the lesion. A hyperkeratotic lesion refers to an overgrowth of skin. The number of lesions treated should be clearly identified in the documentation. Each lesion should be described separately in terms of location and physical characteristics. Although not required for coding, it is advisable to also include the size of the lesion.

Key Terms

Key terms found in the documentation may include:

Cutting

Incision

Paring

Removal of skin tags, multiple fibrocutaneous tags, any area; up to and including 15 lesions (11200)

Removal of skin tags, multiple fibrocutaneous tags, any area; each additional ten lesions, or part thereof (List separately in addition to code for primary procedure) (11201)

Skin or fibrocutaneous tags are benign growths thought to be caused by friction and often are numerous when present. They may be removed by various methods including scissor excision, scalpel, ligature strangulation, and electrosurgical destruction.

Documentation should include the method used, the anatomical location, the size, and the number of lesions removed.

Key Terms

Key terms found in the documentation may include:

Cutting

Electrodessication

Sharp dissection

Skin tags

Shaving of epidermal or dermal lesion, single lesion, trunk, arms or legs (11300–11303)

Shaving of epidermal or dermal lesion, scalp, neck, hands, feet, genitalia (11305–11308)

Shaving of epidermal or dermal lesion, single lesion, face, ears, eyelids, nose, lips, mucous membrane (11310–11313)

Shaving is the sharp removal by transverse incision or horizontal slicing. It is different from excision in that it does not include a full thickness dermal excision and, therefore, does not require suture closure. If documentation notes that suturing is required, the lesion is not shaved but rather excised.

Examine the documentation to determine the site of the lesion as well as the size.

Key Terms

Key terms found in the documentation may include:

Cautery

Horizontal

Shaving

Excision, benign lesion including margins, except skin tag (unless listed elsewhere) trunk, arms or legs (11400–11406)

Excision, benign lesion including margins, except skin tag (unless listed elsewhere) scalp, neck, hand, feet, genitalia (11420–11426)

CPT ALERT

Simple closure when performed is included in the removal and should not be reported separately.

Excision, benign lesion including margins, except skin tag (unless listed elsewhere) face, ears, eyelids, nose, lips, mucous membrane (11440–11446)

Documentation supporting this code assignment will include a pathology report indicating that the lesion is benign, the size of the lesion, the size of the margin, and the anatomical site. Excision of lesions requires a full thickness, through the dermis incision, and may require a suture closure.

Excision, malignant lesion, including margins, trunk, arms or legs (11600–11606)

Excision, malignant lesion, including margins, scalp, neck, hands, feet, genitalia (11620–11626)

CPT ALERT

When a closure other than simple is required, it may be reported separately.

Excision, malignant lesion, including margins, face, ears, eyelids, nose, lips (11640–11646)

Documentation supporting this code assignment will include a pathology report indicating that the lesion is malignant, the size of the lesion, the size of the margin, and the anatomical site. Excision of lesions requires a full thickness, through the dermis incision, and may require a suture closure.

Clinician Documentation Checklist

Clinician documentation should indicate the following:

- Preoperative diagnosis
- Postoperative diagnosis
- Type of lesion
  - benign
  - malignant
  - skin tags
- Anatomical location
- Techniques
  - paring or cutting
  - chemical destruction
  - electrocauterization
  - electrosurgical destruction
  - ligature strangulation
  - removal with anesthesia

  - removal without anesthesia
  - sharp excision or scissoring
  - shaving
- Size of lesion
- Number of lesions
- Type of closure
- Complications

Spinal Disc Disorders (Dorsopathies)

Code Axes

Cervical disc disorders **M5Ø.[Ø-3,8,9]**

Includes subcategories for myelopathy, radiculopathy, disc displacement, disc degeneration, and other and unspecified disc disorders

Thoracic, thoracolumbar, and lumbosacral intervertebral disc disorders **M51.[Ø-4,8,9]**

Includes subcategories for myelopathy, radiculopathy, disc displacement, disc degeneration, Schmorl's nodes, and other and unspecified disc disorders

Spinal instabilities **M53.2X**

Includes subcategories for spinal regions

Radiculopathy **M54.1**

Includes subcategories for spinal regions

Sciatica **M54.3, M54.4**

Includes subcategories for laterality

Clinical Tip

The spinal regions may be defined as follows:

- Occipito-atlanto-axial region: C0-C1-C2
- Mid-cervical region: C4-C5-C6-C7
- Cervicothoracic region: C7-T1
- Thoracic region: T1-T12
- Thoracolumbar region: T9-L2
- Lumbar region: L1-L5
- Lumbosacral region: L1-L5 and S1-S5
- Sacral and sacrococcygeal region: S1-S5 and coccyx

I-10 ALERT

ICD-10-CM contains many more codes for spinal dorsopathies than did ICD-9-CM, and some of the classification axes are different. In some cases, all cervical conditions are together and then all thoracic conditions and then all lumbosacral conditions. Laterality is included, where appropriate, some combination codes are available as well.

CDI ALERT

Not only does the general site of the dorsopathy have to be documented, but the specific vertebral level as well. For example, instead of merely documenting "cervical disc displacement," the information should include one of the following specific areas: occipito-atlanto-axial region, mid-cervical region, cervicothoracic region. The definitions above may also be documented.

Description of Condition

Cervical disc disorders (M5Ø.-)

Includes subcategories for myelopathy, radiculopathy, disc displacement, disc degeneration, and other and unspecified disc disorders

Clinical Tip

The most common cervical disc disorders include the following:

Myelopathy: Most often found with spinal stenosis and involves pinching of the affecting vertebral segment of the spinal cord. It causes a compromise of coordination of the extremities.

I-10 ALERT

There are six different subcategories with various types of cervical disc disorders, each differentiated by the three different cervical regions.

Radiculopathy: When the pinched nerve of myelopathy progresses and involves pain, weakness, numbness, and a "pins and needles" sensation in the arm, it has progressed to radiculopathy.

Disc displacement: Displacement of a cervical intervertebral disc refers to protrusion or herniation of the disc between two adjacent bones (vertebrae) of the cervical spine. The protrusion or herniation may compress the spinal cord or other nerves, causing pain, and changes in sensory, motor, and reflex functions.

Disc degeneration: Refers to a breakdown of the normal architecture of the various components of the spine. The disc no longer provides adequate cushioning between the vertebrae and the bones then come closer and closer together, in some cases impinging on the spinal cord or other nerves.

Key Terms

Key terms found in the documentation for cervical disc disorders may include:

Cervical degenerative disc disease with radiculopathy

Cervical DJD with radiculopathy

Cervical DJD with myelopathy

Cervical myelopathy

Cervical radiculopathy

Cervicothoracic disc disorders with cervicalgia

Cervicothoracic disorders

Clinician Note

Review documentation to determine the site of the disc(s) affected as well as associated disorders such as myelopathy, radiculopathy, or displacement. Coding to the highest specificity may be necessary to get preauthorization for treatments such as physical therapy.

Thoracic, thoracolumbar, and lumbosacral intervertebral disc disorders (M51.-)

Includes subcategories for myelopathy, radiculopathy, disc displacement, disc degeneration, Schmorl's nodes, and other and unspecified disc disorders

Clinical Tip

The most common spinal disc disorders include the following:

Myelopathy: Most often found with spinal stenosis and involves pinching of the affecting vertebral segment of the spinal cord. It causes a compromise of coordination of the extremities.

Radiculopathy: When the pinched nerve of myelopathy progresses and involves pain, weakness, numbness, and a "pins and needles" sensation in the leg, it has progressed to radiculopathy.

Disc displacement: Displacement of a cervical intervertebral disc refers to protrusion or herniation of the disc between two adjacent bones (vertebrae) of the spine. The protrusion or herniation may compress the spinal cord or other nerves, causing pain, and changes in sensory, motor, and reflex functions.

Disc degeneration: Refers to a breakdown of the normal architecture of the various components of the spine. The disc no longer provides adequate cushioning between the vertebrae and the bones then come closer and closer together, in some cases impinging on the spinal cord or other nerves.

Key Terms

Key terms found in the documentation for thoracic, thoracolumbar, and lumbosacral disc disorders may include:

Lumbago due to displacement of intervertebral disc

Sciatica due to intervertebral disc disorder

Clinician Note

Review documentation to determine the site of the disc(s) affected as well as associated disorders such as myelopathy, radiculopathy, or displacement. Coding to the highest specificity may be necessary to get preauthorization for treatments such as physical therapy.

⇨ **I-10 Alert**

In the subcategory for spinal instabilities, there are nine codes, differentiated by spinal region, that represent various instability conditions.

Spinal instabilities (M53.2X-)

Clinical Tip

The term spinal instabilities refers to abnormal movement between one vertebra and another. Disc degeneration may cause loss of the tension or "turgor," which allows the disc to bulge and increases movements between the vertebrae. The loss of disc height causes displacement of the facet joints, which then override beyond their correct congruent alignment. In some cases, this abnormal slipping and overriding of the facet joints induces arthritic overgrowth of the joints and also produces bone spurs around the joint margins.

Clinician Note

Review documentation to determine the site of the disc(s) affected as well as associated disorders such as myelopathy, radiculopathy, or displacement. Coding to the highest specificity may be necessary to get preauthorization for treatments such as physical therapy.

Radiculopathy (M54.1-)

Clinical Tip

The term radiculopathy refers to an abnormally inflamed or pinched nerve, most often involving the nerve root near the spine. Although many radiculopathy conditions are due to an intervertebral disc disorder, some may be caused by other structures in the spinal column, or by an inadequate vascular supply. Most radiculopathy cases involve the cervical (affecting the arm) and lumbar (affecting the leg) spinal regions.

Key Terms

Key terms found in the documentation for radiculopathy may include:

Brachial neuritis or radiculitis

Lumbar neuritis or radiculitis

Lumbosacral neuritis or radiculitis

Radiculitis

Thoracic neuritis or radiculitis

Clinician Note

Review documentation to determine the site of the disc(s) affected as well as associated disorders such as myelopathy or displacement. Coding to the highest specificity may be necessary to get preauthorization for treatments such as physical therapy.

Sciatica (M54.3-, M54.4-)

Clinical Tip

Sciatica refers to a set of symptoms that may include pain, weakness, numbness, or tingling in the leg, referred from an impingement on the sciatic nerve in the lumbar spine. This nerve runs down the back of the leg and controls the muscles on the back of the knee and lower leg and also provides sensation for the back of the thigh, part of the lower leg, and the sole of the foot. It most often affects only one side.

Clinician Note

Ensure that all related conditions (e.g., disc disorders with myelopathy) are documented appropriately.

Clinician Documentation Checklist

Clinician documentation should indicate the following:

- Type
  - degeneration
  - displacement
  - pain
  - panniculitis
  - other specified
  - unspecified
- Severity
  - with myelopathy
  - with radiculopathy
- Anatomic sites
  - cervical
    - C4-C5
    - C5-C6
    - C6-C7

- cervicobrachial
- cervicocranial
- occipito-atlanto-axial
- thoracic
- thoracolumbar
- lumbosacral
- lumbar
- sacral
- sacrococcygeal
- multiple sites (specify sites involved)

Spinal Injection, Drainage, or Aspiration

Code Axes

Spinal puncture, lumbar, diagnostic	**62270**
Spinal puncture, therapeutic, for drainage of cerebrospinal fluid (by needle or catheter)	**62272**

Description of Procedure

Documentation indicating a diagnostic service will specify that a biopsy needle is inserted, fluid is drawn through the needle, and the sample is sent for testing. After the procedure is completed, the wound is dressed.

This is differentiated from a therapeutic service in that for the therapeutic service the L3 and L4 vertebrae are located and local anesthesia is administered. The lumbar puncture needle is inserted. In some cases, spinal fluid is drawn through the needle as in a lumbar puncture test. In other cases, a catheter is inserted and the fluid empties into a reservoir. Pressure reading is performed with a manometer. When the procedure is completed, the needle is removed and the wound is dressed.

Key Terms

Key terms found in the documentation may include:

Spinal tap

Injection(s) of diagnostic or therapeutic substance(s) (including anesthetic, antispasmodic, opioid, steroid, other solution), not including neurolytic substances, including needle or catheter placement, incudes contrast for localization when performed, epidural or subarachnoid (62310–62311)

Documentation will indicate that once the patient is placed in the appropriate position a needle is inserted into the vertebral interspace. Contrast media may be injected to confirm proper needle placement under fluoroscopy. Once location has been confirmed, a solution, other than a neurolytic agent is injected. Documentation may indicate that more than one substance, such as an anesthetic and a steroid, is injected. This procedure is commonly performed to manage chronic pain or to treat chronic spinal conditions.

Key Terms

Key terms found in the documentation may include:

Chronic pain

Epidural injection

Clinician Documentation Checklist

Clinician documentation should indicate the following:

- Medical condition being investigated or treated
  - diagnostic
  - therapeutic
- Anatomical
  - identification of vertebrae
- Anesthesia
- Fluid drawn
- Catheter inserted
- Pressure reading with manometer
- Contrast media used
- Fluoroscopy guidance
- Substance injected

Trigger Point Injections

Code Axes

Injection(s); single or multiple trigger point(s), 1-2 muscle(s)	**20552**
Injection(s); single or multiple trigger point(s), 3 or more muscle(s)	**20553**

Description of Procedure

Trigger points are focal, discrete spots of hypersensitive irritability identified within bands of muscle. These points cause local or referred pain. Trigger points may be formed by acute or repetitive trauma to the muscle tissue, which puts too much stress on the fibers.

These services are often performed for the following conditions:

- Cervicalgia
- Fasciitis
- Myalgia and myositis
- Muscle spasm
- Sciatica
- Tendinitis

Documentation will state that the physician identifies the trigger point injection site by palpation or radiographic imaging and marks the injection site. The needle is inserted and the medicine is injected into the trigger point. The injection may be done under separately reportable image guidance. After withdrawing the needle, the patient is monitored for reactions to the therapeutic agent. The injection procedure is repeated at the other trigger points for multiple sites.

CDI ALERT

Documentation should include details that support the medical necessity in addition to the number of muscles treated and therapies tried prior to this procedure

Key Terms

Trigger point

CDI ALERT

Supplies used when providing this procedure should be clearly documented and may be reported with the appropriate HCPCS Level II code. Check with the specific payer to determine coverage.

Clinician Documentation Checklist

Clinician documentation should indicate the following:

- The medical condition being treated
- Therapies prior to this procedure
- Site of injection
  - single
  - multiple
- Use of image guidance
- Therapeutic agents administered
- Number of muscles treated
- Patient reaction to therapeutic agent

Ulcer — Nonpressure

Code Axes

Non-pressure chronic ulcer of thigh	**L97.1**
Non-pressure chronic ulcer of calf	**L97.2**
Non-pressure chronic ulcer of ankle	**L97.3**
Non-pressure chronic ulcer of heel and midfoot	**L97.4**
Non-pressure chronic ulcer of other part of foot	**L97.5**
Non-pressure chronic ulcer of other part of lower leg	**L97.8**
Non-pressure chronic ulcer of unspecified part of lower leg	**L97.9**
Non-pressure chronic ulcer of skin, not elsewhere classified	**L98.4**
Non-pressure chronic ulcer of buttock	**L98.41**
Non-pressure chronic ulcer of back	**L98.42**
Non-pressure chronic ulcer of skin of other sites	**L98.49**

Description of Condition

Clinical Tip

Chronic skin ulcers initially affect superficial tissues and, depending on the state of the patient's health and other circumstances, may progress to affect muscle and bone. Patients at risk for development of skin ulcers include chronic, debilitating disease with impairment of sensation or impaired immune systems, and delayed healing after injury or trauma. Intrinsic loss of pain and pressure sensations due to nerve damage, poor circulation, and infection contribute to the formation and progression of chronic skin ulcers. In the early stages, with prompt, effective treatment, skin ulcers are reversible. If left untreated or inadequately treated, poorly-healing skin lesions can become extensively infected, necrotic, and ultimately, irreversible.

Key Terms

Key terms found in the documentation include:

Mal perforans ulcer

Nonhealing ulcer of skin

Noninfected sinus of skin

Trophic ulcer

Tropical ulcer

Clinician Note

Document the specific anatomic site and laterality. For multiple skin ulcers, document the specific ulcer depth of each ulcer site, whether a new or (old) healing ulcer.

⇨ I-10 Alert

ICD-10-CM classifies non-pressure skin ulcer by anatomic site, laterality and severity. Paired sites are classified as right, left, or of unspecified laterality.

For example, pressure ulcer of the left ankle with breakdown of skin is classified by site (ankle), by laterality (left), and severity as documented in the record:

L97.321 Non-pressure chronic ulcer of left ankle limited to breakdown of skin

Underlying conditions should be documented and reported first. Skin ulcers due to atherosclerosis (I7Ø.-), diabetes (EØ8.62, EØ9.62, E1Ø.62, E11.62-. E13.62-), varicose ulcers (I83.-) or other causal pathology should be linked appropriately in the documentation to support complete and accurate reporting.

Gangrene (I96.-) is classified separately. When documented with chronic skin ulcer, sequence I96 Gangrene, first to accurately represent severity of condition.

Unlike pressure ulcer (L89), which is reported by stage, chronic non-pressure ulcer of the skin (L97–L98) is reported by severity as documented in the record. For each anatomic site (and laterality), the hierarchy of disease progression is classified as follows in order of progression from mild to severe:

Chronic ulcer:

- Limited to breakdown of skin
- Fat layer exposed
- Necrosis of muscle
- Necrosis of bone

Document any complications with healing, overlapping sites or other changes in the status or nature of the ulcer.

Specify the ulcer depth accurately and thoroughly for each ulcer. For each anatomic site (and laterality), the hierarchy of disease progression is classified as follows in ICD-10-CM in order of progression from mild to severe:

Chronic skin ulcer:

- Limited to breakdown of skin
- Fat layer exposed
- Necrosis of muscle
- Necrosis of bone

Document any change in skin ulcer severity, depth, or healing status during an admission or encounter. For example, if a skin ulcer worsens during an admission, from an exposed fat layer to necrosis of muscle, note the depth progression accordingly.

CDI ALERT

Clinicians (i.e., physicians and other qualified health care practitioners) should document the severity and extent of ulcer as clearly and thoroughly as possible in the record, including any changes in ulcer status or complications associated with the healing process. Although the physician is responsible for documenting the associated diagnoses, nonprovider clinicians should document the depth of non-pressure ulcers and any changes in healing status for each ulcer, by anatomic site.

Clinician Documentation Checklist

Clinician documentation should indicate the following:

- Includes
  - chronic ulcer of skin of lower limb
  - nonhealing ulcer of skin
  - noninfected sinus of skin
  - trophic ulcer
  - tropical ulcer
  - ulcer of skin of lower limb
- Identification of
  - any associated underlying condition
    - atherosclerosis of lower extremities
    - chronic venous hypertension
    - diabetic ulcers
    - postphlebitic syndrome
    - postthrombotic syndrome
    - varicose ulcer
  - any associated gangrene
  - site
    - thigh
    - calf
    - ankle
    - heel and midfoot
      - plantar surface of midfoot
    - other parts of foot
      - toe

⇨ I-10 ALERT

Categories L97 and L98 include valid codes that are six characters in length. These codes include both the site and stage of the ulcer. The following axes of classification describe:

Fourth character:
- Anatomic site or region (skin NEC)

Fifth character:
- Anatomic site
- Anatomic site with laterality

Sixth character:
- Stage (severity, progression status) of ulcer

Do not report unspecified ulcer stage (sixth character 9) if the severity or progression of ulcer is documented in the medical record. Unspecified ulcer (sixth character 9) is only reported when there is **no documentation** regarding the stage, severity, or progression of skin ulcer.

        - other part of lower leg
        - unspecified part of lower leg
    - Laterality of thigh, calf, ankle, heel and midfoot, foot and leg
        - right
        - left
    - extent of nonpressure ulcer
        - limited to breakdown of skin
        - with fat layer exposed
        - with necrosis of muscle
        - with necrosis of bone
        - unspecified severity

Other Disorders of Skin and Subcutaneous Tissue

- Pyogenic granuloma
- Factitial dermatitis
    - neurotic excoriation
- Febrile neutrophilic dermatosis (sweet)
- Eosinophilic cellulitis (wells)
- Nonpressure chronic ulcer of skin
    - identify
        - site
            - buttock
            - back
            - skin of other sites
                - unspecified
        - extent of nonpressure ulcer
            - limited to breakdown of skin
            - with fat layer exposed
            - with necrosis of muscle
            - with necrosis of bone
            - with unspecified severity
- Mucinosis of skin
    - focal mucinosis
    - lichen myxedematosus
    - reticular erythematous mucinosis
- Other infiltrative disorders of skin and subcutaneous tissue
- Other specified disorders of skin and subcutaneous tissue
- Unspecified disorders of skin and subcutaneous tissue

Ulcer — Pressure

Code Axes

Pressure ulcer of elbow	L89.Ø
Pressure ulcer of back	L89.1
Pressure ulcer of hip	L89.2
Pressure ulcer of buttock	L89.3
Pressure ulcer of contiguous sites of back, buttock and hip	L89.4
Pressure ulcer of ankle	L89.5
Pressure ulcer of heel	L89.6
Pressure ulcer of other site	L89.8
Pressure ulcer of unspecified site	L89.9

Description of Condition

Clinical Tip

Pressure ulcers initially affect superficial tissues and, depending on the state of the patient's health and other circumstances, may progress to affect muscle and bone. Patients at risk for development of pressure ulcers include the bedridden, unconscious, or immobile such as stroke patients or those with paralysis and limited motion. Intrinsic loss of pain and pressure sensations, disuse atrophy, malnutrition, anemia, and infection contribute to the formation and progression of decubitus ulcers. In the early stages, the condition is reversible, but left untended, the decubitus ulcer can become extensively infected, necrotic, and ultimately, irreversible.

The National Pressure Ulcer Advisor Panel (NPUAP) has recently updated the definition and staging of pressure ulcers. A pressure ulcer is now defined as a "localized injury to the skin and/or underlying tissue, usually over a bony prominence, as a result of pressure, or pressure in combination with shear and/or friction."

Pressure ulcers are classified by location, shape, depth, and healing status. The depth of the lesion or stage of ulcer is the most important element in clinical measurement:

Unstageable/unspecified stage: lesion inaccessible for evaluation due to nonremovable dressings, eschar, sterile blister, and suspected deep injury in evolution. Deep tissue injury may be difficult to detect in individuals with dark skin tones and, as such, evolution of the wound may progress rapidly. Suspected deep tissue injury may be characterized by purple or maroon discoloration of the skin with or without blistering. Affected tissue may be painful and variant in temperature and texture from surrounding normal tissue.

⇨ I-10 Alert

ICD-10-CM classifies pressure ulcer by anatomic site, laterality, and stage. Paired sites are classified as right, left, or of unspecified laterality. Large areas, such as the back, are further divided into lower and upper regions.

For example, pressure ulcer of the back is divided first by main site (back), by laterality (unspecified, right or left), and subregion (upper, lower):

L89.121 Pressure ulcer of left upper back, stage 1

Category L89 excludes nonpressure ulcers (L97.-), diabetic ulcers (EØ8.62, EØ9.62, E1Ø.62, E11.62-. E13.62-), and varicose ulcers (I83.-). Code and report these conditions separately.

Gangrene (I96.-) is classified separately. When documented with pressure ulcer, sequence I96 Gangrene, first to accurately represent severity of condition.

CDI Alert

These classifications are differentiated by anatomic site, laterality, and severity (stage). Ensure documentation is specific regarding extent or progression of ulcer to avoid misrepresentation of severity.

Ensure documentation of site and laterality is thorough and specific to avoid reporting unspecified codes.

Code I96 should be reported and sequenced first to report gangrene documented with pressure ulcer. Gangrene is an additional severity indicator that poses significant risk for potentially fatal serious systemic infection (sepsis) requiring aggressive treatment.

Documentation should specify any underlying cause, pathology, chronic disease, or disability to explain the patient's immobile or bedridden status.

Stage 1 (I): Non-blanching erythema (a reddened area on the skin).

Stage 2 (II): Abrasion, blister, shallow open crater, or other partial thickness skin loss.

Stage 3 (III): Full thickness skin loss involving damage or necrosis into subcutaneous soft tissues.

Stage 4 (IV): Full thickness skin loss with necrosis of soft tissues through to the muscle, tendons, or tissues around underlying bone.

I-10 ALERT

Category L89 Pressure ulcer, includes valid combination codes that are five or six characters in length. These codes include both the site and stage of the ulcer. The following axes of classification describe:

Fourth character:
 Anatomic region

Fifth character:
 Anatomic site (specified to subregion or laterality)

Sixth character:
 Stage (severity, progression status) of ulcer

Do not confuse unstageable ulcer (sixth character 0) with unspecified ulcer stage (sixth character 9). Unstageable ulcer (sixth character 0) is reported when the stage, severity or progression of ulcer cannot be clinically determined. Unspecified ulcer (sixth character 9) is reported when there is **no documentation** regarding the stage, severity or progression of pressure ulcer.

Key Terms

Key terms found in the documentation include:

Bed sore

Decubitus ulcer

Plaster ulcer

Pressure area

Pressure sore

Clinician Note

Specify the ulcer stage accurately in the diagnosis. Document the specific anatomic site and laterality. For example, the back is separated into upper and lower, right and left quadrants. For paired anatomic sites, specify laterality (right or left).

For example:

L89.131 Pressure ulcer of the right lower back, stage 1

L89.141 Pressure ulcer of the left lower back, stage 1

Document contiguous, overlapping ulcer sites if present.

Document the appropriate clinical stage for "healing" ulcers that accurately reflects the stage of the ulcer during the healing process. For multiple pressure ulcers, document the specific pressure ulcer stage of each ulcer site, whether a new or (old) healing ulcer.

Document any change in pressure ulcer stage (severity or progression) during an admission or encounter. For example, if a pressure ulcer worsens during an admission, from a stage 2 ulcer to stage 3 ulcer, the coder should note the progression in severity accordingly.

CDI ALERT

Clinicians (physicians and other qualified health care practitioners) should document the pressure ulcer stage as clearly and thoroughly as possible in the record, including any changes in ulcer status or complications associated with the healing process. Although the physician is responsible for documenting the associated diagnoses, nonprovider clinicians should document the stage of ulcer, and any changes in healing status for each ulcer, by anatomic site.

Clinician Documentation Checklist

Clinician documentation should indicate the following:

- Includes
  - bed sore
  - decubitus ulcer
  - plaster ulcer
  - pressure area
  - pressure sore

- Identification of
  - pressure ulcer described as healing
  - any associated gangrene
  - site
    - elbow
    - back
      - upper
        - shoulder blade
      - lower
      - unspecified
    - sacral region
      - coccyx
      - tailbone
    - hip
    - buttock
    - contiguous site of back, buttock and hip
    - ankle
    - heel
    - other sites
      - head
        - face
      - other site
    - unspecified site
  - laterality of elbow, hip, buttock, back, ankle and heel
    - right
    - left
  - stage
    - stage 1: pressure pre-ulcer changes limited to persistent focal edema
    - stage 2: pressure ulcer with abrasion, blister, partial thickness skin loss involving epidermis and/or dermis
    - stage 3: pressure ulcer with full thickness skin loss involving damage or necrosis of subcutaneous tissues
    - stage 4: pressure ulcer with necrosis of soft tissues through to underlying muscle, tendon, or bone
    - unspecified stage
    - unstageable: pressure ulcers whose stage cannot be clinically determined
      - ulcer covered by eschar or treated with skin or muscle graft
      - pressure ulcers documented as deep tissue injury and not due to trauma

I-10 ALERT

Although ICD-9-CM codes for ulcerative colitis were differentiated by specific colonic site, they did not involve combination codes indicating the most commonly treated complications. ICD-10-CM codes are similar to Crohn's disease codes and represent those conditions that include rectal bleeding, intestinal obstruction, fistula, abscess, and other and unspecified complications.

Ulcerative Colitis

Code Axes

Note: Sixth characters for subcategories K51.Ø1, K51.21, K51.31, K51.41, K51.51, K51.81, and K51.91 are used to indicate any complications that may be present including rectal bleeding, intestinal obstruction, fistula, abscess, other, and unspecified complications.

Ulcerative (chronic) pancolitis without complications	**K51.ØØ**
Ulcerative (chronic) pancolitis with complications	**K51.Ø1**
Ulcerative (chronic) proctitis without complications	**K51.2Ø**
Ulcerative (chronic) proctitis with complications	**K51.21**
Ulcerative (chronic) rectosigmoiditis without complications	**K51.3Ø**
Ulcerative (chronic) rectosigmoiditis with complications	**K51.31**
Inflammatory polyps of colon without complications	**K51.4Ø**
Inflammatory polyps of colon with complications	**K51.41**
Left-sided colitis without complications	**K51.5Ø**
Left-sided colitis with complications	**K51.51**
Other ulcerative colitis without complications	**K51.8Ø**
Other ulcerative colitis with complications	**K51.81**
Ulcerative colitis, unspecified, without complications	**K51.9Ø**
Ulcerative colitis, unspecified, with complications	**K51.91**

Description of Condition

Clinical Tip

Differentiating ulcerative colitis from Crohn's disease involving the colon is important in these cases because treatment and complications vary significantly between them. Some of the components that help distinguish ulcerative colitis are as follows:

- Nearly always involves the rectum
- Common symptoms are bloody diarrhea, rectal urgency, and tenesmus
- Endoscopy reveals loss of the typical vascular pattern, friability, exudates, ulcerations, and granularity in a continuous, circumferential pattern
- Only the mucosal layer of the bowel is involved
- Fistulae and sinus tracks are rare (they are common in Crohn's disease)

Key Terms
Key terms found in the documentation may include:

Backwash ileitis
Distal ulcerative colitis
Left-sided ulcerative colitis
UC
Ulcerative pancolitis
Ulcerative proctitis
Ulcerative rectosigmoiditis

Clinician Note
Unlike ulcerative colitis, irritable bowel syndrome does not usually cause inflammation of the intestinal mucosa. A code indicating ulcerative colitis should be assigned only when there is documentation substantiating this condition.

CDI ALERT

Ensure that if any of the following complications are present they are clearly documented in the medical record: rectal bleeding, intestinal obstruction, fistula, or abscess. Any other complications that are indicated as being due to ulcerative colitis should also be documented.

Inflammatory polyps of colon without complications (K51.4Ø)

Inflammatory polyps of colon with complications (K51.41-)

Note: Sixth characters for subcategory K51.41 include that for rectal bleeding, intestinal obstruction, fistula, abscess, other and unspecified complications.

Clinical Tip
Inflammatory polyps may be referred to as "pseudopolyps" because in a sense, they are not true polyps, but are reactions to the chronic inflammation in the colon.

Clinician Note
The ICD-10-CM system differentiates between inflammatory and noninflammatory polyps. Documentation should be carefully reviewed to determine appropriate code assignment.

⇨ I-10 ALERT

The identification of the type of polyp is essential for accurate classification in ICD-10-CM. If a polyp is specified as adenomatous, category D12 in the benign neoplasms section of the neoplasms chapter should be reviewed. Polyps for which no specific identification is provided should be classified to code K63.5 Polyp of colon. Inflammatory polyps, which are typically found in inflammatory bowel diseases, are classified in the ulcerative colitis category (K51).

Review endoscopy and pathology reports to ascertain which type of polyp was found.

Left-sided colitis without complications (K51.5Ø)

Left-sided colitis with complications (K51.51-)

Note: Sixth characters for subcategory K51.51 include that for rectal bleeding, intestinal obstruction, fistula, abscess, other and unspecified complications.

Clinical Tip
The vast majority of cases of ulcerative colitis involve the rectum. From there, the inflammation extends up through the sigmoid and descending colon, which are located in the upper left part of the abdomen. When this is the extent of the disease process, it may be referred to as left-sided colitis or left hemicolitis.

Clinician Documentation Checklist

Clinician documentation should indicate the following:

- Identification of manifestation such as pyoderma gangrenosum:
- Type
  - ulcerative (chronic) pancolitis
    - backwash ileitis
  - ulcerative (chronic) proctitis
  - ulcerative (chronic) rectosigmoiditis
  - inflammatory polyps of colon
  - left-sided colitis
    - left hemicolitis
  - other ulcerative colitis
  - unspecified ulcerative colitis
- Associated
  - without complication
  - with complication
    - rectal bleeding
    - intestinal obstruction
    - fistula
    - abscess
    - other complication
    - unspecified complications

Wound Exploration

Code Axes

Wound exploration—trauma (e.g., penetrating gunshot, stab wound) **20100–20103**

Description of Procedure

Documentation will indicate that the physician explores a penetrating wound such as a gunshot, stab wound, or impaling by a foreign body in the operating room. Because code assignment is dependent upon anatomical location, it is critical that the documentation be carefully read to determine the exact site. Documentation will indicate that nerve, organ, and blood vessel integrity was assessed. Enlargement of the wound in order to make this assessment may be recorded.

During the procedure the physician may record that the wound was debrided, that foreign bodies were removed, and the ligation or coagulation of minor blood vessels in the subcutaneous tissues, fascia, and muscle were performed. The wound may be closed or packed open when contaminated by the penetrating body.

Key Terms

Key terms found in the documentation may include:

Assaulted

Gun shot

Knife wound

Stabbing

Clinician Documentation Checklist

Clinician documentation should indicate the following:

- Site(s) of wound(s)
  - neck
  - chest
  - abdomen/flank/back
  - extremity
- Procedures performed
  - debridement
  - expanded dissection of wound for exploration
  - extraction of foreign material
  - open examination
  - tying or coagulation of small vessels

Wound Repair

Code Axes

Repair—simple	**12001–12018**
Repair—intermediate	**12031–12057**
Repair—complex	**13100–13153**

Description of Procedure

Simple wound repair is defined as the closure of wounds involving the epidermis or dermis and may include the subcutaneous tissues without involvement of the deeper tissues. Simple wounds require one layer closure.

An intermediate repair is defined as a wound that requires layered closure of one or more of the deeper layers of subcutaneous tissues and nonmuscular fascia. A heavily contaminated wound that requires extensive cleaning but only single layer closure is also classified as an intermediate repair.

Complex repair is defined as one that requires more than a single layer closure, debridement, undermining, stents, or retention sutures. Documentation will indicate that the physician debrides the wound by removing foreign material or damaged tissue. Irrigation of the wound is performed and antimicrobial solutions are used to decontaminate and cleanse the wound. The physician may trim skin margins with a scalpel or scissors to allow for proper closure. The wound is closed in layers. The physician may perform scar revision, which creates a complex defect requiring repair. Stents or retention sutures may also be used in complex repair of a wound.

Documentation must include the anatomical location, size of wound, depth of wound, and any procedures such as debridement or decontamination when performed. Instrumentation such as the type of suture or glue that was used to accomplish the closure should also be noted.

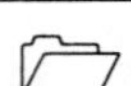

CPT Alert

Reconstructive procedures, such as utilization of local flaps, may be required and are reported separately when complex wound closure is performed.

Key Terms

Key terms found in the documentation may include:

Fascia

Multiple layers

Single layer

Subfascial

Clinician Documentation Checklist

Clinician documentation should indicate the following:

- Type of wound(s)
  - superficial
  - intermediate
  - complicated
- Site(s) of wound(s)
  - wound size
  - length of wound(s)
- Complications
  - dehiscence
- Anesthesia
- Debridement
- Decontamination
- Removal of foreign materials
- Ligation
- Materials
  - sutures
  - staples
  - tissue adhesives
  - stents

Section 4: Terminology Translator

To use the table below, find the term used in the medical record documentation in column one. Column two indicates the term(s) used in the ICD-10-CM system for that condition.

Medical Record Terminology	ICD-10-CM Terminology
Abscess of lung	Gangrene and necrosis of lung
Achalasia and cardiospasm	Achalasia of cardia
Acute coronary occlusion without MI	Acute coronary thrombosis not resulting in MI
Acute infective polyneuritis	Guillain-Barré syndrome
Acute pyelonephritis w/ or w/o lesion of medullary necrosis	Acute tubulo-interstitial nephritis
Acute respiratory failure following trauma and surgery	Postprocedural respiratory failure
Adenocarcinoma of intrahepatic bile duct	Intrahepatic bile duct carcinoma
After-cataract	Other secondary cataract
Allergic alveolitis and pneumonitis	Hypersensitivity pneumonitis (due to: cause)
Allergic rhinitis cause unspecified	Vasomotor rhinitis
Angina decubitus	Other forms of angina pectoris
Asbestosis	Pneumoconiosis due to asbestos and other mineral fibers
Asiderotic anemia	Anemia secondary to blood loss
Atrial flutter	Persistent/Atypical/Typical atrial flutter
Atrophic gastritis	Chronic superficial gastritis
Attacks without alteration of consciousness	Localization-related epilepsy
Autoimmune/Non-autoimmune hemolytic anemias	Drug-induced autoimmune hemolytic anemia
Avian Influenza virus (pneumonia, other resp infection)	Identified novel influenza A virus (with manifestation: pneumonia, other respiratory)
Backwash ileitis	Ulcerative colitis
Bacterial colitis	Bacterial intestinal infection, unspecified
Basilar migraine	Juvenile myoclonic epilepsy
Bed sore	Pressure ulcer
Benign childhood epilepsy with centrotemporal EEG spikes	Localization-related epilepsy
Biliary cirrhosis	Primary biliary cirrhosis Secondary biliary cirrhosis
Blood in stool	Melena
Bloodstream infection [although necessary to differentiate from bacteremia]	Septicemia due to (organism)
Bowen's disease	Carcinoma in situ site unspecified

Medical Record Terminology	ICD-10-CM Terminology
Brachial neuritis or radiculitis	Radiculopathy
Brittle diabetes	Type I diabetes mellitus
C. difficile colitis	Enterocolitis due to Clostridium difficile
Cancrum oris	Necrotizing ulcerative stomatitis
Cataracta brunescens	Age-related cataract
Cataracta complicate	Complicated cataract
Cerebrospinal fluid rhinorrhea	Cerebral spinal fluid leak
Cervical degenerative disc disease with radiculopathy	Cervical disc disorder
Cervical DJD with myelopathy	Cervical disc disorder
Cervical DJD with radiculopathy	Cervical disc disorder
Cervical myelopathy	Cervical disc disorder
Cervical radiculopathy	Cervical disc disorder
Cervical spondylosis with myelopathy	Vertebral artery compression syndromes
Cervicothoracic disc disorders with cervicalgia	Cervical disc disorder
Cervicothoracic disorders	Cervical disc disorder
Cheyne-Stokes respiration	Periodic breathing
Childhood epilepsy with occipital EEG paroxysms	Localization-related epilepsy
Chlorosis	Anemia secondary to blood loss
Cholangiocarcinoma	Liver cell carcinoma
Chronic airway obstruction, NEC	Chronic obstructive pulmonary disease
Chronic cold hemagglutinin disease	Other autoimmune hemolytic anemia
Chronic hypotension	Idiopathic hypotension
Chronic lymphadenitis	Chronic lymphadenitis, except mesenteric
Chronic nonalcoholic liver disease	Nonalcoholic steatohepatitis (NASH) Fatty liver, NEC
Classical migraine	Juvenile myoclonic epilepsy
Coccidiosis	Isosporiasis
Cold agglutinin disease	Other autoimmune hemolytic anemia
Cold agglutinin hemoglobinuria	Other autoimmune hemolytic anemia
Cold type (secondary) (symptomatic) hemolytic anemia	Other autoimmune hemolytic anemia
Collapsed vertebra NOS	Collapsed vertebra
Colloid carcinoma of breast	Malignant neoplasm of breast
Complications of surgical and medical care, not elsewhere classified	Complications of surgical and medical care, not elsewhere classified
Compression fracture	Collapsed vertebra
Condyloma acuminatum	Anogenital (venereal) warts
Congenital factor (VII/IX/XI) deficiency	Hereditary factor VII deficiency Hereditary factor IX deficiency Hereditary factor XI deficiency
Congestive heart failure, unspecified	Heart failure, unspecified

Medical Record Terminology	ICD-10-CM Terminology
Coronary atherosclerosis of (native) (bypass) (transplant) vessel	Atherosclerotic heart disease of (native) (bypass) (transplant) with or w/o angina (type)
Coronary cataract	Age-related cataract
Coronary slow flow syndrome	Angina
Cranial neuritis	Other neurologic disorders in Lyme disease
Cyst of thyroid	Nontoxic single thyroid nodule
Decubitus ulcer	Pressure ulcer
Defibrination syndrome	Disseminated intravascular coagulation
Degenerative cataract	Complicated cataract
Diabetes due to autoimmune process	Type I diabetes mellitus
Diabetes due to immune mediated pancreatic islet beta-cell destruction	Type I diabetes mellitus
Diabetes due to insulin secretory defect	Type II diabetes mellitus
Diabetes mellitus due to genetic defects in insulin action	Other specified diabetes
Diabetes mellitus due to genetic defects of beta-cell function	Other specified diabetes
Diabetes NOS	Type II diabetes mellitus
Diabetes w/o complication type I (juvenile) controlled	Type 1 diabetes mellitus without complications
Diabetes w/o complication type I (juvenile) uncontrolled	Type 1 diabetes with hyperglycemia
Diabetes w/o complication type II controlled	Type 2 diabetes mellitus without complications Other specified diabetes mellitus without complications
Diabetes w/o complications type II uncontrolled	Type 2 diabetes mellitus with hyperglycemia
Diffusely adherent E. coli	Escherichia coli, enteropathogenic
Ductal carcinoma in situ	Carcinoma in situ of breast
E. coli O157:H7	Enterohemorrhagic Escherichia coli infections
Empyema	Pyothorax (with or without: fistula)
Epilepsia partialis continua [Kozhevnikov]	Localization-related epilepsy
Epithelioid hemangioendothelioma	Other sarcomas of liver
Erythema chronicum migrans	Lyme disease
Erythroplasia	Carcinoma in situ site unspecified
External hemorrhoids without complication	Residual hemorrhoidal skin tags
External thrombosed hemorrhoids	Perianal venous thrombosis
Extracapillary glomerulonephritis	Recurrent and persistent hematuria
Familial migraine	Hemiplegic migraine
Fibrosarcoma	Other sarcomas of liver
Flatulence eructation and gas pain	Abdominal distension (gaseous)
Focal epilepsy	Intractable epilepsy

Medical Record Terminology	ICD-10-CM Terminology
Food poisoning (due to organism)	Foodborne (organism) intoxication
Foot and mouth disease	Other viral infections with skin and mucous membrane lesions
Frozen shoulder	Adhesive capsulitis
Glaucoma: Use additional code for stage	Glaucoma: [Diagnoses specify type/laterality] Stage included in seventh character
Glaucomatous flecks	Complicated cataract
Glaukomflecken	Complicated cataract
Glomerulonephritis – mesangial proliferative	Recurrent and persistent hematuria
Grade III intraepithelial neoplasia	Carcinoma in situ site unspecified
Granulomatous colitis	Crohn's disease
HCC	Intrahepatic bile duct carcinoma
Hemangioendothelioma	Angiosarcoma of liver
Hemoglobinuria due to hemolysis from external causes	Paroxysmal nocturnal hemoglobinuria
Hemophagocytic syndromes	Hemophagocytic lymphohistiocytosis
Hepatic angiosarcoma	Angiosarcoma of liver
Hepatitis (unspecified)	[Diagnosis includes type, causal factors and complications:] Toxic liver disease (specify complications) Nonspecific reactive hepatitis Peliosis hepatitis
Hepatocellular carcinoma	Liver cell carcinoma
Hepatoma	Intrahepatic bile duct carcinoma
Hereditary peripheral neuropathy	Hereditary motor and sensory neuropathy
Herpangina	Enteroviral vesicular pharyngitis
Hypermature cataract	Age-related cataract
Hyperpotassemia	
Hypertrophy of prostate	Enlarged prostate
Hypochromic anemia	Anemia secondary to blood loss
Hypochromic microcytic anemia	Anemia secondary to blood loss
Hypochromic or microcytic anemia	Anemia secondary to blood loss
Hypoferric anemia	Anemia secondary to blood loss
Hypoparathyroidism	Idiopathic hypoparathyroidism Other hypoparathyroidism Hypoparathyroidism, unspecified Postprocedural hypoparathyroidism
Hypopotassemia	Hyperkalemia
Iatrogenic thyroiditis	Drug-induced thyroiditis
Idiopathic diabetes	Type I diabetes mellitus
Idiopathic myocarditis	Isolated myocarditis
Idiopathic osteoporosis with current pathological fracture	Drug-induced osteoporosis
Immature cataract	Age-related cataract

Medical Record Terminology	ICD-10-CM Terminology
Immune complex hemolytic anemia	Other autoimmune hemolytic anemia
Immunohemolytic anemia	Other autoimmune hemolytic anemia
Incipient cataract	Age-related cataract
Inclusion conjunctivitis	Chlamydial conjunctivitis
Indolent cataract	Age-related cataract
Infiltrating lobular carcinoma of the breast	Malignant neoplasm of breast
Inflammatory breast cancer (IBC)	Malignant neoplasm of breast
Inflammatory cataract	Complicated cataract
Insulin resistant diabetes	Type II diabetes mellitus
Intermediate coronary syndrome	Angina
Intermediate coronary syndrome	Unstable angina
Intracholangiocarcinoma	Liver cell carcinoma
Invasive cribriform carcinoma of the breast	Malignant neoplasm of breast
Invasive ductal carcinoma (IDC) of breast	Malignant neoplasm of breast
Invasive lobular carcinoma of the breast	Malignant neoplasm of breast
Invasive papillary carcinoma of the breast	Malignant neoplasm of breast
Involutional osteoporosis with current pathological fracture	Age-related osteoporosis
Iodine hypothyroidism	Hypothyroidism due to meds and other exogenous substances
Ischemic chest pain	Angina
Janz syndrome	Juvenile myoclonic epilepsy
Juvenile onset diabetes	Type I diabetes mellitus
Kelly-Paterson syndrome	Anemia secondary to blood loss
Ketosis-prone diabetes	Type I diabetes mellitus
Kupffer cell sarcoma	Angiosarcoma of liver
Left bundle branch hemiblock	Left anterior fascicular block Left posterior fascicular block Other/unspecified fascicular block
Left heart failure	Left ventricular failure
Leiomyosarcoma	Other sarcomas of liver
Letterer-Siwe disease	Malignant mast cell tumor
Leukemic reticuloendotheliosis	Hairy cell leukemia
Leukocytopenia unspecified	Decreased white blood cell count, unspecified
Lobular carcinoma in situ (LCIS)	Carcinoma in situ of breast
Localization-related idiopathic epilepsy and epileptic syndromes with seizures of localized onset	Localization-related epilepsy
Lown-Ganong-Levine syndrome	Pre-excitation syndrome
Lumbago due to displacement of intervertebral disc	Lumbar disc disorder Lumbosacral disc disorder
Lumbar neuritis or radiculitis	Radiculopathy
Lumbosacral neuritis or radiculitis	Radiculopathy

Medical Record Terminology	ICD-10-CM Terminology
Lupus erythematosus (non-systemic)	Discoid lupus erythematosus Subacute cutaneous lupus erythematosus Other local lupus erythematosus
Lyme disease meningoencephalitis	Other neurologic disorders in Lyme disease
Lyme disease myopericarditis	Other conditions associated with Lyme disease
Lyme disease polyencephalitis	Other neurologic disorders in Lyme disease
Lymphosarcoma	Lymphoblastic lymphoma
Malignant fibrous histiocytoma	Other sarcomas of liver
Malignant hepatoma	Intrahepatic bile duct carcinoma
Malignant histiocytoma	Other sarcomas of liver
Malignant histiocytosis	Histiocytic sarcoma
Malignant neoplasm of other specified sites (of site)	Malignant neoplasm of overlapping sites (of site)
Malignant phyllodes tumors of the breast	Malignant neoplasm of breast
Marginal zone lymphoma	Other non-follicular lymphoma Extranodal marginal zone B-cell lymphoma of mucosa associated lymphatic tissue
Mechanical complication of esophagostomy	[Diagnoses specify type of complication:] Esophagostomy hemorrhage Esophagostomy malfunction
Medullary carcinoma of breast	Malignant neoplasm of breast
Membranous glomerulopathy	Recurrent and persistent hematuria
Membranous nephritis	Recurrent and persistent hematuria
Membranous nephropathy	Recurrent and persistent hematuria
Meningitis due to coxsackie virus/Echo virus	Enteroviral meningitis
Mesangial proliferative GN	Recurrent and persistent hematuria
Mucinous carcinoma of breast	Malignant neoplasm of breast
Necrosis of artery	Necrotizing vasculopathy
Neovascularization cataract	Complicated cataract
Nodular lymphoma	Follicular lymphoma (specify grade/site) Cutaneous follicle center lymphoma specify grade/site) Other/unspecified follicular lymphoma
Noise-induced hearing loss	Noise effects on (specify laterality) inner ear
Non-healing ulcer of skin	Chronic skin ulcer
Non-infected sinus of skin	Chronic skin ulcer
Nontransmural myocardial infarction	Non nontransmural myocardial infarction
Nuclear cataract, nonsenile	Infantile and juvenile nuclear cataract
Nuclear sclerosis	Age-related cataract
Nuclear sclerosis cataract	Age-related cataract
Occlusion and stenosis (cerebral/precerebral artery) w/Infarction	Cerebral infarction due to (thrombosis, embolism, occlusion)
Osteoporosis NOS with current pathological fracture	Age-related osteoporosis

Medical Record Terminology	ICD-10-CM Terminology
Osteoporosis of disuse with current pathological fracture	Drug-induced osteoporosis
Osteoporosis with current fragility fracture	Age-related osteoporosis
Osteoporotic fracture	Age-related osteoporosis
Paget's disease of the breast	Malignant neoplasm of breast
Paget's disease of the nipple	Malignant neoplasm of breast
Pain in or around eye	Ocular pain
Painful arc syndrome	Shoulder impingement syndrome
Painful respiration	Chest pain on breathing Pleurodynia
Paralysis agitans	Parkinson's disease Vascular parkinsonism
Paraplegia	Tropical spastic paraplegia Paraplegia unspecified Paraplegia, complete Paraplegia, incomplete
Paroxysmal supraventricular tachycardia	Supraventricular tachycardia Junctional premature depolarization
Paroxysmal ventricular tachycardia	Re-entry ventricular arrhythmia Ventricular tachycardia
Pars planitis	Posterior cyclitis (specify laterality)
Partial tear of rotator cuff	Incomplete rotator cuff tear/rupture of shoulder, nontraumatic (specify laterality)
Periarthritis of shoulder	Adhesive capsulitis
Pernicious anemia	Vitamin B12 deficiency anemia due to intrinsic factor deficiency
Pharmacoresistant (pharmacologically) resistant epilepsy	Intractable epilepsy
Plaster ulcer	Pressure ulcer
Pleurisy w/o effusion	Pyothorax without fistula Pleural plaque (w/ or w/o asbestos) Fibrothorax
Plummer-Vinson syndrome	Anemia secondary to blood loss
Pneumonia due to other virus	Human metapneumovirus pneumonia
Pneumonia in aspergillosis	Invasive pulmonary aspergillosis
Poorly controlled epilepsy	Intractable epilepsy
Post-traumatic osteoporosis with current pathological fracture	Drug-induced osteoporosis
Posthemorrhagic anemia (chronic)	Anemia secondary to blood loss
Postmenopausal osteoporosis with current pathological fracture	Age-related osteoporosis
Postmyocardial infarction syndrome	Dressler's syndrome
Postoophorectomy osteoporosis with current pathological fracture	Drug-induced osteoporosis
Postpancreatectomy diabetes mellitus	Other specified diabetes
Postprocedural diabetes mellitus	Other specified diabetes

Medical Record Terminology	ICD-10-CM Terminology
Postsurgical malabsorption osteoporosis with current pathological fracture	Drug-induced osteoporosis
Preinfarction syndrome	Angina
Pressure area	Pressure ulcer
Pressure sore	Pressure ulcer
Primary hepatic sarcoma	Other sarcomas of liver
Primary hypercoagulable state	Activated protein C resistance Prothrombin gene mutation Other primary thrombophilia Antiphospholipid syndrome Lupus anticoagulant syndrome
Primary liver carcinoma	Intrahepatic bile duct carcinoma
Primary liver cell carcinoma	Intrahepatic bile duct carcinoma
Prinzmetal angina	Angina pectoris with documented spasm
Progressive muscular atrophy	Amyotrophic lateral sclerosis
Pseudomembranous colitis (C. difficile)	Enterocolitis due to Clostridium difficile
Pseudopolyposis	Inflammatory polyps [Combination diagnoses specify assoc. complications:] Inflammatory polyps with rectal bleeding Inflammatory polyps with intestinal obstruction Inflammatory polyps of colon with fistula Inflammatory polyps with abscess
Pulmonary collapse	Atelectasis Other pulmonary collapse
Pulmonary congestion and hypostasis	Hypostatic pneumonia
Punctate cataract	Age-related cataract
Queyrat's erythroplasia	Carcinoma in situ site unspecified
Radiculitis	Radiculopathy
Red cell aplasia acquired adult with thymoma	Acquired pure red cell aplasia (specify as:) acute , chronic, transient
Reflex sympathetic dystrophy (site)	Complex regional pain syndrome (site)
Reflux esophagitis	Gastro-esophageal reflux disease with esophagitis
Refractory (medically) epilepsy	Intractable epilepsy
Regional enteritis	Crohn's disease
Reticulosarcoma	Diffuse large B-cell lymphoma
Retinal migraine	Juvenile myoclonic epilepsy
Right bundle branch block	Right fascicular block Other/unspecified right bundle branch block
Right bundle branch block and (right) (left) (anterior) (posterior) fascicular block	Bifascicular block
Roseola infantum due to human herpesvirus 6	Exanthema subitum [sixth disease] due to human herpesvirus 6
Rotator cuff syndrome	Rotator cuff tear

Medical Record Terminology	ICD-10-CM Terminology
Sciatica due to intervertebral disc disorder	Lumbar disc disorder Lumbosacral disc disorder
Secondary diabetes mellitus NEC	Other specified diabetes
Senile	Age-related
Senile cataract	Age-related cataract
Senile osteoporosis	Age-related osteoporosis w/o current pathological fracture
Senile osteoporosis with current pathological fracture	Age-related osteoporosis
Senility	Age-related cognitive decline
Senility without mention of psychosis	Age-related cognitive decline Age-related physical debility
Septic intoxication	Septicemia due to (organism)
Septic myocarditis	Infective myocarditis
Septic syndrome	Septicemia due to (organism)
Septicemia	Sepsis due to (organism)
Septicemia due to (organism)	Sepsis due to (organism)
Sideropenic dysphagia	Sideropenic dysphagia (iron deficiency anemia)
Simple partial seizures developing into secondarily generalized seizures	Localization-related epilepsy
Sinoatrial node dysfunction	Sick sinus syndrome
Sporadic migraine	Hemiplegic migraine
STEMI	ST elevation myocardial infarction
Stress fracture, spinal	Fatigue fracture of vertebra
Sub capsular flecks	Complicated cataract
Subsequent (refers to episode of care)	Subsequent (refers to consecutive AMIs)
Supraspinatus syndrome	Shoulder impingement syndrome
Supraspinatus syndrome	Rotator cuff tear
Supraspinatus tear or rupture, not specified as traumatic	Rotator cuff tear
Supraventricular premature beats	Atrial premature depolarization
Swimmer's shoulder	Shoulder impingement syndrome
Swyer-James-MacLeod syndrome	Unilateral pulmonary emphysema
Thoracic neuritis or radiculitis	Radiculopathy
Thrower's shoulder	Shoulder impingement syndrome
Tick born fever	Colorado fever
Toxemia	Septicemia due to (organism)
Toxic cataract	Drug-induced cataract
Tracheoesophageal fistula	Pyothorax with fistula
Transmural Q-wave infarction	ST elevation myocardial infarction
Traveler's diarrhea	Other intestinal Escherichia coli infections
Treatment resistant epilepsy	Intractable epilepsy
Trophic ulcer	Chronic skin ulcer

Medical Record Terminology	ICD-10-CM Terminology
Tropical ulcer	Chronic skin ulcer
Tubular carcinoma of breast	Malignant neoplasm of breast
Undifferentiated embryonal sarcoma of the liver	Other sarcomas of liver
Undifferentiated liver sarcoma	Other sarcomas of liver
Unilateral hyperlucent lung syndrome	Unilateral pulmonary emphysema
Unilateral pulmonary artery functional hypoplasia	Unilateral pulmonary emphysema
Unilateral transparency of lung	Unilateral pulmonary emphysema
Universal ulcerative colitis	Ulcerative pancolitis
Unspecified chronic pulmonary heart disease	Cor pulmonale (chronic)
Unspecified sudden hearing loss	Sudden idiopathic hearing loss
Urosepsis [antiquated term; necessary to differentiate from UTI]	Septicemia due to (organism)
Ventilation pneumonitis	Air conditioner and humidifier lung
Warm type (secondary) (symptomatic) hemolytic anemia	Other autoimmune hemolytic anemia
Water clefts	Age-related cataract
Wedging of vertebra NOS	Collapsed vertebra
Word deafness	Auditory processing disorder

Appendix 1: Physician Query Samples

The major purpose of queries is to obtain clarification when documentation in the health record impacts an externally reportable data element and is illegible, incomplete, unclear, inconsistent, or imprecise. As noted earlier in this manual, queries should not be leading by eliciting a specific response, introduce new information not documented elsewhere, be "yes/no" in format, or appear to question a provider's clinical judgment.

The query examples that follow here are intended to provide those actively working with physicians in clinical documentation improvement activities, to encourage accurate and appropriate documentation.

Pressure Ulcer Clarification

Dr. Walker:

You documented a diagnosis of sacral pressure ulcer for this patient, but did not specify the stage of pressure ulcer. A dressing change was performed on 7/5. The nurse noted "breakdown of skin with clean, circumscribed edges." Nursing documentation is unclear whether this indicates a partial (Stage II) or full (Stage III) thickness skin ulcer.

Can this patient's pressure ulcer be specified to The National Pressure Ulcer Advisor Panel (NPUAP) stage as:

- Unstageable/unspecified stage
- Stage I: non-blanching erythema (a reddened area on the skin).
- Stage II: abrasion, blister, shallow open crater, or other partial thickness skin loss.
- Stage III: full thickness skin loss involving damage or necrosis into subcutaneous soft tissues.
- Stage IV: full thickness skin loss with necrosis of soft tissues through to the muscle, tendons, or tissues around underlying bone.

Undetermined or Unknown: ______________________________

If so, please document the ulcer stage in the progress notes.

Signature______________________________

Date ______________________________

Thank you!

Cathy Coder

X 5437

Pneumonia Clarification

Dr. Miller:

This patient's final diagnosis is documented as "Pneumonia." Can the pneumonia be further specified to causal organism or type?

Pneumonia due to (Causal type/organism):______________________________

The following clinical indicators support this query for further information:

- The 7/5 Gram stain is positive for predominance of Gram negative rods.
- Your 7/5 progress note documents, "sputum culture invalid due to antibiotic therapy, patient unable to produce adequate sample."
- The patient was treated with third generation cephalosporin, which you link in your treatment plan to his immunocompromised status from steroid-dependent chronic obstructive asthma.

If so, please document the type/etiology of the pneumonia in the progress notes.

Undetermined or Unknown: ______________________________

Signature ______________________________

Date ______________________________

Thanks!

CDI Dan

Extension 435

Respiratory Diagnosis Clarification

Dr. Smith:

This patient's final diagnosis is documented as "respiratory distress." Your H&P indicates that the patient was admitted with COPD exacerbation and on admission she had 85 percent oxygen saturation on room air, respiratory rate of 28, and arterial blood gas (ABG) results were: pO_2 47, pCO_2 52, pH 7.34. Admission orders included oxygen and BiPAP.

Can your final diagnosis documentation of respiratory distress be further clarified?:

Acute respiratory failure: ______________________________

Acute on chronic respiratory failure: ______________________________

Acute respiratory insufficiency: ______________________________

Another cause of respiratory distress: ______________________________

Other: ______________________________

Unable to determine: ______________________________

Not Applicable: ______________________________

Signature______________________________

Date ______________________________

Thank you,

Elaine Record

X7676

Diagnosis Linkage Clarification

Dr. Jones:

The H&P for this patient indicates the presence of diabetes mellitus type 2 and peripheral vascular disease with gangrene.

If possible, can you please clarify whether or not these conditions are believed to be associated?

Please document any associated or unrelated status in the progress notes.

Unable to determine: ______________________________

Not Applicable: ______________________________

Signature ______________________________

Date ______________________________

Thank you,

Mary Med

X9043

Anemia Clarification

Dr. Davis:

This patient was admitted with a duodenal bleed per your admission note. At that time, her hemoglobin was 7.4gm/dl and her hematocrit was 22.6 percent . The H&P states "anemia." After admission, the patient was treated with two units packed red blood cells (PRBC).

Can your diagnosis of anemia be further specified to any of the following?:

Acute blood loss anemia: ________________________________

Chronic blood loss anemia: ________________________________

Other type of anemia: ________________________________

Unable to determine: ________________________________

Please document any clarification in the progress notes or on the discharge summary.

Signature________________________________

Date ________________________________

Thank you,

John Jay

X349

Intracerebral Bleeding Clarification

Dr. Santos:

In your progress note of October 31, you documented "subarachnoid hemorrhage." Can you please clarify the specific vessel involved?

Anterior Communicating Artery ____________________

Basilar Artery ____________________

Carotid Siphon & Bifurcation ____________________

Middle Cerebral Artery ____________________

Posterior Communicating Artery ____________________

Other Intracranial Artery ____________________

Vertebral Artery ____________________

Cannot determine ____________________

Also, please specify the underlying cause and laterality:

Traumatic ____________________

Non-traumatic ____________________

Cannot determine ____________________

Right Brain ____________________

Left Brain ____________________

Cannot determine ____________________

Please document this information in the progress notes.

Signature ____________________

Date ____________________

Thanks very much!

Tom Terry, CDI Specialist, 3 North Unit

X6676

Chest Pain Clarification

Dr. Ellis:

The admitting diagnosis in the progress notes for this patient indicates "unspecified chest pain."

Please review the following list of potential diagnoses and clarify the underlying cause, if known.

Note: for hospital admissions, the final diagnosis may be presumptive. Terms such as "probable," "likely," or "suspected" may be used.

Cardiac arrhythmia (please specify type, if known) ____________________

Coronary artery disease (specify with or w/o unstable angina) __________

Costochondritis ____________________

Gastroesophageal reflux ____________________

Pleuritic ____________________

Psychogenic causes ____________________

Stress and/or anxiety ____________________

Other cause ____________________

Chest pain, cause undetermined ____________________

Please document this information in the progress notes or discharge summary.

Thanks,

Hannah Hospital

X9989

Confirmation Request for Pathology Findings

ATTENTION: THIS FORM IS A PERMANENT PART OF THE MEDICAL RECORD

Dr. Green (attending physician):

This patient had surgery on ________ (date) and the corresponding pathology report indicated an abnormal finding of ______________.

Abnormal findings of this nature are not allowed as reportable conditions unless substantiated by an authorized provider, indicating their clinical significance.

Please specify below:

I concur with this finding/diagnosis ______________________________

I do not concur with this finding/diagnosis _________________________

I am unable to concur at this time (unable to determine)_______________

There is no clinical significance to this finding _______________________

Other diagnosis based on these findings___________________________

____

____

____

____

Attending signature ____

Date: ____

Appendix 2: ICD-10-CM Official Guidelines for Coding and Reporting 2017

Narrative changes appear in bold text

Items underlined have been moved within the guidelines since the FY 2016 version

***Italics* are used to indicate revisions to heading changes**

The Centers for Medicare and Medicaid Services (CMS) and the National Center for Health Statistics (NCHS), two departments within the U.S. Federal Government's Department of Health and Human Services (DHHS) provide the following guidelines for coding and reporting using the International Classification of Diseases, 10th Revision, Clinical Modification (ICD-10-CM). These guidelines should be used as a companion document to the official version of the ICD-10-CM as published on the NCHS website. The ICD-10-CM is a morbidity classification published by the United States for classifying diagnoses and reason for visits in all health care settings. The ICD-10-CM is based on the ICD-10, the statistical classification of disease published by the World Health Organization (WHO).

These guidelines have been approved by the four organizations that make up the Cooperating Parties for the ICD-10-CM: the American Hospital Association (AHA), the American Health Information Management Association (AHIMA), CMS, and NCHS.

These guidelines are a set of rules that have been developed to accompany and complement the official conventions and instructions provided within the ICD-10-CM itself. The instructions and conventions of the classification take precedence over guidelines. These guidelines are based on the coding and sequencing instructions in the Tabular List and Alphabetic Index of ICD-10-CM, but provide additional instruction. Adherence to these guidelines when assigning ICD-10-CM diagnosis codes is required under the Health Insurance Portability and Accountability Act (HIPAA). The diagnosis codes (Tabular List and Alphabetic Index) have been adopted under HIPAA for all healthcare settings. A joint effort between the healthcare provider and the coder is essential to achieve complete and accurate documentation, code assignment, and reporting of diagnoses and procedures. These guidelines have been developed to assist both the healthcare provider and the coder in identifying those diagnoses that are to be reported. The importance of consistent, complete documentation in the medical record cannot be overemphasized. Without such documentation accurate coding cannot be achieved. The entire record should be reviewed to determine the specific reason for the encounter and the conditions treated.

The term encounter is used for all settings, including hospital admissions. In the context of these guidelines, the term provider is used throughout the guidelines to mean physician or any qualified health care practitioner who is legally accountable for establishing the patient's diagnosis. Only this set of guidelines, approved by the Cooperating Parties, is official.

The guidelines are organized into sections. Section I includes the structure and conventions of the classification and general guidelines that apply to the entire classification, and chapter-specific guidelines that correspond to the chapters as they are arranged in the classification. Section II includes guidelines for selection of principal diagnosis for non-outpatient settings. Section III includes guidelines for reporting additional diagnoses in non-outpatient settings. Section IV is for outpatient coding and reporting. It is necessary to review all sections of the guidelines to fully understand all of the rules and instructions needed to code properly.

Section I. Conventions, general coding guidelines and chapter specific guidelines

The conventions, general guidelines and chapter-specific guidelines are applicable to all health care settings unless otherwise indicated. The conventions and instructions of the classification take precedence over guidelines.

A. Conventions for the ICD-10-CM

The conventions for the ICD-10-CM are the general rules for use of the classification independent of the guidelines. These conventions are incorporated within the Alphabetic Index and Tabular List of the ICD-10-CM as instructional notes.

1. The Alphabetic Index and Tabular List

The ICD-10-CM is divided into the Alphabetic Index, an alphabetical list of terms and their corresponding code, and the Tabular List, a structured list of codes divided into chapters based on body system or condition. The Alphabetic Index consists of the following parts: the Index of Diseases and Injury, the Index of External Causes of Injury, the Table of Neoplasms and the Table of Drugs and Chemicals.

See Section I.C2. General guidelines

See Section I.C.19. Adverse effects, poisoning, underdosing and toxic effects

2. Format and Structure:

The ICD-10-CM Tabular List contains categories, subcategories and codes. Characters for categories, subcategories and codes may be either a letter or a number. All categories are 3 characters. A three-character category that has no further subdivision is equivalent to a code. Subcategories are either 4 or 5 characters. Codes may be 3, 4, 5, 6 or 7 characters. That is, each level of subdivision after a category is a subcategory. The final level of subdivision is a code. Codes that have applicable 7th characters are still referred to as codes, not subcategories. A code that has an applicable 7th character is considered invalid without the 7th character.

The ICD-10-CM uses an indented format for ease in reference.

3. **Use of codes for reporting purposes**
For reporting purposes only codes are permissible, not categories or subcategories, and any applicable 7th character is required.

4. **Placeholder character**
The ICD-10-CM utilizes a placeholder character "X". The "X" is used as a placeholder at certain codes to allow for future expansion. An example of this is at the poisoning, adverse effect and underdosing codes, categories T36-T5Ø.

Where a placeholder exists, the X must be used in order for the code to be considered a valid code.

5. **7th Characters**
Certain ICD-10-CM categories have applicable 7th characters. The applicable 7th character is required for all codes within the category, or as the notes in the Tabular List instruct. The 7th character must always be the 7th character in the data field. If a code that requires a 7th character is not 6 characters, a placeholder X must be used to fill in the empty characters.

6. **Abbreviations**

a. **Alphabetic Index abbreviations**

NEC "Not elsewhere classifiable"
This abbreviation in the Alphabetic Index represents "other specified." When a specific code is not available for a condition, the Alphabetic Index directs the coder to the "other specified" code in the Tabular List.

NOS "Not otherwise specified"
This abbreviation is the equivalent of unspecified.

b. **Tabular List abbreviations**

NEC "Not elsewhere classifiable"
This abbreviation in the Tabular List represents "other specified". When a specific code is not available for a condition, the Tabular List includes an NEC entry under a code to identify the code as the "other specified" code.

NOS "Not otherwise specified"
This abbreviation is the equivalent of unspecified.

7. **Punctuation**

[ ] Brackets are used in the Tabular List to enclose synonyms, alternative wording or explanatory phrases. Brackets are used in the Alphabetic Index to identify manifestation codes.

( ) Parentheses are used in both the Alphabetic Index and Tabular List to enclose supplementary words that may be present or absent in the statement of a disease or procedure without affecting the code number to which it is assigned. The terms within the parentheses are referred to as nonessential modifiers. The nonessential modifiers in the Alphabetic Index to Diseases apply to subterms following a main term except when a nonessential modifier and a subentry are mutually exclusive, the subentry takes precedence. For example, in the ICD-1Ø-CM Alphabetic Index under the main term Enteritis, "acute" is a nonessential modifier and "chronic" is a subentry. In this case, the nonessential modifier "acute" does not apply to the subentry "chronic".

: Colons are used in the Tabular List after an incomplete term which needs one or more of the modifiers following the colon to make it assignable to a given category.

8. Use of "and".

See Section I.A.14. Use of the term "And"

9. Other and Unspecified codes

a. "Other" codes

Codes titled "other" or "other specified" are for use when the information in the medical record provides detail for which a specific code does not exist. Alphabetic Index entries with NEC in the line designate "other" codes in the Tabular List. These Alphabetic Index entries represent specific disease entities for which no specific code exists so the term is included within an "other" code.

b. "Unspecified" codes

Codes titled "unspecified" are for use when the information in the medical record is insufficient to assign a more specific code. For those categories for which an unspecified code is not provided, the "other specified" code may represent both other and unspecified.

See Section I.B.18 Use of Signs/Symptom/Unspecified Codes

10. Includes Notes

This note appears immediately under a three character code title to further define, or give examples of, the content of the category.

11. Inclusion terms

List of terms is included under some codes. These terms are the conditions for which that code is to be used. The terms may be synonyms of the code title, or, in the case of "other specified" codes, the terms are a list of the various conditions assigned to that code. The inclusion terms are not necessarily exhaustive. Additional terms found only in the Alphabetic Index may also be assigned to a code.

12. Excludes Notes

The ICD-10-CM has two types of excludes notes. Each type of note has a different definition for use but they are all similar in that they indicate that codes excluded from each other are independent of each other.

a. Excludes1

A type 1 Excludes note is a pure excludes note. It means "NOT CODED HERE!" An Excludes1 note indicates that the code excluded should never be used at the same time as the code above the Excludes1 note. An Excludes1 is used when two conditions cannot occur together, such as a congenital form versus an acquired form of the same condition.

An exception to the Excludes1 definition is the circumstance when the two conditions are unrelated to each other. If it is not clear whether the two conditions involving an Excludes1 note are related or not, query the provider. For example, code F45.8, Other somatoform disorders, has an Excludes1 note for "sleep related teeth grinding (G47.63)," because "teeth grinding" is an inclusion term under F45.8. Only one of these two codes should be assigned for teeth grinding. However psychogenic dysmenorrhea is also an inclusion term under F45.8, and a patient could have both this condition and sleep related teeth grinding. In this case, the two conditions are clearly unrelated to each other, and so it would be appropriate to report F45.8 and G47.63 together.

b. Excludes2

A type 2 Excludes note represents "Not included here." An excludes2 note indicates that the condition excluded is not part of the condition represented by the code, but a patient may have both conditions at the same time. When an Excludes2 note appears under a code, it is acceptable to use both the code and the excluded code together, when appropriate.

13. Etiology/manifestation convention ("code first", "use additional code" and "in diseases classified elsewhere" notes)

Certain conditions have both an underlying etiology and multiple body system manifestations due to the underlying etiology. For such conditions, the ICD-10-CM has a coding convention that requires the underlying condition be sequenced first, **if applicable,** followed by the manifestation. Wherever such a combination exists, there is a "use additional code" note at the etiology code, and a "code first" note at the manifestation code. These instructional notes indicate the proper sequencing order of the codes, etiology followed by manifestation.

In most cases the manifestation codes will have in the code title, "in diseases classified elsewhere." Codes with this title are a component of the etiology/ manifestation convention. The code title indicates that it is a manifestation code. "In diseases classified elsewhere" codes are never permitted to be used as first-listed or principal diagnosis codes. They must be used in conjunction with an underlying condition code and they must be listed following the underlying condition. See category F02, Dementia in other diseases classified elsewhere, for an example of this convention.

There are manifestation codes that do not have "in diseases classified elsewhere" in the title. For such codes, there is a "use additional code" note at the etiology code and a "code first" note at the manifestation code, and the rules for sequencing apply.

In addition to the notes in the Tabular List, these conditions also have a specific Alphabetic Index entry structure. In the Alphabetic Index both conditions are listed together with the etiology code first followed by the manifestation codes in brackets. The code in brackets is always to be sequenced second.

An example of the etiology/manifestation convention is dementia in Parkinson's disease. In the Alphabetic Index, code G20 is listed first, followed by code FØ2.8Ø or FØ2.81 in brackets. Code G20 represents the underlying etiology, Parkinson's disease, and must be sequenced first, whereas codes FØ2.8Ø and FØ2.81 represent the manifestation of dementia in diseases classified elsewhere, with or without behavioral disturbance.

"Code first" and "Use additional code" notes are also used as sequencing rules in the classification for certain codes that are not part of an etiology/ manifestation combination.

See Section I.B.7. Multiple coding for a single condition.

14. "And"

The word "and" should be interpreted to mean either "and" or "or" when it appears in a title.

For example, cases of "tuberculosis of bones", "tuberculosis of joints" and "tuberculosis of bones and joints" are classified to subcategory A18.Ø, Tuberculosis of bones and joints.

15. "With"

The word "with" should be interpreted to mean "associated with" or "due to" when it appears in a code title, the Alphabetic Index, or an instructional note in the Tabular List. **The classification presumes a causal relationship between the two conditions linked by these terms in the Alphabetic Index or Tabular List. These conditions should be coded as related even in the absence of provider documentation explicitly linking them, unless the documentation clearly states the conditions are unrelated. For conditions not specifically linked by these relational terms in the classification, provider documentation must link the conditions in order to code them as related.** The word "with" in the Alphabetic Index is sequenced immediately following the main term, not in alphabetical order.

16. "See" and "See Also"
The "see" instruction following a main term in the Alphabetic Index indicates that another term should be referenced. It is necessary to go to the main term referenced with the "see" note to locate the correct code.

A "see also" instruction following a main term in the Alphabetic Index instructs that there is another main term that may also be referenced that may provide additional Alphabetic Index entries that may be useful. It is not necessary to follow the "see also" note when the original main term provides the necessary code.

17. "Code also" note
A "code also" note instructs that two codes may be required to fully describe a condition, but this note does not provide sequencing direction.

18. Default codes
A code listed next to a main term in the ICD-10-CM Alphabetic Index is referred to as a default code. The default code represents that condition that is most commonly associated with the main term, or is the unspecified code for the condition. If a condition is documented in a medical record (for example, appendicitis) without any additional information, such as acute or chronic, the default code should be assigned.

19. Code assignment and Clinical Criteria
The assignment of a diagnosis code is based on the provider's diagnostic statement that the condition exists. The provider's statement that the patient has a particular condition is sufficient. Code assignment is not based on clinical criteria used by the provider to establish the diagnosis.

B. General Coding Guidelines

1. **Locating a code in the ICD-10-CM**
To select a code in the classification that corresponds to a diagnosis or reason for visit documented in a medical record, first locate the term in the Alphabetic Index, and then verify the code in the Tabular List. Read and be guided by instructional notations that appear in both the Alphabetic Index and the Tabular List.

It is essential to use both the Alphabetic Index and Tabular List when locating and assigning a code. The Alphabetic Index does not always provide the full code. Selection of the full code, including laterality and any applicable 7th character can only be done in the Tabular List. A dash (-) at the end of an Alphabetic Index entry indicates that additional characters are required. Even if a dash is not included at the Alphabetic Index entry, it is necessary to refer to the Tabular List to verify that no 7th character is required.

2. **Level of Detail in Coding**
Diagnosis codes are to be used and reported at their highest number of characters available.

ICD-10-CM diagnosis codes are composed of codes with 3, 4, 5, 6 or 7 characters. Codes with three characters are included in ICD-10-CM as the heading of a category of codes that may be further subdivided by the use of fourth and/or fifth characters and/or sixth characters, which provide greater detail.

A three-character code is to be used only if it is not further subdivided. A code is invalid if it has not been coded to the full number of characters required for that code, including the 7th character, if applicable.

3. **Code or codes from A00.0 through T88.9, Z00-Z99.8**
The appropriate code or codes from A00.0 through T88.9, Z00-Z99.8 must be used to identify diagnoses, symptoms, conditions, problems, complaints or other reason(s) for the encounter/visit.

4. Signs and symptoms

Codes that describe symptoms and signs, as opposed to diagnoses, are acceptable for reporting purposes when a related definitive diagnosis has not been established (confirmed) by the provider. Chapter 18 of ICD-10-CM, Symptoms, Signs, and Abnormal Clinical and Laboratory Findings, Not Elsewhere Classified (codes RØØ.Ø - R99) contains many, but not all, codes for symptoms.

See Section I.B.18 Use of Signs/Symptom/Unspecified Codes

5. Conditions that are an integral part of a disease process

Signs and symptoms that are associated routinely with a disease process should not be assigned as additional codes, unless otherwise instructed by the classification.

6. Conditions that are not an integral part of a disease process

Additional signs and symptoms that may not be associated routinely with a disease process should be coded when present.

7. Multiple coding for a single condition

In addition to the etiology/manifestation convention that requires two codes to fully describe a single condition that affects multiple body systems, there are other single conditions that also require more than one code. "Use additional code" notes are found in the Tabular List at codes that are not part of an etiology/manifestation pair where a secondary code is useful to fully describe a condition. The sequencing rule is the same as the etiology/manifestation pair, "use additional code" indicates that a secondary code should be added.

For example, for bacterial infections that are not included in chapter 1, a secondary code from category B95, Streptococcus, Staphylococcus, and Enterococcus, as the cause of diseases classified elsewhere, or B96, Other bacterial agents as the cause of diseases classified elsewhere, may be required to identify the bacterial organism causing the infection. A "use additional code" note will normally be found at the infectious disease code, indicating a need for the organism code to be added as a secondary code.

"Code first" notes are also under certain codes that are not specifically manifestation codes but may be due to an underlying cause. When there is a "code first" note and an underlying condition is present, the underlying condition should be sequenced first.

"Code, if applicable, any causal condition first" notes indicate that this code may be assigned as a principal diagnosis when the causal condition is unknown or not applicable. If a causal condition is known, then the code for that condition should be sequenced as the principal or first-listed diagnosis.

Multiple codes may be needed for sequela, complication codes and obstetric codes to more fully describe a condition. See the specific guidelines for these conditions for further instruction.

8. Acute and Chronic Conditions

If the same condition is described as both acute (subacute) and chronic, and separate subentries exist in the Alphabetic Index at the same indentation level, code both and sequence the acute (subacute) code first.

9. Combination Code

A combination code is a single code used to classify:
Two diagnoses, or
A diagnosis with an associated secondary process (manifestation)
A diagnosis with an associated complication

Combination codes are identified by referring to subterm entries in the Alphabetic Index and by reading the inclusion and exclusion notes in the Tabular List.

Assign only the combination code when that code fully identifies the diagnostic conditions involved or when the Alphabetic Index so directs. Multiple coding should not be used when the classification provides a combination code that clearly identifies all of the elements documented in the diagnosis. When the combination code lacks necessary specificity in describing the manifestation or complication, an additional code should be used as a secondary code.

10. Sequela (Late Effects)
A sequela is the residual effect (condition produced) after the acute phase of an illness or injury has terminated. There is no time limit on when a sequela code can be used. The residual may be apparent early, such as in cerebral infarction, or it may occur months or years later, such as that due to a previous injury. Examples of sequela include: scar formation resulting from a burn, deviated septum due to a nasal fracture, and infertility due to tubal occlusion from old tuberculosis. Coding of sequela generally requires two codes sequenced in the following order: the condition or nature of the sequela is sequenced first. The sequela code is sequenced second.

An exception to the above guidelines are those instances where the code for the sequela is followed by a manifestation code identified in the Tabular List and title, or the sequela code has been expanded (at the fourth, fifth or sixth character levels) to include the manifestation(s). The code for the acute phase of an illness or injury that led to the sequela is never used with a code for the late effect.

See Section I.C.9. Sequelae of cerebrovascular disease

See Section I.C.15. Sequelae of complication of pregnancy, childbirth and the puerperium

See Section I.C.19. Application of 7th characters for Chapter 19

11. Impending or Threatened Condition
Code any condition described at the time of discharge as "impending" or "threatened" as follows:

If it did occur, code as confirmed diagnosis.
If it did not occur, reference the Alphabetic Index to determine if the condition has a subentry term for "impending" or "threatened" and also reference main term entries for "Impending" and for "Threatened."
If the subterms are listed, assign the given code.
If the subterms are not listed, code the existing underlying condition(s) and not the condition described as impending or threatened.

12. Reporting Same Diagnosis Code More than Once
Each unique ICD-10-CM diagnosis code may be reported only once for an encounter. This applies to bilateral conditions when there are no distinct codes identifying laterality or two different conditions classified to the same ICD-10-CM diagnosis code.

13. Laterality
Some ICD-10-CM codes indicate laterality, specifying whether the condition occurs on the left, right or is bilateral. If no bilateral code is provided and the condition is bilateral, assign separate codes for both the left and right side. If the side is not identified in the medical record, assign the code for the unspecified side.

When a patient has a bilateral condition and each side is treated during separate encounters, assign the "bilateral" code (as the condition still exists on both sides), including for the encounter to treat the first side. For the second encounter for treatment after one side has previously been treated and the condition no longer exists on that side, assign the appropriate unilateral code for the side where the condition still exists (e.g., cataract surgery performed on each eye in separate encounters). The bilateral code would not be assigned for the subsequent encounter, as the patient no longer has the condition in the previously-treated site. If the treatment on the first side did not completely resolve the condition, then the bilateral code would still be appropriate.

14. Documentation for BMI, *Depth of* Non-pressure ulcers, Pressure Ulcer Stages, Coma Scale, *and NIH Stroke Scale*

For the Body Mass Index (BMI**),** depth of non-pressure chronic ulcers, pressure ulcer stage, **coma scale, and NIH stroke scale (NIHSS) codes**, code assignment may be based on medical record documentation from clinicians who are not the patient's provider (i.e., physician or other qualified healthcare practitioner legally accountable for establishing the patient's diagnosis), since this information is typically documented by other clinicians involved in the care of the patient (e.g., a dietitian often documents the BMI, a nurse often documents the pressure ulcer stages, **and an emergency medical technician often documents the coma scale**). However, the associated diagnosis (such as overweight, obesity, **acute stroke,** or pressure ulcer) must be documented by the patient's provider. If there is conflicting medical record documentation, either from the same clinician or different clinicians, the patient's attending provider should be queried for clarification.

The BMI, **coma scale, and NIHSS** codes should only be reported as secondary diagnoses.

15. Syndromes

Follow the Alphabetic Index guidance when coding syndromes. In the absence of Alphabetic Index guidance, assign codes for the documented manifestations of the syndrome. Additional codes for manifestations that are not an integral part of the disease process may also be assigned when the condition does not have a unique code.

16. Documentation of Complications of Care

Code assignment is based on the provider's documentation of the relationship between the condition and the care or procedure**, unless otherwise instructed by the classification**. The guideline extends to any complications of care, regardless of the chapter the code is located in. It is important to note that not all conditions that occur during or following medical care or surgery are classified as complications. There must be a cause-and-effect relationship between the care provided and the condition, and an indication in the documentation that it is a complication. Query the provider for clarification, if the complication is not clearly documented.

17. Borderline Diagnosis

If the provider documents a "borderline" diagnosis at the time of discharge, the diagnosis is coded as confirmed, unless the classification provides a specific entry (e.g., borderline diabetes). If a borderline condition has a specific index entry in ICD-10-CM, it should be coded as such. Since borderline conditions are not uncertain diagnoses, no distinction is made between the care setting (inpatient versus outpatient). Whenever the documentation is unclear regarding a borderline condition, coders are encouraged to query for clarification.

18. Use of Sign/Symptom/Unspecified Codes

Sign/symptom and "unspecified" codes have acceptable, even necessary, uses. While specific diagnosis codes should be reported when they are supported by the available medical record documentation and clinical knowledge of the patient's health condition, there are instances when signs/symptoms or unspecified codes are the best choices for accurately reflecting the healthcare encounter. Each healthcare encounter should be coded to the level of certainty known for that encounter.

If a definitive diagnosis has not been established by the end of the encounter, it is appropriate to report codes for sign(s) and/or symptom(s) in lieu of a definitive diagnosis. When sufficient clinical information isn't known or available about a particular health condition to assign a more specific code, it is acceptable to report the appropriate "unspecified" code (e.g., a diagnosis of pneumonia has been determined, but not the specific type). Unspecified codes should be reported when they are the codes that most accurately reflect what is known about the patient's condition at the time of that particular encounter. It would be inappropriate to select a specific code that is not supported by the medical record documentation or conduct medically unnecessary diagnostic testing in order to determine a more specific code.

C. Chapter-Specific Coding Guidelines

In addition to general coding guidelines, there are guidelines for specific diagnoses and/or conditions in the classification. Unless otherwise indicated, these guidelines apply to all health care settings. Please refer to Section II for guidelines on the selection of principal diagnosis.

1. Chapter 1: Certain Infectious and Parasitic Diseases (AØØ-B99)

a. Human Immunodeficiency Virus (HIV) Infections

1) Code only confirmed cases

Code only confirmed cases of HIV infection/illness. This is an exception to the hospital inpatient guideline Section II, H.

In this context, "confirmation" does not require documentation of positive serology or culture for HIV; the provider's diagnostic statement that the patient is HIV positive, or has an HIV-related illness is sufficient.

2) Selection and sequencing of HIV codes

(a) Patient admitted for HIV-related condition

If a patient is admitted for an HIV-related condition, the principal diagnosis should be B20, Human immunodeficiency virus [HIV] disease followed by additional diagnosis codes for all reported HIV-related conditions.

(b) Patient with HIV disease admitted for unrelated condition

If a patient with HIV disease is admitted for an unrelated condition (such as a traumatic injury), the code for the unrelated condition (e.g., the nature of injury code) should be the principal diagnosis. Other diagnoses would be B20 followed by additional diagnosis codes for all reported HIV-related conditions.

(c) Whether the patient is newly diagnosed

Whether the patient is newly diagnosed or has had previous admissions/encounters for HIV conditions is irrelevant to the sequencing decision.

(d) Asymptomatic human immunodeficiency virus

Z21, Asymptomatic human immunodeficiency virus [HIV] infection status, is to be applied when the patient without any documentation of symptoms is listed as being "HIV positive," "known HIV," "HIV test positive," or similar terminology. Do not use this code if the term "AIDS" is used or if the patient is treated for any HIV-related illness or is described as having any condition(s) resulting from his/her HIV positive status; use B20 in these cases.

(e) Patients with inconclusive HIV serology

Patients with inconclusive HIV serology, but no definitive diagnosis or manifestations of the illness, may be assigned code R75, Inconclusive laboratory evidence of human immunodeficiency virus [HIV].

(f) Previously diagnosed HIV-related illness

Patients with any known prior diagnosis of an HIV-related illness should be coded to B2Ø. Once a patient has developed an HIV-related illness, the patient should always be assigned code B2Ø on every subsequent admission/encounter. Patients previously diagnosed with any HIV illness (B20) should never be assigned to R75 or Z21, Asymptomatic human immunodeficiency virus [HIV] infection status.

(g) HIV Infection in Pregnancy, Childbirth and the Puerperium

During pregnancy, childbirth or the puerperium, a patient admitted (or presenting for a health care encounter) because of an HIV-related illness should receive a principal diagnosis code of O98.7-, Human immunodeficiency [HIV] disease complicating pregnancy, childbirth and the puerperium, followed by B2Ø and the code(s) for the HIV-related illness(es). Codes from Chapter 15 always take sequencing priority.

Patients with asymptomatic HIV infection status admitted (or presenting for a health care encounter) during pregnancy, childbirth, or the puerperium should receive codes of O98.7- and Z21.

(h) Encounters for testing for HIV

If a patient is being seen to determine his/her HIV status, use code Z11.4, Encounter for screening for human immunodeficiency virus [HIV]. Use additional codes for any associated high risk behavior.

If a patient with signs or symptoms is being seen for HIV testing, code the signs and symptoms. An additional counseling code Z71.7, Human immunodeficiency virus [HIV] counseling, may be used if counseling is provided during the encounter for the test.

When a patient returns to be informed of his/her HIV test results and the test result is negative, use code Z71.7, Human immunodeficiency virus [HIV] counseling.

If the results are positive, see previous guidelines and assign codes as appropriate.

b. Infectious agents as the cause of diseases classified to other chapters

Certain infections are classified in chapters other than Chapter 1 and no organism is identified as part of the infection code. In these instances, it is necessary to use an additional code from Chapter 1 to identify the organism. A code from category B95, Streptococcus, Staphylococcus, and Enterococcus as the cause of diseases classified to other chapters, B96, Other bacterial agents as the cause of diseases classified to other chapters, or B97, Viral agents as the cause of diseases classified to other chapters, is to be used as an additional code to identify the organism. An instructional note will be found at the infection code advising that an additional organism code is required.

c. Infections resistant to antibiotics

Many bacterial infections are resistant to current antibiotics. It is necessary to identify all infections documented as antibiotic resistant. Assign a code from category Z16, Resistance to antimicrobial drugs, following the infection code only if the infection code does not identify drug resistance.

d. Sepsis, Severe Sepsis, and Septic Shock

1) Coding of Sepsis and Severe Sepsis

(a) Sepsis

For a diagnosis of sepsis, assign the appropriate code for the underlying systemic infection. If the type of infection or causal organism is not further specified, assign code A41.9, Sepsis, unspecified organism.

A code from subcategory R65.2, Severe sepsis, should not be assigned unless severe sepsis or an associated acute organ dysfunction is documented.

(i) Negative or inconclusive blood cultures and sepsis

Negative or inconclusive blood cultures do not preclude a diagnosis of sepsis in patients with clinical evidence of the condition; however, the provider should be queried.

(ii) Urosepsis

The term urosepsis is a nonspecific term. It is not to be considered synonymous with sepsis. It has no default code in the Alphabetic

Index. Should a provider use this term, he/she must be queried for clarification.

(iii) Sepsis with organ dysfunction

If a patient has sepsis and associated acute organ dysfunction or multiple organ dysfunction (MOD), follow the instructions for coding severe sepsis.

(iv) Acute organ dysfunction that is not clearly associated with the sepsis

If a patient has sepsis and an acute organ dysfunction, but the medical record documentation indicates that the acute organ dysfunction is related to a medical condition other than the sepsis, do not assign a code from subcategory R65.2, Severe sepsis. An acute organ dysfunction must be associated with the sepsis in order to assign the severe sepsis code. If the documentation is not clear as to whether an acute organ dysfunction is related to the sepsis or another medical condition, query the provider.

(b) Severe sepsis

The coding of severe sepsis requires a minimum of 2 codes: first a code for the underlying systemic infection, followed by a code from subcategory R65.2, Severe sepsis. If the causal organism is not documented, assign code A41.9, Sepsis, unspecified organism, for the infection. Additional code(s) for the associated acute organ dysfunction are also required.

Due to the complex nature of severe sepsis, some cases may require querying the provider prior to assignment of the codes.

2) Septic shock

(a) Septic shock generally refers to circulatory failure associated with severe sepsis, and therefore, it represents a type of acute organ dysfunction.

For cases of septic shock, the code for the systemic infection should be sequenced first, followed by code R65.21, Severe sepsis with septic shock or code T81.12, Postprocedural septic shock. Any additional codes for the other acute organ dysfunctions should also be assigned. As noted in the sequencing instructions in the Tabular List, the code for septic shock cannot be assigned as a principal diagnosis.

3) Sequencing of severe sepsis

If severe sepsis is present on admission, and meets the definition of principal diagnosis, the underlying systemic infection should be assigned as principal diagnosis followed by the appropriate code from subcategory R65.2 as required by the sequencing rules in the Tabular List. A code from subcategory R65.2 can never be assigned as a principal diagnosis.

When severe sepsis develops during an encounter (it was not present on admission), the underlying systemic infection and the appropriate code from subcategory R65.2 should be assigned as secondary diagnoses.

Severe sepsis may be present on admission, but the diagnosis may not be confirmed until sometime after admission. If the documentation is not clear whether severe sepsis was present on admission, the provider should be queried.

4) Sepsis and severe sepsis with a localized infection

If the reason for admission is both sepsis or severe sepsis and a localized infection, such as pneumonia or cellulitis, a code(s) for the underlying systemic infection should be assigned first and the code for the localized infection should be assigned as a secondary diagnosis. If the patient has severe sepsis, a code from subcategory R65.2 should also be assigned as a secondary diagnosis. If the patient is admitted with a localized infection, such as pneumonia, and sepsis/severe sepsis doesn't develop until after admission, the localized infection should be assigned first, followed by the appropriate sepsis/severe sepsis codes.

5) Sepsis due to a postprocedural infection

(a) Documentation of causal relationship

As with all postprocedural complications, code assignment is based on the provider's documentation of the relationship between the infection and the procedure.

(b) Sepsis due to a postprocedural infection

For such cases, the postprocedural infection code, such as T80.2, Infections following infusion, transfusion, and therapeutic injection, T81.4, Infection following a procedure, T88.0, Infection following immunization, or O86.0, Infection of obstetric surgical wound, should be coded first, followed by the code for the specific infection. If the patient has severe sepsis, the appropriate code from subcategory R65.2 should also be assigned with the additional code(s) for any acute organ dysfunction.

(c) Postprocedural infection and postprocedural septic shock

In cases where a postprocedural infection has occurred and has resulted in severe sepsis the code for the precipitating complication such as code T81.4, Infection following a procedure, or O86.0, Infection of obstetrical surgical wound should be coded first followed by code R65.20, Severe sepsis without septic shock. A code for the systemic infection should also be assigned.

If a postprocedural infection has resulted in postprocedural septic shock, the code for the precipitating complication such as code T81.4, Infection following a procedure, or O86.0, Infection of obstetrical surgical wound should be coded first followed by code T81.12-, Postprocedural septic shock. A code for the systemic infection should also be assigned.

6) Sepsis and severe sepsis associated with a noninfectious process (condition)

In some cases a noninfectious process (condition), such as trauma, may lead to an infection which can result in sepsis or severe sepsis. If sepsis or severe sepsis is documented as associated with a noninfectious condition, such as a burn or serious injury, and this condition meets the definition for principal diagnosis, the code for the noninfectious condition should be sequenced first, followed by the code for the resulting infection. If severe sepsis is present, a code from subcategory

R65.2 should also be assigned with any associated organ dysfunction(s) codes. It is not necessary to assign a code from subcategory R65.1, Systemic inflammatory response syndrome (SIRS) of non-infectious origin, for these cases.

If the infection meets the definition of principal diagnosis, it should be sequenced before the non-infectious condition. When both the associated non-infectious condition and the infection meet the definition of principal diagnosis, either may be assigned as principal diagnosis.

Only one code from category R65, Symptoms and signs specifically associated with systemic inflammation and infection, should be assigned. Therefore, when a non-infectious condition leads to an infection resulting in severe sepsis, assign the appropriate code from subcategory R65.2, Severe sepsis. Do not additionally assign a code from subcategory R65.1, Systemic inflammatory response syndrome (SIRS) of non-infectious origin.

See Section I.C.18. SIRS due to non-infectious process

7) Sepsis and septic shock complicating abortion, pregnancy, childbirth, and the puerperium
See Section I.C.15. Sepsis and septic shock complicating abortion, pregnancy, childbirth and the puerperium

8) Newborn sepsis
See Section I.C.16. f. Bacterial sepsis of Newborn

e. Methicillin Resistant *Staphylococcus aureus* (MRSA) Conditions

1) Selection and sequencing of MRSA codes

(a) Combination codes for MRSA infection
When a patient is diagnosed with an infection that is due to methicillin resistant Staphylococcus aureus (MRSA), and that infection has a combination code that includes the causal organism (e.g., sepsis, pneumonia) assign the appropriate combination code for the condition (e.g., code A41.Ø2, Sepsis due to Methicillin resistant Staphylococcus aureus or code J15.212, Pneumonia due to Methicillin resistant Staphylococcus aureus). Do not assign code B95.62, Methicillin resistant Staphylococcus aureus infection as the cause of diseases classified elsewhere, as an additional code, because the combination code includes the type of infection and the MRSA organism. Do not assign a code from subcategory Z16.11, Resistance to penicillins, as an additional diagnosis.

See Section C.1. for instructions on coding and sequencing of sepsis and severe sepsis.

(b) Other codes for MRSA infection
When there is documentation of a current infection (e.g., wound infection, stitch abscess, urinary tract infection) due to MRSA, and that infection does not have a combination code that includes the causal organism, assign the appropriate code to identify the condition along with code B95.62, Methicillin resistant Staphylococcus aureus infection as the cause of diseases classified elsewhere for the MRSA infection. Do not assign a code from subcategory Z16.11, Resistance to penicillins.

(c) Methicillin susceptible Staphylococcus aureus (MSSA) and MRSA colonization
The condition or state of being colonized or carrying MSSA or MRSA is called colonization or carriage, while an individual person is described as being colonized or being a carrier. Colonization means that MSSA or MSRA is present on or in the body without necessarily causing illness. A positive MRSA colonization test might be documented by the provider as "MRSA screen positive" or "MRSA nasal swab positive".

Assign code Z22.322, Carrier or suspected carrier of Methicillin resistant Staphylococcus aureus, for patients documented as having MRSA colonization. Assign code Z22.321, Carrier or suspected carrier of Methicillin susceptible Staphylococcus aureus, for patient documented as having MSSA colonization. Colonization is not necessarily indicative of a disease process or as the cause of a specific condition the patient may have unless documented as such by the provider.

(d) MRSA colonization and infection
If a patient is documented as having both MRSA colonization and infection during a hospital admission, code Z22.322, Carrier or suspected carrier of Methicillin resistant Staphylococcus aureus, and a code for the MRSA infection may both be assigned.

f. Zika virus infections

1) Code only confirmed cases
Code only a confirmed diagnosis of Zika virus (A92.5, Zika virus disease) as documented by the provider. This is an exception to the hospital inpatient guideline Section II, H.

In this context, "confirmation" does not require documentation of the type of test performed; the physician's diagnostic statement that the condition is confirmed is sufficient. This code should be assigned regardless of the stated mode of transmission.

If the provider documents "suspected", "possible" or "probable" Zika, do not assign code A92.5. Assign a code(s) explaining the reason for encounter (such as fever, rash, or joint pain) or Z20.828, Contact with and (suspected) exposure to other viral communicable diseases.

2. Chapter 2: Neoplasms (C00-D49)
General guidelines

Chapter 2 of the ICD-10-CM contains the codes for most benign and all malignant neoplasms. Certain benign neoplasms, such as prostatic adenomas, may be found in the specific body system chapters. To properly code a neoplasm it is necessary to determine from the record if the neoplasm is benign, in-situ, malignant, or of uncertain histologic behavior. If malignant, any secondary (metastatic) sites should also be determined.

Primary malignant neoplasms overlapping site boundaries

A primary malignant neoplasm that overlaps two or more contiguous (next to each other) sites should be classified to the subcategory/code .8 ('overlapping lesion'), unless the combination is specifically indexed elsewhere. For multiple neoplasms of the same site that are not contiguous such as tumors in different quadrants of the same breast, codes for each site should be assigned.

Malignant neoplasm of ectopic tissue

Malignant neoplasms of ectopic tissue are to be coded to the site of origin mentioned, e.g., ectopic pancreatic malignant neoplasms involving the stomach are coded to pancreas, unspecified (C25.9).

The neoplasm table in the Alphabetic Index should be referenced first. However, if the histological term is documented, that term should be referenced first, rather than going immediately to the Neoplasm Table, in order to determine which column in the Neoplasm Table is appropriate. For example, if the documentation indicates "adenoma," refer to the term in the Alphabetic Index to review the entries under this term and the instructional note to "see also neoplasm, by site, benign." The table provides the proper code based on the type of neoplasm and the site. It is important to select the proper column in the table that corresponds to the type of neoplasm. The Tabular List should then be referenced to verify that the correct code has been selected from the table and that a more specific site code does not exist.

See Section I.C.21. Factors influencing health status and contact with health services, Status, for information regarding Z15.0, codes for genetic susceptibility to cancer.

a. Treatment directed at the malignancy
If the treatment is directed at the malignancy, designate the malignancy as the principal diagnosis.

The only exception to this guideline is if a patient admission/encounter is solely for the administration of chemotherapy, immunotherapy or radiation therapy, assign the appropriate Z51.-- code as the first-listed or principal diagnosis, and the diagnosis or problem for which the service is being performed as a secondary diagnosis.

b. Treatment of secondary site
When a patient is admitted because of a primary neoplasm with metastasis and treatment is directed toward the secondary site only, the secondary neoplasm is designated as the principal diagnosis even though the primary malignancy is still present.

c. Coding and sequencing of complications
Coding and sequencing of complications associated with the malignancies or with the therapy thereof are subject to the following guidelines:

1) Anemia associated with malignancy
When admission/encounter is for management of an anemia associated with the malignancy, and the treatment is only for anemia, the appropriate code for the malignancy is sequenced as the principal or first-listed diagnosis followed by the appropriate code for the anemia (such as code D63.0, Anemia in neoplastic disease**).**

2) Anemia associated with chemotherapy, immunotherapy and radiation therapy
When the admission/encounter is for management of an anemia associated with an adverse effect of the administration of chemotherapy or immunotherapy and the only treatment is for the anemia, the anemia code is sequenced first followed by the appropriate codes for the neoplasm and the adverse effect (T45.1X5, Adverse effect of antineoplastic and immunosuppressive drugs).

When the admission/encounter is for management of an anemia associated with an adverse effect of radiotherapy, the anemia code should be sequenced first, followed by the appropriate neoplasm code and code Y84.2, Radiological procedure and radiotherapy as the cause of abnormal reaction of the patient, or of later complication, without mention of misadventure at the time of the procedure.

3) Management of dehydration due to the malignancy
When the admission/encounter is for management of dehydration due to the malignancy and only the dehydration is being treated (intravenous rehydration), the dehydration is sequenced first, followed by the code(s) for the malignancy.

4) Treatment of a complication resulting from a surgical procedure
When the admission/encounter is for treatment of a complication resulting from a surgical procedure, designate the complication as the principal or first-listed diagnosis if treatment is directed at resolving the complication.

d. Primary malignancy previously excised
When a primary malignancy has been previously excised or eradicated from its site and there is no further treatment directed to that site and there is no evidence of any existing primary malignancy, a code from category Z85, Personal history of malignant neoplasm, should be used to indicate the former site of the malignancy. Any mention of extension, invasion, or metastasis to another site is coded as a secondary malignant neoplasm to that site. The secondary site may be the principal or first-listed with the Z85 code used as a secondary code.

e. Admissions/Encounters involving chemotherapy, immunotherapy and radiation therapy

1) Episode of care involves surgical removal of neoplasm
When an episode of care involves the surgical removal of a neoplasm, primary or secondary site, followed by adjunct chemotherapy or radiation treatment during the same episode of care, the code for the neoplasm should be assigned as principal or first-listed diagnosis**.**

2) Patient admission/encounter solely for administration of chemotherapy, immunotherapy and radiation therapy
If a patient admission/encounter is solely for the administration of chemotherapy, immunotherapy or radiation therapy assign code Z51.Ø, Encounter for antineoplastic radiation therapy, or Z51.11, Encounter for antineoplastic chemotherapy, or Z51.12, Encounter for antineoplastic immunotherapy as the first-listed or principal diagnosis. If a patient receives more than one of these therapies during the same admission more than one of these codes may be assigned, in any sequence.

The malignancy for which the therapy is being administered should be assigned as a secondary diagnosis.

3) Patient admitted for radiation therapy, chemotherapy or immunotherapy and develops complications
When a patient is admitted for the purpose of radiotherapy, immunotherapy or chemotherapy and develops complications such as uncontrolled nausea and vomiting or dehydration, the principal or first-listed diagnosis is Z51.Ø, Encounter for antineoplastic radiation therapy, or Z51.11, Encounter for antineoplastic chemotherapy, or Z51.12, Encounter for antineoplastic immunotherapy followed by any codes for the complications.

f. Admission/encounter to determine extent of malignancy
When the reason for admission/encounter is to determine the extent of the malignancy, or for a procedure such as paracentesis or thoracentesis, the primary malignancy or appropriate metastatic site is designated as the principal or first-listed diagnosis, even though chemotherapy or radiotherapy is administered.

g. Symptoms, signs, and abnormal findings listed in Chapter 18 associated with neoplasms
Symptoms, signs, and ill-defined conditions listed in Chapter 18 characteristic of, or associated with, an existing primary or secondary site malignancy cannot be used to replace the malignancy as principal or first-listed diagnosis, regardless of the number of admissions or encounters for treatment and care of the neoplasm.

See section I.C.21. Factors influencing health status and contact with health services, Encounter for prophylactic organ removal.

h. Admission/encounter for pain control/management
See Section I.C.6. for information on coding admission/encounter for pain control/management.

i. Malignancy in two or more noncontiguous sites
A patient may have more than one malignant tumor in the same organ. These tumors may represent different primaries or metastatic disease, depending on the site. Should the documentation be unclear, the provider should be queried as to the status of each tumor so that the correct codes can be assigned.

j. Disseminated malignant neoplasm, unspecified
Code C80.0, Disseminated malignant neoplasm, unspecified, is for use only in those cases where the patient has advanced metastatic disease and no known primary or secondary sites are specified. It should not be used in place of assigning codes for the primary site and all known secondary sites.

k. Malignant neoplasm without specification of site
Code C80.1, Malignant (primary) neoplasm, unspecified, equates to Cancer, unspecified. This code should only be used when no determination can be made as to the primary site of a malignancy. This code should rarely be used in the inpatient setting.

l. Sequencing of neoplasm codes

1) Encounter for treatment of primary malignancy
If the reason for the encounter is for treatment of a primary malignancy, assign the malignancy as the principal/first-listed diagnosis. The primary site is to be sequenced first, followed by any metastatic sites.

2) Encounter for treatment of secondary malignancy
When an encounter is for a primary malignancy with metastasis and treatment is directed toward the metastatic (secondary) site(s) only, the metastatic site(s) is designated as the principal/first-listed diagnosis. The primary malignancy is coded as an additional code.

3) Malignant neoplasm in a pregnant patient
When a pregnant woman has a malignant neoplasm, a code from subcategory O9A.1-, Malignant neoplasm complicating pregnancy, childbirth, and the puerperium, should be sequenced first, followed by the appropriate code from Chapter 2 to indicate the type of neoplasm.

4) Encounter for complication associated with a neoplasm
When an encounter is for management of a complication associated with a neoplasm, such as dehydration, and the treatment is only for the complication, the complication is coded first, followed by the appropriate code(s) for the neoplasm.

The exception to this guideline is anemia. When the admission/encounter is for management of an anemia associated with the malignancy, and the treatment is only for anemia, the appropriate code for the malignancy is sequenced as the principal or first-listed diagnosis followed by code D63.Ø, Anemia in neoplastic disease.

5) Complication from surgical procedure for treatment of a neoplasm
When an encounter is for treatment of a complication resulting from a surgical procedure performed for the treatment of the neoplasm, designate the complication as the principal/first-listed diagnosis. See guideline regarding the coding of a current malignancy versus personal history to determine if the code for the neoplasm should also be assigned.

6) Pathologic fracture due to a neoplasm
When an encounter is for a pathological fracture due to a neoplasm, and the focus of treatment is the fracture, a code from subcategory M84.5, Pathological fracture in neoplastic disease, should be sequenced first, followed by the code for the neoplasm.

If the focus of treatment is the neoplasm with an associated pathological fracture, the neoplasm code should be sequenced first, followed by a code from M84.5 for the pathological fracture.

m. Current malignancy versus personal history of malignancy
When a primary malignancy has been excised but further treatment, such as an additional surgery for the malignancy, radiation therapy or chemotherapy is directed to that site, the primary malignancy code should be used until treatment is completed.

When a primary malignancy has been previously excised or eradicated from its site, there is no further treatment (of the malignancy) directed to that site, and there is no evidence of any existing primary malignancy, a code from category Z85, Personal history of malignant neoplasm, should be used to indicate the former site of the malignancy.

See Section I.C.21. Factors influencing health status and contact with health services, History (of)

n. Leukemia, Multiple Myeloma, and Malignant Plasma Cell Neoplasms in remission versus personal history

The categories for leukemia, and category C9Ø, Multiple myeloma and malignant plasma cell neoplasms, have codes indicating whether or not the leukemia has achieved remission. There are also codes Z85.6, Personal history of leukemia, and Z85.79, Personal history of other malignant neoplasms of lymphoid, hematopoietic and related tissues. If the documentation is unclear as to whether the leukemia has achieved remission, the provider should be queried.

See Section I.C.21. Factors influencing health status and contact with health services, History (of)

o. Aftercare following surgery for neoplasm

See Section I.C.21. Factors influencing health status and contact with health services, Aftercare

p. Follow-up care for completed treatment of a malignancy

See Section I.C.21. Factors influencing health status and contact with health services, Follow-up

q. Prophylactic organ removal for prevention of malignancy

See Section I.C. 21, Factors influencing health status and contact with health services, Prophylactic organ removal

r. Malignant neoplasm associated with transplanted organ

A malignant neoplasm of a transplanted organ should be coded as a transplant complication. Assign first the appropriate code from category T86.-, Complications of transplanted organs and tissue, followed by code C8Ø.2, Malignant neoplasm associated with transplanted organ. Use an additional code for the specific malignancy.

3. Chapter 3: Disease of the blood and blood-forming organs and certain disorders involving the immune mechanism (D5Ø-D89)

Reserved for future guideline expansion

4. Chapter 4: Endocrine, Nutritional, and Metabolic Diseases (EØØ-E89)

a. Diabetes mellitus

The diabetes mellitus codes are combination codes that include the type of diabetes mellitus, the body system affected, and the complications affecting that body system. As many codes within a particular category as are necessary to describe all of the complications of the disease may be used. They should be sequenced based on the reason for a particular encounter. Assign as many codes from categories EØ8 – E13 as needed to identify all of the associated conditions that the patient has.

1) Type of diabetes

The age of a patient is not the sole determining factor, though most type 1 diabetics develop the condition before reaching puberty. For this reason type 1 diabetes mellitus is also referred to as juvenile diabetes.

2) Type of diabetes mellitus not documented

If the type of diabetes mellitus is not documented in the medical record the default is E11.-, Type 2 diabetes mellitus.

3) Diabetes mellitus and the use of insulin and oral hypoglycemics

If the documentation in a medical record does not indicate the type of diabetes but does indicate that the patient uses insulin, code E11, Type 2 diabetes mellitus, should be assigned. Code Z79.4, Long-term (current) use of insulin, **or Z79.84, Long term (current) use of oral hypoglycemic drugs**, should also be assigned to indicate that the patient uses insulin **or hypoglycemic drugs**. Code Z79.4 should not be assigned if insulin is given temporarily to bring a type 2 patient's blood sugar under control during an encounter.

4) Diabetes mellitus in pregnancy and gestational diabetes
See Section I.C.15. Diabetes mellitus in pregnancy.

See Section I.C.15. Gestational (pregnancy induced) diabetes

5) Complications due to insulin pump malfunction

(a) Underdose of insulin due to insulin pump failure
An underdose of insulin due to an insulin pump failure should be assigned to a code from subcategory T85.6, Mechanical complication of other specified internal and external prosthetic devices, implants and grafts, that specifies the type of pump malfunction, as the principal or first-listed code, followed by code T38.3X6-, Underdosing of insulin and oral hypoglycemic [antidiabetic] drugs. Additional codes for the type of diabetes mellitus and any associated complications due to the underdosing should also be assigned.

(b) Overdose of insulin due to insulin pump failure
The principal or first-listed code for an encounter due to an insulin pump malfunction resulting in an overdose of insulin, should also be T85.6-, Mechanical complication of other specified internal and external prosthetic devices, implants and grafts, followed by code T38.3X1-, Poisoning by insulin and oral hypoglycemic [antidiabetic] drugs, accidental (unintentional).

6) Secondary diabetes mellitus
Codes under categories EØ8, Diabetes mellitus due to underlying condition, EØ9, Drug or chemical induced diabetes mellitus, and E13, Other specified diabetes mellitus, identify complications/manifestations associated with secondary diabetes mellitus. Secondary diabetes is always caused by another condition or event (e.g., cystic fibrosis, malignant neoplasm of pancreas, pancreatectomy, adverse effect of drug, or poisoning).

(a) Secondary diabetes mellitus and the use of insulin or hypoglycemic drugs
For patients who routinely use insulin **or hypoglycemic drugs**, *code Z79.4, Long-term (current) use of insulin,* **or Z79.84, Long term (current) use of oral hypoglycemic drugs** *should also be assigned. Code Z79.4 should not be assigned if insulin is given temporarily to bring a patient's blood sugar under control during an encounter.*

(b) Assigning and sequencing secondary diabetes codes and its causes
The sequencing of the secondary diabetes codes in relationship to codes for the cause of the diabetes is based on the Tabular List instructions for categories EØ8, EØ9 and E13.

(i) Secondary diabetes mellitus due to pancreatectomy
For postpancreatectomy diabetes mellitus (lack of insulin due to the surgical removal of all or part of the pancreas), assign code E89.1, Postprocedural hypoinsulinemia. Assign a code from

category E13 and a code from subcategory Z90.41-, Acquired absence of pancreas, as additional codes.

(ii) Secondary diabetes due to drugs

Secondary diabetes may be caused by an adverse effect of correctly administered medications, poisoning or sequela of poisoning.

See section I.C.19.e for coding of adverse effects and poisoning, and section I.C.20 for external cause code reporting.

5. Chapter 5: Mental, Behavioral and Neurodevelopmental disorders (F01 – F99)

a. Pain disorders related to psychological factors

Assign code F45.41, for pain that is exclusively related to psychological disorders. As indicated by the Excludes 1 note under category G89, a code from category G89 should not be assigned with code F45.41.

Code F45.42, Pain disorders with related psychological factors, should be used with a code from category G89, Pain, not elsewhere classified, if there is documentation of a psychological component for a patient with acute or chronic pain.

See Section I.C.6. Pain

b. Mental and behavioral disorders due to psychoactive substance use

1) In Remission

Selection of codes for "in remission" for categories F10-F19, Mental and behavioral disorders due to psychoactive substance use (categories F10-F19 with -.21) requires the provider's clinical judgment. The appropriate codes for "in remission" are assigned only on the basis of provider documentation (as defined in the Official Guidelines for Coding and Reporting).

2) Psychoactive Substance Use, Abuse And Dependence

When the provider documentation refers to use, abuse and dependence of the same substance (e.g. alcohol, opioid, cannabis, etc.), only one code should be assigned to identify the pattern of use based on the following hierarchy:

- If both use and abuse are documented, assign only the code for abuse
- If both abuse and dependence are documented, assign only the code for dependence
- If use, abuse and dependence are all documented, assign only the code for dependence
- If both use and dependence are documented, assign only the code for dependence.

3) Psychoactive Substance Use

As with all other diagnoses, the codes for psychoactive substance use (F10.9-, F11.9-, F12.9-, F13.9-, F14.9-, F15.9-, F16.9-) should only be assigned based on provider documentation and when they meet the definition of a reportable diagnosis (see Section III, Reporting Additional Diagnoses). The codes are to be used only when the psychoactive substance use is associated with a mental or behavioral disorder, and such a relationship is documented by the provider.

6. Chapter 6: Diseases of the Nervous System (G00-G99)

a. Dominant/nondominant side

Codes from category G81, Hemiplegia and hemiparesis, and subcategories G83.1, Monoplegia of lower limb, G83.2, Monoplegia of upper limb, and G83.3, Monoplegia, unspecified, identify whether the dominant or nondominant side is affected. Should the affected side be documented, but not specified as dominant or nondominant, and the classification system does not indicate a default, code selection is as follows:

- For ambidextrous patients, the default should be dominant.
- If the left side is affected, the default is non-dominant.
- If the right side is affected, the default is dominant.

b. Pain - Category G89

1) General coding information

Codes in category G89, Pain, not elsewhere classified, may be used in conjunction with codes from other categories and chapters to provide more detail about acute or chronic pain and neoplasm-related pain, unless otherwise indicated below.

If the pain is not specified as acute or chronic, post-thoracotomy, postprocedural, or neoplasm-related, do not assign codes from category G89.

A code from category G89 should not be assigned if the underlying (definitive) diagnosis is known, unless the reason for the encounter is pain control/ management and not management of the underlying condition.

When an admission or encounter is for a procedure aimed at treating the underlying condition (e.g., spinal fusion, kyphoplasty), a code for the underlying condition (e.g., vertebral fracture, spinal stenosis) should be assigned as the principal diagnosis. No code from category G89 should be assigned.

(a) Category G89 Codes as Principal or First-Listed Diagnosis

Category G89 codes are acceptable as principal diagnosis or the first-listed code:

- When pain control or pain management is the reason for the admission/encounter (e.g., a patient with displaced intervertebral disc, nerve impingement and severe back pain presents for injection of steroid into the spinal canal). The underlying cause of the pain should be reported as an additional diagnosis, if known.
- When a patient is admitted for the insertion of a neurostimulator for pain control, assign the appropriate pain code as the principal or first-listed diagnosis. When an admission or encounter is for a procedure aimed at treating the underlying condition and a neurostimulator is inserted for pain control during the same admission/encounter, a code for the underlying condition should be assigned as the principal diagnosis and the appropriate pain code should be assigned as a secondary diagnosis.

(b) Use of Category G89 Codes in Conjunction with Site Specific Pain Codes

(i) Assigning Category G89 and Site-Specific Pain Codes

Codes from category G89 may be used in conjunction with codes that identify the site of pain (including codes from chapter 18) if the category G89 code provides additional information. For example, if the code describes the site of the pain, but does not fully describe whether the pain is acute or chronic, then both codes should be assigned.

(ii) Sequencing of Category G89 Codes with Site-Specific Pain Codes

The sequencing of category G89 codes with site-specific pain codes (including chapter 18 codes), is dependent on the circumstances of the encounter/admission as follows:

- If the encounter is for pain control or pain management, assign the code from category G89 followed by the code identifying the specific site of pain (e.g., encounter for pain management for acute neck pain from trauma is assigned code G89.11, Acute pain due to trauma, followed by code M54.2, Cervicalgia, to identify the site of pain).

- If the encounter is for any other reason except pain control or pain management, and a related definitive diagnosis has not been established (confirmed) by the provider, assign the code for the specific site of pain first, followed by the appropriate code from category G89.

2) Pain due to devices, implants and grafts

See Section I.C.19. Pain due to medical devices

3) Postoperative Pain

The provider's documentation should be used to guide the coding of postoperative pain, as well as *Section III. Reporting Additional Diagnoses* and *Section IV. Diagnostic Coding and Reporting in the Outpatient Setting.*

The default for post-thoracotomy and other postoperative pain not specified as acute or chronic is the code for the acute form.

Routine or expected postoperative pain immediately after surgery should not be coded.

(a) Postoperative pain not associated with specific postoperative complication

Postoperative pain not associated with a specific postoperative complication is assigned to the appropriate postoperative pain code in category G89.

(b) Postoperative pain associated with specific postoperative complication

Postoperative pain associated with a specific postoperative complication (such as painful wire sutures) is assigned to the appropriate code(s) found in Chapter 19, Injury, poisoning, and certain other consequences of external causes. If appropriate, use additional code(s) from category G89 to identify acute or chronic pain (G89.18 or G89.28).

4) Chronic pain

Chronic pain is classified to subcategory G89.2. There is no time frame defining when pain becomes chronic pain. The provider's documentation should be used to guide use of these codes.

5) Neoplasm Related Pain

Code G89.3 is assigned to pain documented as being related, associated or due to cancer, primary or secondary malignancy, or tumor. This code is assigned regardless of whether the pain is acute or chronic.

This code may be assigned as the principal or first-listed code when the stated reason for the admission/encounter is documented as pain control/pain management. The underlying neoplasm should be reported as an additional diagnosis.

When the reason for the admission/encounter is management of the neoplasm and the pain associated with the neoplasm is also documented, code G89.3 may be assigned as an additional diagnosis. It is not necessary to assign an additional code for the site of the pain.

See Section I.C.2 for instructions on the sequencing of neoplasms for all other stated reasons for the admission/encounter (except for pain control/pain management).

6) Chronic pain syndrome

Central pain syndrome (G89.Ø) and chronic pain syndrome (G89.4) are different than the term "chronic pain," and therefore codes should only be used when the provider has specifically documented this condition.

See Section I.C.5. Pain disorders related to psychological factors

7. Chapter 7: Diseases of the Eye and Adnexa (HØØ-H59)

a. Glaucoma

1) Assigning Glaucoma Codes
Assign as many codes from category H4Ø, Glaucoma, as needed to identify the type of glaucoma, the affected eye, and the glaucoma stage.

2) Bilateral glaucoma with same type and stage
When a patient has bilateral glaucoma and both eyes are documented as being the same type and stage, and there is a code for bilateral glaucoma, report only the code for the type of glaucoma, bilateral, with the seventh character for the stage.

When a patient has bilateral glaucoma and both eyes are documented as being the same type and stage, and the classification does not provide a code for bilateral glaucoma (i.e. subcategories H4Ø.1Ø, H4Ø.11 and H4Ø.2Ø) report only one code for the type of glaucoma with the appropriate seventh character for the stage.

3) Bilateral glaucoma stage with different types or stages
When a patient has bilateral glaucoma and each eye is documented as having a different type or stage, and the classification distinguishes laterality, assign the appropriate code for each eye rather than the code for bilateral glaucoma.

When a patient has bilateral glaucoma and each eye is documented as having a different type, and the classification does not distinguish laterality (i.e. subcategories H4Ø.1Ø, H4Ø.11 and H4Ø.2Ø), assign one code for each type of glaucoma with the appropriate seventh character for the stage.

When a patient has bilateral glaucoma and each eye is documented as having the same type, but different stage, and the classification does not distinguish laterality (i.e. subcategories H4Ø.1Ø, H4Ø.11 and H4Ø.2Ø), assign a code for the type of glaucoma for each eye with the seventh character for the specific glaucoma stage documented for each eye.

4) Patient admitted with glaucoma and stage evolves during the admission
If a patient is admitted with glaucoma and the stage progresses during the admission, assign the code for highest stage documented.

5) Indeterminate stage glaucoma
Assignment of the seventh character "4" for "indeterminate stage" should be based on the clinical documentation. The seventh character "4" is used for glaucomas whose stage cannot be clinically determined. This seventh character should not be confused with the seventh character "0", unspecified, which should be assigned when there is no documentation regarding the stage of the glaucoma.

8. Chapter 8: Diseases of the Ear and Mastoid Process (H6Ø-H95)
Reserved for future guideline expansion

9. Chapter 9: Diseases of the Circulatory System (IØØ-I99)

a. Hypertension
The classification presumes a causal relationship between hypertension and heart involvement and between hypertension and kidney involvement, as the two conditions are linked by the term "with" in the Alphabetic Index. These conditions should be coded as related even in the absence of provider documentation explicitly linking them, unless the documentation clearly states the conditions are unrelated.

For hypertension and conditions not specifically linked by relational terms such as "with," "associated with" or "due to" in the classification, provider documentation must link the conditions in order to code them as related.

1) **Hypertension with Heart Disease**
Hypertension with heart conditions classified to I5Ø.- or I51.4-I51.9, are assigned to a code from category I11, Hypertensive heart disease. Use an additional code from category I5Ø, Heart failure, to identify the type of heart failure in those patients with heart failure.

The same heart conditions (I5Ø.-, I51.4-I51.9) with hypertension are coded separately **if the provider has specifically documented a different cause**. Sequence according to the circumstances of the admission/encounter.

2) **Hypertensive Chronic Kidney Disease**
Assign codes from category I12, Hypertensive chronic kidney disease, when both hypertension and a condition classifiable to category N18, Chronic kidney disease (CKD), are present. **CKD should not be coded as hypertensive if the physician has specifically documented a different cause.**

The appropriate code from category N18 should be used as a secondary code with a code from category I12 to identify the stage of chronic kidney disease.

See Section I.C.14. Chronic kidney disease.

If a patient has hypertensive chronic kidney disease and acute renal failure, an additional code for the acute renal failure is required.

3) **Hypertensive Heart and Chronic Kidney Disease**
Assign codes from combination category I13, Hypertensive heart and chronic kidney disease, when **there is hypertension with both heart and kidney involvement.** If heart failure is present, assign an additional code from category I5Ø to identify the type of heart failure.

The appropriate code from category N18, Chronic kidney disease, should be used as a secondary code with a code from category I13 to identify the stage of chronic kidney disease.

See Section I.C.14. Chronic kidney disease.

The codes in category I13, Hypertensive heart and chronic kidney disease, are combination codes that include hypertension, heart disease and chronic kidney disease. The Includes note at I13 specifies that the conditions included at I11 and I12 are included together in I13. If a patient has hypertension, heart disease and chronic kidney disease, then a code from I13 should be used, not individual codes for hypertension, heart disease and chronic kidney disease, or codes from I11 or I12.

For patients with both acute renal failure and chronic kidney disease, an additional code for acute renal failure is required.

4) **Hypertensive Cerebrovascular Disease**
For hypertensive cerebrovascular disease, first assign the appropriate code from categories I6Ø-I69, followed by the appropriate hypertension code.

5) **Hypertensive Retinopathy**
Subcategory H35.Ø, Background retinopathy and retinal vascular changes, should be used with a code from category I1Ø – I15, Hypertensive disease to include the systemic hypertension. The sequencing is based on the reason for the encounter.

6) **Hypertension, Secondary**
Secondary hypertension is due to an underlying condition. Two codes are required: one to identify the underlying etiology and one from category I15 to identify the hypertension. Sequencing of codes is determined by the reason for admission/encounter.

7) **Hypertension, Transient**
Assign code R03.0, Elevated blood pressure reading without diagnosis of hypertension, unless patient has an established diagnosis of hypertension. Assign code O13.-, Gestational [pregnancy-induced] hypertension without significant proteinuria, or O14.-, Pre-eclampsia, for transient hypertension of pregnancy.

8) **Hypertension, Controlled**
This diagnostic statement usually refers to an existing state of hypertension under control by therapy. Assign the appropriate code from categories I1Ø-I15, Hypertensive diseases.

9) **Hypertension, Uncontrolled**
Uncontrolled hypertension may refer to untreated hypertension or hypertension not responding to current therapeutic regimen. In either case, assign the appropriate code from categories I1Ø-I15, Hypertensive diseases.

1Ø) **Hypertensive Crisis**
Assign a code from category I16, Hypertensive crisis, for documented hypertensive urgency, hypertensive emergency or unspecified hypertensive crisis. Code also any identified hypertensive disease (I1Ø-I15). The sequencing is based on the reason for the encounter.

b. **Atherosclerotic Coronary Artery Disease and Angina**
ICD-10-CM has combination codes for atherosclerotic heart disease with angina pectoris. The subcategories for these codes are I25.11, Atherosclerotic heart disease of native coronary artery with angina pectoris and I25.7, Atherosclerosis of coronary artery bypass graft(s) and coronary artery of transplanted heart with angina pectoris.

When using one of these combination codes it is not necessary to use an additional code for angina pectoris. A causal relationship can be assumed in a patient with both atherosclerosis and angina pectoris, unless the documentation indicates the angina is due to something other than the atherosclerosis.

If a patient with coronary artery disease is admitted due to an acute myocardial infarction (AMI), the AMI should be sequenced before the coronary artery disease.

See Section I.C.9. Acute myocardial infarction (AMI)

c. **Intraoperative and Postprocedural Cerebrovascular Accident**
Medical record documentation should clearly specify the cause- and-effect relationship between the medical intervention and the cerebrovascular accident in order to assign a code for intraoperative or postprocedural cerebrovascular accident.

Proper code assignment depends on whether it was an infarction or hemorrhage and whether it occurred intraoperatively or postoperatively. If it was a cerebral hemorrhage, code assignment depends on the type of procedure performed.

d. **Sequelae of Cerebrovascular Disease**

1) **Category I69, Sequelae of Cerebrovascular disease**
Category I69 is used to indicate conditions classifiable to categories I6Ø-I67 as the causes of sequela (neurologic deficits), themselves classified elsewhere. These "late effects" include neurologic deficits that

persist after initial onset of conditions classifiable to categories I60-I67. The neurologic deficits caused by cerebrovascular disease may be present from the onset or may arise at any time after the onset of the condition classifiable to categories I6Ø-I67.

Codes from category I69, Sequelae of cerebrovascular disease, that specify hemiplegia, hemiparesis and monoplegia identify whether the dominant or nondominant side is affected. Should the affected side be documented, but not specified as dominant or nondominant, and the classification system does not indicate a default, code selection is as follows:

- For ambidextrous patients, the default should be dominant.
- If the left side is affected, the default is non-dominant.
- If the right side is affected, the default is dominant.

2) **Codes from category I69 with codes from I6Ø-I67**
Codes from category I69 may be assigned on a health care record with codes from I6Ø-I67, if the patient has a current cerebrovascular disease and deficits from an old cerebrovascular disease.

3) **Codes from category I69 and Personal history of transient ischemic attack (TIA) and cerebral infarction (Z86.73)**
Codes from category I69 should not be assigned if the patient does not have neurologic deficits.

See Section I.C.21. 4. History (of) for use of personal history codes

e. **Acute myocardial infarction (AMI)**

1) **ST elevation myocardial infarction (STEMI) and non ST elevation myocardial infarction (NSTEMI)**
The ICD-10-CM codes for acute myocardial infarction (AMI) identify the site, such as anterolateral wall or true posterior wall. Subcategories I21.Ø-I21.2 and code I21.3 are used for ST elevation myocardial infarction (STEMI). Code I21.4, Non-ST elevation (NSTEMI) myocardial infarction, is used for non ST elevation myocardial infarction (NSTEMI) and nontransmural MIs.

If NSTEMI evolves to STEMI, assign the STEMI code. If STEMI converts to NSTEMI due to thrombolytic therapy, it is still coded as STEMI.

For encounters occurring while the myocardial infarction is equal to, or less than, four weeks old, including transfers to another acute setting or a postacute setting, and the myocardial infarction **meets the definition for "other diagnoses" (see Section III, Reporting Additional Diagnoses)**, codes from category I21 may continue to be reported. For encounters after the 4 week time frame and the patient is still receiving care related to the myocardial infarction, the appropriate aftercare code should be assigned, rather than a code from category I21. For old or healed myocardial infarctions not requiring further care, code I25.2, Old myocardial infarction, may be assigned.

2) **Acute myocardial infarction, unspecified**
Code I21.3, ST elevation (STEMI) myocardial infarction of unspecified site, is the default for unspecified acute myocardial infarction. If only STEMI or transmural MI without the site is documented, assign code I21.3.

3) **AMI documented as nontransmural or subendocardial but site provided**
If an AMI is documented as nontransmural or subendocardial, but the site is provided, it is still coded as a subendocardial AMI.

See Section I.C.21.3 for information on coding status post administration of tPA in a different facility within the last 24 hours.

4) **Subsequent acute myocardial infarction**
A code from category I22, Subsequent ST elevation (STEMI) and non ST elevation (NSTEMI) myocardial infarction, is to be used when a patient who has suffered an AMI has a new AMI within the 4 week time frame of the initial AMI. A code from category I22 must be used in conjunction with a code from category I21. The sequencing of the I22 and I21 codes depends on the circumstances of the encounter.

10. Chapter 10: Diseases of the Respiratory System (JØØ-J99)

a. **Chronic Obstructive Pulmonary Disease [COPD] and Asthma**

1) **Acute exacerbation of chronic obstructive bronchitis and asthma**
The codes in categories J44 and J45 distinguish between uncomplicated cases and those in acute exacerbation. An acute exacerbation is a worsening or a decompensation of a chronic condition. An acute exacerbation is not equivalent to an infection superimposed on a chronic condition, though an exacerbation may be triggered by an infection.

b. **Acute Respiratory Failure**

1) **Acute respiratory failure as principal diagnosis**
A code from subcategory J96.Ø, Acute respiratory failure, or subcategory J96.2, Acute and chronic respiratory failure, may be assigned as a principal diagnosis when it is the condition established after study to be chiefly responsible for occasioning the admission to the hospital, and the selection is supported by the Alphabetic Index and Tabular List. However, chapter-specific coding guidelines (such as obstetrics, poisoning, HIV, newborn) that provide sequencing direction take precedence.

2) **Acute respiratory failure as secondary diagnosis**
Respiratory failure may be listed as a secondary diagnosis if it occurs after admission, or if it is present on admission, but does not meet the definition of principal diagnosis.

3) **Sequencing of acute respiratory failure and another acute condition**
When a patient is admitted with respiratory failure and another acute condition, (e.g., myocardial infarction, cerebrovascular accident, aspiration pneumonia), the principal diagnosis will not be the same in every situation. This applies whether the other acute condition is a respiratory or nonrespiratory condition. Selection of the principal diagnosis will be dependent on the circumstances of admission. If both the respiratory failure and the other acute condition are equally responsible for occasioning the admission to the hospital, and there are no chapter-specific sequencing rules, the guideline regarding two or more diagnoses that equally meet the definition for principal diagnosis *(Section II, C.)* may be applied in these situations.

If the documentation is not clear as to whether acute respiratory failure and another condition are equally responsible for occasioning the admission, query the provider for clarification.

c. **Influenza due to certain identified influenza viruses**
Code only confirmed cases of influenza due to certain identified influenza viruses (category JØ9), and due to other identified influenza virus (category J10). This is an exception to the hospital inpatient guideline Section II, H. (Uncertain Diagnosis).

In this context, "confirmation" does not require documentation of positive laboratory testing specific for avian or other novel influenza A or other identified influenza virus. However, coding should be based on the provider's diagnostic statement that the patient has avian influenza, or other novel influenza A, for category JØ9, or has another particular identified strain of influenza, such as H1N1 or H3N2, but not identified as novel or variant, for category J1Ø.

If the provider records "suspected" or "possible" or "probable" avian influenza, or novel influenza, or other identified influenza, then the appropriate influenza code from category J11, Influenza due to unidentified influenza virus, should be assigned. A code from category JØ9, Influenza due to certain identified influenza viruses, should not be assigned nor should a code from category J1Ø, Influenza due to other identified influenza virus.

d. Ventilator associated Pneumonia

1) Documentation of Ventilator associated Pneumonia
As with all procedural or postprocedural complications, code assignment is based on the provider's documentation of the relationship between the condition and the procedure.

Code J95.851, Ventilator associated pneumonia, should be assigned only when the provider has documented ventilator associated pneumonia (VAP). An additional code to identify the organism (e.g., Pseudomonas aeruginosa, code B96.5) should also be assigned. Do not assign an additional code from categories J12-J18 to identify the type of pneumonia.

Code J95.851 should not be assigned for cases where the patient has pneumonia and is on a mechanical ventilator and the provider has not specifically stated that the pneumonia is ventilator-associated pneumonia. If the documentation is unclear as to whether the patient has a pneumonia that is a complication attributable to the mechanical ventilator, query the provider.

2) Ventilator associated Pneumonia Develops after Admission
A patient may be admitted with one type of pneumonia (e.g., code J13, Pneumonia due to Streptococcus pneumonia) and subsequently develop VAP. In this instance, the principal diagnosis would be the appropriate code from categories J12-J18 for the pneumonia diagnosed at the time of admission. Code J95.851, Ventilator associated pneumonia, would be assigned as an additional diagnosis when the provider has also documented the presence of ventilator associated pneumonia.

11. Chapter 11: Diseases of the Digestive System (KØØ-K95)
Reserved for future guideline expansion

12. Chapter 12: Diseases of the Skin and Subcutaneous Tissue (LØØ-L99)

a. Pressure ulcer stage codes

1) Pressure ulcer stages
Codes from category L89, Pressure ulcer, identify the site of the pressure ulcer as well as the stage of the ulcer.

The ICD-10-CM classifies pressure ulcer stages based on severity, which is designated by stages 1-4, unspecified stage and unstageable.

Assign as many codes from category L89 as needed to identify all the pressure ulcers the patient has, if applicable.

2) Unstageable pressure ulcers
Assignment of the code for unstageable pressure ulcer (L89.--Ø) should be based on the clinical documentation. These codes are used for pressure ulcers whose stage cannot be clinically determined (e.g., the ulcer is covered by eschar or has been treated with a skin or muscle graft) and pressure ulcers that are documented as deep tissue injury but not documented as due to trauma. This code should not be confused with the codes for unspecified stage (L89.--9). When there is no

documentation regarding the stage of the pressure ulcer, assign the appropriate code for unspecified stage (L89.--9).

3) **Documented pressure ulcer stage**
Assignment of the pressure ulcer stage code should be guided by clinical documentation of the stage or documentation of the terms found in the Alphabetic Index. For clinical terms describing the stage that are not found in the Alphabetic Index, and there is no documentation of the stage, the provider should be queried.

4) **Patients admitted with pressure ulcers documented as healed**
No code is assigned if the documentation states that the pressure ulcer is completely healed.

5) **Patients admitted with pressure ulcers documented as healing**
Pressure ulcers described as healing should be assigned the appropriate pressure ulcer stage code based on the documentation in the medical record. If the documentation does not provide information about the stage of the healing pressure ulcer, assign the appropriate code for unspecified stage.

If the documentation is unclear as to whether the patient has a current (new) pressure ulcer or if the patient is being treated for a healing pressure ulcer, query the provider.

For ulcers that were present on admission but healed at the time of discharge, assign the code for the site and stage of the pressure ulcer at the time of admission.

6) **Patient admitted with pressure ulcer evolving into another stage during the admission**
If a patient is admitted with a pressure ulcer at one stage and it progresses to a higher stage, **two separate codes should be assigned: one code for the site and stage of the ulcer on admission and a second code for the same ulcer site and the highest stage reported during the stay.**

13. Chapter 13: Diseases of the Musculoskeletal System and Connective Tissue (MØØ-M99)

a. Site and laterality
Most of the codes within Chapter 13 have site and laterality designations. The site represents the bone, joint or the muscle involved. For some conditions where more than one bone, joint or muscle is usually involved, such as osteoarthritis, there is a "multiple sites" code available. For categories where no multiple site code is provided and more than one bone, joint or muscle is involved, multiple codes should be used to indicate the different sites involved.

1) **Bone versus joint**
For certain conditions, the bone may be affected at the upper or lower end, (e.g., avascular necrosis of bone, M87, Osteoporosis, M8Ø, M81). Though the portion of the bone affected may be at the joint, the site designation will be the bone, not the joint.

b. Acute traumatic versus chronic or recurrent musculoskeletal conditions
Many musculoskeletal conditions are a result of previous injury or trauma to a site, or are recurrent conditions. Bone, joint or muscle conditions that are the result of a healed injury are usually found in chapter 13. Recurrent bone, joint or muscle conditions are also usually found in chapter 13. Any current, acute injury should be coded to the appropriate injury code from chapter 19. Chronic or recurrent conditions should generally be coded with a code from chapter 13. If it is difficult to determine from the documentation in the record which code is best to describe a condition, query the provider.

c. Coding of Pathologic Fractures

7th character A is for use as long as the patient is receiving active treatment for the fracture. While the patient may be seen by a new or different provider over the course of treatment for a pathological fracture, assignment of the 7th character is based on whether the patient is undergoing active treatment and not whether the provider is seeing the patient for the first time.

7th character D is to be used for encounters after the patient has completed active treatment. The other 7th characters, listed under each subcategory in the Tabular List, are to be used for subsequent encounters for **routine care of fractures during the healing and recovery phase as well as** treatment of problems associated with the healing, such as malunions, nonunions, and sequelae.

Care for complications of surgical treatment for fracture repairs during the healing or recovery phase should be coded with the appropriate complication codes.

See Section I.C.19. Coding of traumatic fractures.

d. Osteoporosis

Osteoporosis is a systemic condition, meaning that all bones of the musculoskeletal system are affected. Therefore, site is not a component of the codes under category M81, Osteoporosis without current pathological fracture. The site codes under category M8Ø, Osteoporosis with current pathological fracture, identify the site of the fracture, not the osteoporosis.

1) Osteoporosis without pathological fracture

Category M81, Osteoporosis without current pathological fracture, is for use for patients with osteoporosis who do not currently have a pathologic fracture due to the osteoporosis, even if they have had a fracture in the past. For patients with a history of osteoporosis fractures, status code Z87.31Ø, Personal history of (healed) osteoporosis fracture, should follow the code from M81.

2) Osteoporosis with current pathological fracture

Category M8Ø, Osteoporosis with current pathological fracture, is for patients who have a current pathologic fracture at the time of an encounter. The codes under M8Ø identify the site of the fracture. A code from category M8Ø, not a traumatic fracture code, should be used for any patient with known osteoporosis who suffers a fracture, even if the patient had a minor fall or trauma, if that fall or trauma would not usually break a normal, healthy bone.

14. Chapter 14: Diseases of Genitourinary System (NØØ-N99)

a. Chronic kidney disease

1) Stages of chronic kidney disease (CKD)

The ICD-10-CM classifies CKD based on severity. The severity of CKD is designated by stages 1-5. Stage 2, code N18.2, equates to mild CKD; stage 3, code N18.3, equates to moderate CKD; and stage 4, code N18.4, equates to severe CKD. Code N18.6, End stage renal disease (ESRD), is assigned when the provider has documented end-stage-renal disease (ESRD).

If both a stage of CKD and ESRD are documented, assign code N18.6 only.

2) Chronic kidney disease and kidney transplant status

Patients who have undergone kidney transplant may still have some form of chronic kidney disease (CKD) because the kidney transplant may not fully restore kidney function. Therefore, the presence of CKD alone does not constitute a transplant complication. Assign the appropriate N18 code for the patient's stage of CKD and code Z94.Ø, Kidney transplant status. If a transplant complication such as failure or rejection or other transplant complication is documented, see section I.C.19.g for information on coding complications of a kidney transplant. If the documentation is unclear as to whether the patient has a complication of the transplant, query the provider.

3) **Chronic kidney disease with other conditions**
Patients with CKD may also suffer from other serious conditions, most commonly diabetes mellitus and hypertension. The sequencing of the CKD code in relationship to codes for other contributing conditions is based on the conventions in the Tabular List.

See I.C.9. Hypertensive chronic kidney disease.

See I.C.19. Chronic kidney disease and kidney transplant complications.

15. Chapter 15: Pregnancy, Childbirth, and the Puerperium (OØØ-O9A)

a. General Rules for Obstetric Cases

1) **Codes from chapter 15 and sequencing priority**
Obstetric cases require codes from chapter 15, codes in the range O00-O9A, Pregnancy, Childbirth, and the Puerperium. Chapter 15 codes have sequencing priority over codes from other chapters. Additional codes from other chapters may be used in conjunction with chapter 15 codes to further specify conditions. Should the provider document that the pregnancy is incidental to the encounter, then code Z33.1, Pregnant state, incidental, should be used in place of any chapter 15 codes. It is the provider's responsibility to state that the condition being treated is not affecting the pregnancy.

2) **Chapter 15 codes used only on the maternal record**
Chapter 15 codes are to be used only on the maternal record, never on the record of the newborn.

3) **Final character for trimester**
The majority of codes in Chapter 15 have a final character indicating the trimester of pregnancy. The timeframes for the trimesters are indicated at the beginning of the chapter. If trimester is not a component of a code, it is because the condition always occurs in a specific trimester, or the concept of trimester of pregnancy is not applicable. Certain codes have characters for only certain trimesters because the condition does not occur in all trimesters, but it may occur in more than just one. Assignment of the final character for trimester should be based on the provider's documentation of the trimester (or number of weeks) for the current admission/encounter. This applies to the assignment of trimester for pre-existing conditions as well as those that develop during or are due to the pregnancy. The provider's documentation of the number of weeks may be used to assign the appropriate code identifying the trimester.

Whenever delivery occurs during the current admission, and there is an "in childbirth" option for the obstetric complication being coded, the "in childbirth" code should be assigned.

4) **Selection of trimester for inpatient admissions that encompass more than one trimester**
In instances when a patient is admitted to a hospital for complications of pregnancy during one trimester and remains in the hospital into a subsequent trimester, the trimester character for the antepartum complication code should be assigned on the basis of the trimester when the complication developed, not the trimester of the discharge. If the condition developed prior to the current admission/encounter or represents a pre-existing condition, the trimester character for the trimester at the time of the admission/encounter should be assigned.

5) Unspecified trimester
Each category that includes codes for trimester has a code for "unspecified trimester." The "unspecified trimester" code should rarely be used, such as when the documentation in the record is insufficient to determine the trimester and it is not possible to obtain clarification.

6) 7th character for Fetus Identification
Where applicable, a 7th character is to be assigned for certain categories (O31, O32, O33.3 - O33.6, O35, O36, O4Ø, O41, O6Ø.1, O6Ø.2, O64, and O69) to identify the fetus for which the complication code applies.

Assign 7th character "Ø":

- For single gestations
- When the documentation in the record is insufficient to determine the fetus affected and it is not possible to obtain clarification.
- When it is not possible to clinically determine which fetus is affected.

b. Selection of OB Principal or First-listed Diagnosis

1) Routine outpatient prenatal visits
For routine outpatient prenatal visits when no complications are present, a code from category Z34, Encounter for supervision of normal pregnancy, should be used as the first-listed diagnosis. These codes should not be used in conjunction with chapter 15 codes.

2) Supervision of High-Risk Pregnancy
Codes from category OØ9, Supervision of high-risk pregnancy, are intended for use only during the prenatal period. For complications during the labor or delivery episode as a result of a high-risk pregnancy, assign the applicable complication codes from Chapter 15. If there are no complications during the labor or delivery episode, assign code O8Ø, Encounter for full-term uncomplicated delivery.

For routine prenatal outpatient visits for patients with high-risk pregnancies, a code from category OØ9, Supervision of high-risk pregnancy, should be used as the first-listed diagnosis. Secondary chapter 15 codes may be used in conjunction with these codes if appropriate.

3) Episodes when no delivery occurs
In episodes when no delivery occurs, the principal diagnosis should correspond to the principal complication of the pregnancy which necessitated the encounter. Should more than one complication exist, all of which are treated or monitored, any of the complications codes may be sequenced first.

4) When a delivery occurs
When an obstetric patient is admitted and delivers during that admission, the condition that prompted the admission should be sequenced as the principal diagnosis. If multiple conditions prompted the admission, sequence the one most related to the delivery as the principal diagnosis. A code for any complication of the delivery should be assigned as an additional diagnosis. In cases of cesarean delivery, if the patient was admitted with a condition that resulted in the performance of a cesarean procedure, that condition should be selected as the principal diagnosis. If the reason for the admission was unrelated to the condition resulting in the cesarean delivery, the condition related to the reason for the admission should be selected as the principal diagnosis.

5) Outcome of delivery
A code from category Z37, Outcome of delivery, should be included on every maternal record when a delivery has occurred. These codes are not to be used on subsequent records or on the newborn record.

c. Pre-existing conditions versus conditions due to the pregnancy
Certain categories in Chapter 15 distinguish between conditions of the mother that existed prior to pregnancy (pre-existing) and those that are a direct result of pregnancy. When assigning codes from Chapter 15, it is important to assess if a condition was pre-existing prior to pregnancy or developed during or due to the pregnancy in order to assign the correct code.

Categories that do not distinguish between pre-existing and pregnancy-related conditions may be used for either. It is acceptable to use codes specifically for the puerperium with codes complicating pregnancy and childbirth if a condition arises postpartum during the delivery encounter.

d. Pre-existing hypertension in pregnancy
Category O1Ø, Pre-existing hypertension complicating pregnancy, childbirth and the puerperium, includes codes for hypertensive heart and hypertensive chronic kidney disease. When assigning one of the O1Ø codes that includes hypertensive heart disease or hypertensive chronic kidney disease, it is necessary to add a secondary code from the appropriate hypertension category to specify the type of heart failure or chronic kidney disease.

See Section I.C.9. Hypertension.

e. Fetal Conditions Affecting the Management of the Mother

1) Codes from categories O35 and O36
Codes from categories O35, Maternal care for known or suspected fetal abnormality and damage, and O36, Maternal care for other fetal problems, are assigned only when the fetal condition is actually responsible for modifying the management of the mother, i.e., by requiring diagnostic studies, additional observation, special care, or termination of pregnancy. The fact that the fetal condition exists does not justify assigning a code from this series to the mother's record.

2) In utero surgery
In cases when surgery is performed on the fetus, a diagnosis code from category O35, Maternal care for known or suspected fetal abnormality and damage, should be assigned identifying the fetal condition. Assign the appropriate procedure code for the procedure performed.

No code from Chapter 16, the perinatal codes, should be used on the mother's record to identify fetal conditions. Surgery performed in utero on a fetus is still to be coded as an obstetric encounter.

f. HIV Infection in Pregnancy, Childbirth and the Puerperium
During pregnancy, childbirth or the puerperium, a patient admitted because of an HIV-related illness should receive a principal diagnosis from subcategory O98.7-, Human immunodeficiency [HIV] disease complicating pregnancy, childbirth and the puerperium, followed by the code(s) for the HIV-related illness(es).

Patients with asymptomatic HIV infection status admitted during pregnancy, childbirth, or the puerperium should receive codes of O98.7- and Z21, Asymptomatic human immunodeficiency virus [HIV] infection status.

g. Diabetes mellitus in pregnancy
Diabetes mellitus is a significant complicating factor in pregnancy. Pregnant women who are diabetic should be assigned a code from category O24, Diabetes mellitus in pregnancy, childbirth, and the puerperium, first, followed by the appropriate diabetes code(s) (EØ8-E13) from Chapter 4.

h. Long term use of insulin and oral hypoglycemics

Code Z79.4, Long-term (current) use of insulin, or **code Z79.84, Long-term (current) use of oral hypoglycemic drugs,** should also be assigned if the diabetes mellitus is being treated with insulin **or oral medications. If the patient is treated with both oral medications and insulin, only the code for insulin-controlled should be assigned.**

i. Gestational (pregnancy induced) diabetes

Gestational (pregnancy induced) diabetes can occur during the second and third trimester of pregnancy in women who were not diabetic prior to pregnancy. Gestational diabetes can cause complications in the pregnancy similar to those of pre-existing diabetes mellitus. It also puts the woman at greater risk of developing diabetes after the pregnancy. Codes for gestational diabetes are in subcategory O24.4, Gestational diabetes mellitus. No other code from category O24, Diabetes mellitus in pregnancy, childbirth, and the puerperium, should be used with a code from O24.4.

The codes under subcategory O24.4 include diet controlled**,** insulin controlled**, and controlled by oral hypoglycemic drugs**. If a patient with gestational diabetes is treated with both diet and insulin, only the code for insulin-controlled is required. **If a patient with gestational diabetes is treated with both diet and oral hypoglycemic medications, only the code for "controlled by oral hypoglycemic drugs" is required.** Code Z79.4, Long-term (current) use of insulin **or code Z79.84, Long-term (current) use of oral hypoglycemic drugs,** should not be assigned with codes from subcategory O24.4.

An abnormal glucose tolerance in pregnancy is assigned a code from subcategory O99.81, Abnormal glucose complicating pregnancy, childbirth, and the puerperium.

j. Sepsis and septic shock complicating abortion, pregnancy, childbirth and the puerperium

When assigning a chapter 15 code for sepsis complicating abortion, pregnancy, childbirth, and the puerperium, a code for the specific type of infection should be assigned as an additional diagnosis. If severe sepsis is present, a code from subcategory R65.2, Severe sepsis, and code(s) for associated organ dysfunction(s) should also be assigned as additional diagnoses.

k. Puerperal sepsis

Code O85, Puerperal sepsis, should be assigned with a secondary code to identify the causal organism (e.g., for a bacterial infection, assign a code from category B95-B96, Bacterial infections in conditions classified elsewhere). A code from category A4Ø, Streptococcal sepsis, or A41, Other sepsis, should not be used for puerperal sepsis. If applicable, use additional codes to identify severe sepsis (R65.2-) and any associated acute organ dysfunction.

l. Alcohol and tobacco use during pregnancy, childbirth and the puerperium

1) Alcohol use during pregnancy, childbirth and the puerperium

Codes under subcategory O99.31, Alcohol use complicating pregnancy, childbirth, and the puerperium, should be assigned for any pregnancy case when a mother uses alcohol during the pregnancy or postpartum. A secondary code from category F1Ø, Alcohol related disorders, should also be assigned to identify manifestations of the alcohol use.

2) Tobacco use during pregnancy, childbirth and the puerperium

Codes under subcategory O99.33, Smoking (tobacco) complicating pregnancy, childbirth, and the puerperium, should be assigned for any pregnancy case when a mother uses any type of tobacco product during the pregnancy or postpartum. A secondary code from category F17, Nicotine dependence, should also be assigned to identify the type of nicotine dependence.

m. Poisoning, toxic effects, adverse effects and underdosing in a pregnant patient

A code from subcategory O9A.2, Injury, poisoning and certain other consequences of external causes complicating pregnancy, childbirth, and the puerperium, should be sequenced first, followed by the appropriate injury, poisoning, toxic effect, adverse effect or underdosing code, and then the additional code(s) that specifies the condition caused by the poisoning, toxic effect, adverse effect or underdosing.

See Section I.C.19. Adverse effects, poisoning, underdosing and toxic effects.

n. Normal Delivery, Code O8Ø

1) Encounter for full term uncomplicated delivery

Code O80 should be assigned when a woman is admitted for a full-term normal delivery and delivers a single, healthy infant without any complications antepartum, during the delivery, or postpartum during the delivery episode. Code O8Ø is always a principal diagnosis. It is not to be used if any other code from chapter 15 is needed to describe a current complication of the antenatal, delivery, or perinatal period. Additional codes from other chapters may be used with code O8Ø if they are not related to or are in any way complicating the pregnancy.

2) Uncomplicated delivery with resolved antepartum complication

Code O80 may be used if the patient had a complication at some point during the pregnancy, but the complication is not present at the time of the admission for delivery.

3) Outcome of delivery for O8Ø

Z37.Ø, Single live birth, is the only outcome of delivery code appropriate for use with O8Ø.

o. The Peripartum and Postpartum Periods

1) Peripartum and Postpartum periods

The postpartum period begins immediately after delivery and continues for six weeks following delivery. The peripartum period is defined as the last month of pregnancy to five months postpartum.

2) Peripartum and postpartum complication

A postpartum complication is any complication occurring within the six-week period.

3) Pregnancy-related complications after 6 week period

Chapter 15 codes may also be used to describe pregnancy-related complications after the peripartum or postpartum period if the provider documents that a condition is pregnancy related.

4) Admission for routine postpartum care following delivery outside hospital

When the mother delivers outside the hospital prior to admission and is admitted for routine postpartum care and no complications are noted, code Z39.Ø, Encounter for care and examination of mother immediately after delivery, should be assigned as the principal diagnosis.

5) Pregnancy associated cardiomyopathy

Pregnancy associated cardiomyopathy, code O9Ø.3, is unique in that it may be diagnosed in the third trimester of pregnancy but may continue to progress months after delivery. For this reason, it is referred to as peripartum cardiomyopathy. Code O9Ø.3 is only for use when the cardiomyopathy develops as a result of pregnancy in a woman who did not have pre-existing heart disease.

p. Code O94, Sequelae of complication of pregnancy, childbirth, and the puerperium

1) Code O94
Code O94, Sequelae of complication of pregnancy, childbirth, and the puerperium, is for use in those cases when an initial complication of a pregnancy develops a sequelae requiring care or treatment at a future date.

2) After the initial postpartum period
This code may be used at any time after the initial postpartum period.

3) Sequencing of Code O94
This code, like all sequela codes, is to be sequenced following the code describing the sequelae of the complication.

q. *Termination of Pregnancy and Spontaneous abortions*

1) Abortion with Liveborn Fetus
When an attempted termination of pregnancy results in a liveborn fetus, assign code Z33.2, Encounter for elective termination of pregnancy and a code from category Z37, Outcome of Delivery.

2) Retained Products of Conception following an abortion
Subsequent encounters for retained products of conception following a spontaneous abortion or elective termination of pregnancy are assigned the appropriate code from category O03, Spontaneous abortion, or codes O07.4, Failed attempted termination of pregnancy without complication and Z33.2, Encounter for elective termination of pregnancy. This advice is appropriate even when the patient was discharged previously with a discharge diagnosis of complete abortion.

3) Complications leading to abortion
Codes from Chapter 15 may be used as additional codes to identify any documented complications of the pregnancy in conjunction with codes in categories in O07 and O08.

r. Abuse in a pregnant patient
For suspected or confirmed cases of abuse of a pregnant patient, a code(s) from subcategories O9A.3, Physical abuse complicating pregnancy, childbirth, and the puerperium, O9A.4, Sexual abuse complicating pregnancy, childbirth, and the puerperium, and O9A.5, Psychological abuse complicating pregnancy, childbirth, and the puerperium, should be sequenced first, followed by the appropriate codes (if applicable) to identify any associated current injury due to physical abuse, sexual abuse, and the perpetrator of abuse.

See Section I.C.19. Adult and child abuse, neglect and other maltreatment.

16. Chapter 16: Certain Conditions Originating in the Perinatal Period (P00-P96)
For coding and reporting purposes the perinatal period is defined as before birth through the 28th day following birth. The following guidelines are provided for reporting purposes.

a. General Perinatal Rules

1) Use of Chapter 16 Codes
Codes in this chapter are never for use on the maternal record. Codes from Chapter 15, the obstetric chapter, are never permitted on the newborn record. Chapter 16 codes may be used throughout the life of the patient if the condition is still present.

2) Principal Diagnosis for Birth Record
When coding the birth episode in a newborn record, assign a code from category Z38, Liveborn infants according to place of birth and type of delivery, as the principal diagnosis. A code from category Z38 is assigned

only once, to a newborn at the time of birth. If a newborn is transferred to another institution, a code from category Z38 should not be used at the receiving hospital.

A code from category Z38 is used only on the newborn record, not on the mother's record.

3) **Use of Codes from other Chapters with Codes from Chapter 16**
Codes from other chapters may be used with codes from chapter 16 if the codes from the other chapters provide more specific detail. Codes for signs and symptoms may be assigned when a definitive diagnosis has not been established. If the reason for the encounter is a perinatal condition, the code from chapter 16 should be sequenced first.

4) **Use of Chapter 16 Codes after the Perinatal Period**
Should a condition originate in the perinatal period, and continue throughout the life of the patient, the perinatal code should continue to be used regardless of the patient's age.

5) **Birth process or community acquired conditions**
If a newborn has a condition that may be either due to the birth process or community acquired and the documentation does not indicate which it is, the default is due to the birth process and the code from Chapter 16 should be used. If the condition is community-acquired, a code from Chapter 16 should not be assigned.

6) **Code all clinically significant conditions**
All clinically significant conditions noted on routine newborn examination should be coded. A condition is clinically significant if it requires:

- clinical evaluation; or
- therapeutic treatment; or
- diagnostic procedures; or
- extended length of hospital stay; or
- increased nursing care and/or monitoring; or
- has implications for future health care needs

Note: The perinatal guidelines listed above are the same as the general coding guidelines for "additional diagnoses", except for the final point regarding implications for future health care needs. Codes should be assigned for conditions that have been specified by the provider as having implications for future health care needs.

b. **Observation and Evaluation of Newborns for Suspected Conditions not Found**

1) **Assign a code from category Z05, Observation and evaluation of newborns and infants for suspected conditions ruled out, to identify those instances when a healthy newborn is evaluated for a suspected condition that is determined after study not to be present. Do not use a code from category Z05 when the patient has identified signs or symptoms of a suspected problem; in such cases code the sign or symptom.**

2) **A code from category Z05 may also be assigned as a principal or first-listed code for readmissions or encounters when the code from category Z38 code no longer applies. Codes from category Z05 are for use only for healthy newborns and infants for which no condition after study is found to be present.**

3) **Z05 on a birth record**
A code from category Z05 is to be used as a secondary code after the code from category Z38, Liveborn infants according to place of birth and type of delivery.

c. Coding Additional Perinatal Diagnoses

1) Assigning codes for conditions that require treatment
Assign codes for conditions that require treatment or further investigation, prolong the length of stay, or require resource utilization.

2) Codes for conditions specified as having implications for future health care needs
Assign codes for conditions that have been specified by the provider as having implications for future health care needs.

Note: This guideline should not be used for adult patients.

d. Prematurity and Fetal Growth Retardation
Providers utilize different criteria in determining prematurity. A code for prematurity should not be assigned unless it is documented. Assignment of codes in categories PØ5, Disorders of newborn related to slow fetal growth and fetal malnutrition, and PØ7, Disorders of newborn related to short gestation and low birth weight, not elsewhere classified, should be based on the recorded birth weight and estimated gestational age. Codes from category P05 should not be assigned with codes from category PØ7.

When both birth weight and gestational age are available, two codes from category PØ7 should be assigned, with the code for birth weight sequenced before the code for gestational age.

e. Low birth weight and immaturity status
Codes from category PØ7, Disorders of newborn related to short gestation and low birth weight, not elsewhere classified, are for use for a child or adult who was premature or had a low birth weight as a newborn and this is affecting the patient's current health status.

See Section I.C.21. Factors influencing health status and contact with health services, Status.

f. Bacterial Sepsis of Newborn
Category P36, Bacterial sepsis of newborn, includes congenital sepsis. If a perinate is documented as having sepsis without documentation of congenital or community acquired, the default is congenital and a code from category P36 should be assigned. If the P36 code includes the causal organism, an additional code from category B95, Streptococcus, Staphylococcus, and Enterococcus as the cause of diseases classified elsewhere, or B96, Other bacterial agents as the cause of diseases classified elsewhere, should not be assigned. If the P36 code does not include the causal organism, assign an additional code from category B96. If applicable, use additional codes to identify severe sepsis (R65.2-) and any associated acute organ dysfunction.

g. Stillbirth
Code P95, Stillbirth, is only for use in institutions that maintain separate records for stillbirths. No other code should be used with P95. Code P95 should not be used on the mother's record.

17. Chapter 17: Congenital malformations, deformations, and chromosomal abnormalities (QØØ-Q99)
Assign an appropriate code(s) from categories QØØ-Q99, Congenital malformations, deformations, and chromosomal abnormalities when a malformation/deformation or chromosomal abnormality is documented. A malformation/deformation/or chromosomal abnormality may be the principal/first-listed diagnosis on a record or a secondary diagnosis.

When a malformation/deformation or chromosomal abnormality does not have a unique code assignment, assign additional code(s) for any manifestations that may be present.

When the code assignment specifically identifies the malformation/deformation or chromosomal abnormality, manifestations that are an inherent component of the anomaly should not be coded separately. Additional codes should be assigned for manifestations that are not an inherent component.

Codes from Chapter 17 may be used throughout the life of the patient. If a congenital malformation or deformity has been corrected, a personal history code should be used to identify the history of the malformation or deformity. Although present at birth, malformation/deformation/or chromosomal abnormality may not be identified until later in life. Whenever the condition is diagnosed by the physician, it is appropriate to assign a code from codes Q00-Q99.For the birth admission, the appropriate code from category Z38, Liveborn infants, according to place of birth and type of delivery, should be sequenced as the principal diagnosis, followed by any congenital anomaly codes, Q00- Q99.

18. Chapter 18: Symptoms, signs, and abnormal clinical and laboratory findings, not elsewhere classified (R00-R99)

Chapter 18 includes symptoms, signs, abnormal results of clinical or other investigative procedures, and ill-defined conditions regarding which no diagnosis classifiable elsewhere is recorded. Signs and symptoms that point to a specific diagnosis have been assigned to a category in other chapters of the classification.

a. Use of symptom codes

Codes that describe symptoms and signs are acceptable for reporting purposes when a related definitive diagnosis has not been established (confirmed) by the provider.

b. Use of a symptom code with a definitive diagnosis code

Codes for signs and symptoms may be reported in addition to a related definitive diagnosis when the sign or symptom is not routinely associated with that diagnosis, such as the various signs and symptoms associated with complex syndromes. The definitive diagnosis code should be sequenced before the symptom code.

Signs or symptoms that are associated routinely with a disease process should not be assigned as additional codes, unless otherwise instructed by the classification.

c. Combination codes that include symptoms

ICD-10-CM contains a number of combination codes that identify both the definitive diagnosis and common symptoms of that diagnosis. When using one of these combination codes, an additional code should not be assigned for the symptom.

d. Repeated falls

Code R29.6, Repeated falls, is for use for encounters when a patient has recently fallen and the reason for the fall is being investigated.

Code Z91.81, History of falling, is for use when a patient has fallen in the past and is at risk for future falls. When appropriate, both codes R29.6 and Z91.81 may be assigned together.

e. Coma scale

The coma scale codes (R40.2-) can be used in conjunction with traumatic brain injury codes, acute cerebrovascular disease or sequelae of cerebrovascular disease codes. These codes are primarily for use by trauma registries, but they may be used in any setting where this information is collected. **The coma scale may also be used to assess the status of the central nervous system for other non-trauma conditions, such as monitoring patients in the intensive care unit regardless of medical condition.** The coma scale codes should be sequenced after the diagnosis code(s).

These codes, one from each subcategory, are needed to complete the scale. The 7th character indicates when the scale was recorded. The 7th character should match for all three codes.

At a minimum, report the initial score documented on presentation at your facility. This may be a score from the emergency medicine technician (EMT) or in the emergency department. If desired, a facility may choose to capture multiple coma scale scores.

Assign code R40.24, Glasgow coma scale, total score, when only the total score is documented in the medical record and not the individual score(s).

f. **Functional quadriplegia**
Functional quadriplegia (code R53.2) is the lack of ability to use one's limbs or to ambulate due to extreme debility. It is not associated with neurologic deficit or injury, and code R53.2 should not be used for cases of neurologic quadriplegia. It should only be assigned if functional quadriplegia is specifically documented in the medical record.

g. **SIRS due to Non-Infectious Process**
The systemic inflammatory response syndrome (SIRS) can develop as a result of certain non-infectious disease processes, such as trauma, malignant neoplasm, or pancreatitis. When SIRS is documented with a noninfectious condition, and no subsequent infection is documented, the code for the underlying condition, such as an injury, should be assigned, followed by code R65.10, Systemic inflammatory response syndrome (SIRS) of non-infectious origin without acute organ dysfunction, or code R65.11, Systemic inflammatory response syndrome (SIRS) of non-infectious origin with acute organ dysfunction. If an associated acute organ dysfunction is documented, the appropriate code(s) for the specific type of organ dysfunction(s) should be assigned in addition to code R65.11. If acute organ dysfunction is documented, but it cannot be determined if the acute organ dysfunction is associated with SIRS or due to another condition (e.g., directly due to the trauma), the provider should be queried.

h. **Death NOS**
Code R99, Ill-defined and unknown cause of mortality, is only for use in the very limited circumstance when a patient who has already died is brought into an emergency department or other healthcare facility and is pronounced dead upon arrival. It does not represent the discharge disposition of death.

i. **NIHSS Stroke Scale**
The NIH stroke scale (NIHSS) codes (R29.7- -) can be used in conjunction with acute stroke codes (I63) to identify the patient's neurological status and the severity of the stroke. The stroke scale codes should be sequenced after the acute stroke diagnosis code(s).

At a minimum, report the initial score documented. If desired, a facility may choose to capture multiple stroke scale scores.

See Section I.B.14. for information concerning the medical record documentation that may be used for assignment of the NIHSS codes.

19. Chapter 19: Injury, poisoning, and certain other consequences of external causes (S00-T88)

a. **Application of 7th Characters in Chapter 19**
Most categories in chapter 19 have a 7th character requirement for each applicable code. Most categories in this chapter have three 7th character values (with the exception of fractures): A, initial encounter, D, subsequent encounter and S, sequela. Categories for traumatic fractures have additional 7th character values. While the patient may be seen by a new or different provider over the course of treatment for an injury, assignment of the 7th character is based on whether the patient is undergoing active treatment and not whether the provider is seeing the patient for the first time.

For complication codes, active treatment refers to treatment for the condition described by the code, even though it may be related to an earlier precipitating problem. For example, code T84.50XA, Infection and inflammatory reaction due to unspecified internal joint prosthesis, initial encounter, is used when active treatment is provided for the infection, even though the condition relates to the prosthetic device, implant or graft that was placed at a previous encounter.

7th character "A", initial encounter is used **for each encounter where** the patient is receiving active treatment for the condition.

7th character "D" subsequent encounter is used for encounters after the patient has **completed** active treatment of the condition and is receiving routine care for the condition during the healing or recovery phase.

The aftercare Z codes should not be used for aftercare for conditions such as injuries or poisonings, where 7th characters are provided to identify subsequent care. For example, for aftercare of an injury, assign the acute injury code with the 7th character "D" (subsequent encounter).

7th character "S", sequela, is for use for complications or conditions that arise as a direct result of a condition, such as scar formation after a burn. The scars are sequelae of the burn. When using 7th character "S", it is necessary to use both the injury code that precipitated the sequela and the code for the sequela itself. The "S" is added only to the injury code, not the sequela code. The 7th character "S" identifies the injury responsible for the sequela. The specific type of sequela (e.g. scar) is sequenced first, followed by the injury code.

See Section I.B.10 Sequelae, (Late Effects)

b. Coding of Injuries

When coding injuries, assign separate codes for each injury unless a combination code is provided, in which case the combination code is assigned. Code TØ7, Unspecified multiple injuries should not be assigned in the inpatient setting unless information for a more specific code is not available. Traumatic injury codes (SØØ-T14.9) are not to be used for normal, healing surgical wounds or to identify complications of surgical wounds.

The code for the most serious injury, as determined by the provider and the focus of treatment, is sequenced first.

1) Superficial injuries

Superficial injuries such as abrasions or contusions are not coded when associated with more severe injuries of the same site.

2) Primary injury with damage to nerves/blood vessels

When a primary injury results in minor damage to peripheral nerves or blood vessels, the primary injury is sequenced first with additional code(s) for injuries to nerves and spinal cord (such as category SØ4), and/or injury to blood vessels (such as category S15). When the primary injury is to the blood vessels or nerves, that injury should be sequenced first.

c. Coding of Traumatic Fractures

The principles of multiple coding of injuries should be followed in coding fractures. Fractures of specified sites are coded individually by site in accordance with both the provisions within categories SØ2, S12, S22, S32, S42, S49, S52, S59, S62, S72, S79, S82, S89, S92 and the level of detail furnished by medical record content.

A fracture not indicated as open or closed should be coded to closed. A fracture not indicated whether displaced or not displaced should be coded to displaced.

More specific guidelines are as follows:

1) Initial vs. Subsequent Encounter for Fractures

Traumatic fractures are coded using the appropriate 7th character for initial encounter (A, B, C) **for each encounter where** the patient is receiving active treatment for the fracture. The appropriate 7th character for initial encounter should also be assigned for a patient who delayed seeking treatment for the fracture or nonunion.

Fractures are coded using the appropriate 7th character for subsequent care for encounters after the patient has completed active treatment of the fracture and is receiving routine care for the fracture during the healing or recovery phase.

Care for complications of surgical treatment for fracture repairs during the healing or recovery phase should be coded with the appropriate complication codes.

Care of complications of fractures, such as malunion and nonunion, should be reported with the appropriate 7th character for subsequent care with nonunion (K, M, N,) or subsequent care with malunion (P, Q, R).

Malunion/nonunion: The appropriate 7th character for initial encounter should also be assigned for a patient who delayed seeking treatment for the fracture or nonunion.

The open fracture designations in the assignment of the 7th character for fractures of the forearm, femur and lower leg, including ankle are based on the Gustilo open fracture classification. When the Gustilo classification type is not specified for an open fracture, the 7th character for open fracture type I or II should be assigned (B, E, H, M, Q).

A code from category M8Ø, not a traumatic fracture code, should be used for any patient with known osteoporosis who suffers a fracture, even if the patient had a minor fall or trauma, if that fall or trauma would not usually break a normal, healthy bone.

See Section I.C.13. Osteoporosis.

The aftercare Z codes should not be used for aftercare for traumatic fractures. For aftercare of a traumatic fracture, assign the acute fracture code with the appropriate 7th character.

2) Multiple fractures sequencing
Multiple fractures are sequenced in accordance with the severity of the fracture.

d. Coding of Burns and Corrosions
The ICD-10-CM makes a distinction between burns and corrosions. The burn codes are for thermal burns, except sunburns, that come from a heat source, such as a fire or hot appliance. The burn codes are also for burns resulting from electricity and radiation. Corrosions are burns due to chemicals. The guidelines are the same for burns and corrosions.

Current burns (T2Ø-T25) are classified by depth, extent and by agent (X code). Burns are classified by depth as first degree (erythema), second degree (blistering), and third degree (full-thickness involvement). Burns of the eye and internal organs (T26-T28) are classified by site, but not by degree.

1) Sequencing of burn and related condition codes
Sequence first the code that reflects the highest degree of burn when more than one burn is present.

a. When the reason for the admission or encounter is for treatment of external multiple burns, sequence first the code that reflects the burn of the highest degree.

b. When a patient has both internal and external burns, the circumstances of admission govern the selection of the principal diagnosis or first-listed diagnosis.

c. When a patient is admitted for burn injuries and other related conditions such as smoke inhalation and/or respiratory failure, the circumstances of admission govern the selection of the principal or first-listed diagnosis.

2) **Burns of the same local site**
Classify burns of the same local site (three-character category level, T2Ø-T28) but of different degrees to the subcategory identifying the highest degree recorded in the diagnosis.

3) **Non-healing burns**
Non-healing burns are coded as acute burns.

Necrosis of burned skin should be coded as a non-healed burn.

4) **Infected Burn**
For any documented infected burn site, use an additional code for the infection.

5) **Assign separate codes for each burn site**
When coding burns, assign separate codes for each burn site. Category T30, Burn and corrosion, body region unspecified is extremely vague and should rarely be used.

6) **Burns and Corrosions Classified According to Extent of Body Surface Involved**
Assign codes from category T31, Burns classified according to extent of body surface involved, or T32, Corrosions classified according to extent of body surface involved, when the site of the burn is not specified or when there is a need for additional data. It is advisable to use category T31 as additional coding when needed to provide data for evaluating burn mortality, such as that needed by burn units. It is also advisable to use category T31 as an additional code for reporting purposes when there is mention of a third-degree burn involving 20 percent or more of the body surface.

Categories T31 and T32 are based on the classic "rule of nines" in estimating body surface involved: head and neck are assigned nine percent, each arm nine percent, each leg 18 percent, the anterior trunk 18 percent, posterior trunk 18 percent, and genitalia one percent. Providers may change these percentage assignments where necessary to accommodate infants and children who have proportionately larger heads than adults, and patients who have large buttocks, thighs, or abdomen that involve burns.

7) **Encounters for treatment of sequela of burns**
Encounters for the treatment of the late effects of burns or corrosions (i.e., scars or joint contractures) should be coded with a burn or corrosion code with the 7th character "S" for sequela.

8) **Sequelae with a late effect code and current burn**
When appropriate, both a code for a current burn or corrosion with 7th character "A" or "D" and a burn or corrosion code with 7th character "S" may be assigned on the same record (when both a current burn and sequelae of an old burn exist). Burns and corrosions do not heal at the same rate and a current healing wound may still exist with sequela of a healed burn or corrosion.

See Section I.B.10 Sequela (Late Effects)

9) **Use of an external cause code with burns and corrosions**
An external cause code should be used with burns and corrosions to identify the source and intent of the burn, as well as the place where it occurred.

e. Adverse Effects, Poisoning, Underdosing and Toxic Effects

Codes in categories T36-T65 are combination codes that include the substance that was taken as well as the intent. No additional external cause code is required for poisonings, toxic effects, adverse effects and underdosing codes.

1) Do not code directly from the Table of Drugs

Do not code directly from the Table of Drugs and Chemicals. Always refer back to the Tabular List.

2) Use as many codes as necessary to describe

Use as many codes as necessary to describe completely all drugs, medicinal or biological substances.

3) If the same code would describe the causative agent

If the same code would describe the causative agent for more than one adverse reaction, poisoning, toxic effect or underdosing, assign the code only once.

4) If two or more drugs, medicinal or biological substances

If two or more drugs, medicinal or biological substances are reported, code each individually unless a combination code is listed in the Table of Drugs and Chemicals.

5) The occurrence of drug toxicity is classified in ICD-10-CM as follows:

(a) Adverse Effect

When coding an adverse effect of a drug that has been correctly prescribed and properly administered, assign the appropriate code for the nature of the adverse effect followed by the appropriate code for the adverse effect of the drug (T36-T5Ø). The code for the drug should have a 5th or 6th character "5" (for example T36.ØX5-) Examples of the nature of an adverse effect are tachycardia, delirium, gastrointestinal hemorrhaging, vomiting, hypokalemia, hepatitis, renal failure, or respiratory failure.

(b) Poisoning

When coding a poisoning or reaction to the improper use of a medication (e.g., overdose, wrong substance given or taken in error, wrong route of administration), first assign the appropriate code from categories T36-T5Ø. The poisoning codes have an associated intent as their 5th or 6th character (accidental, intentional self-harm, assault and undetermined. **If the intent of the poisoning is unknown or unspecified, code the intent as accidental intent. The undetermined intent is only for use if the documentation in the record specifies that the intent cannot be determined.** *Use additional code(s) for all manifestations of poisonings.*

If there is also a diagnosis of abuse or dependence of the substance, the abuse or dependence is assigned as an additional code.

Examples of poisoning include:

(i) Error was made in drug prescription

Errors made in drug prescription or in the administration of the drug by provider, nurse, patient, or other person.

(ii) Overdose of a drug intentionally taken

If an overdose of a drug was intentionally taken or administered and resulted in drug toxicity, it would be coded as a poisoning.

(iii) Nonprescribed drug taken with correctly prescribed and properly administered drug

If a nonprescribed drug or medicinal agent was taken in combination with a correctly prescribed and properly administered drug, any drug toxicity or other reaction resulting from the interaction of the two drugs would be classified as a poisoning.

(iv) Interaction of drug(s) and alcohol

When a reaction results from the interaction of a drug(s) and alcohol, this would be classified as poisoning.

See Section I.C.4. if poisoning is the result of insulin pump malfunctions.

(c) Underdosing

Underdosing refers to taking less of a medication than is prescribed by a provider or a manufacturer's instruction. For underdosing, assign the code from categories T36-T5Ø (fifth or sixth character "6").

Codes for underdosing should never be assigned as principal or first-listed codes. If a patient has a relapse or exacerbation of the medical condition for which the drug is prescribed because of the reduction in dose, then the medical condition itself should be coded.

Noncompliance (Z91.12-, Z91.13-) or complication of care (Y63.6-Y63.9) codes are to be used with an underdosing code to indicate intent, if known.

(d) Toxic Effects

When a harmful substance is ingested or comes in contact with a person, this is classified as a toxic effect. The toxic effect codes are in categories T51-T65.

Toxic effect codes have an associated intent: accidental, intentional self-harm, assault and undetermined.

f. Adult and child abuse, neglect and other maltreatment

Sequence first the appropriate code from categories T74.- (Adult and child abuse, neglect and other maltreatment, confirmed) or T76.- (Adult and child abuse, neglect and other maltreatment, suspected) for abuse, neglect and other maltreatment, followed by any accompanying mental health or injury code(s).

If the documentation in the medical record states abuse or neglect it is coded as confirmed (T74.-). It is coded as suspected if it is documented as suspected (T76.-).

For cases of confirmed abuse or neglect an external cause code from the assault section (X92-YØ9) should be added to identify the cause of any physical injuries. A perpetrator code (Y07) should be added when the perpetrator of the abuse is known. For suspected cases of abuse or neglect, do not report external cause or perpetrator code.

If a suspected case of abuse, neglect or mistreatment is ruled out during an encounter code ZØ4.71, Encounter for examination and observation following alleged physical adult abuse, ruled out, or code ZØ4.72, Encounter for examination and observation following alleged child physical abuse, ruled out, should be used, not a code from T76.

If a suspected case of alleged rape or sexual abuse is ruled out during an encounter code ZØ4.41, Encounter for examination and observation following alleged **adult rape** or code ZØ4.42, Encounter for examination and observation following alleged **child** rape, should be used, not a code from T76.

See Section I.C.15. Abuse in a pregnant patient.

g. Complications of care

1) General guidelines for complications of care

(a) Documentation of complications of care

See Section I.B.16. for information on documentation of complications of care.

2) Pain due to medical devices

Pain associated with devices, implants or grafts left in a surgical site (for example painful hip prosthesis) is assigned to the appropriate code(s) found in Chapter 19, Injury, poisoning, and certain other consequences of external causes. Specific codes for pain due to medical devices are found in the T code section of the ICD-10-CM. Use additional code(s) from category G89 to identify acute or chronic pain due to presence of the device, implant or graft (G89.18 or G89.28).

3) Transplant complications

(a) Transplant complications other than kidney

Codes under category T86, Complications of transplanted organs and tissues, are for use for both complications and rejection of transplanted organs. A transplant complication code is only assigned if the complication affects the function of the transplanted organ. Two codes are required to fully describe a transplant complication: the appropriate code from category T86 and a secondary code that identifies the complication.

Pre-existing conditions or conditions that develop after the transplant are not coded as complications unless they affect the function of the transplanted organs.

See I.C.21. for transplant organ removal status

See I.C.2. for malignant neoplasm associated with transplanted organ.

(b) Kidney transplant complications

Patients who have undergone kidney transplant may still have some form of chronic kidney disease (CKD) because the kidney transplant may not fully restore kidney function. Code T86.1- should be assigned for documented complications of a kidney transplant, such as transplant failure or rejection or other transplant complication. Code T86.1- should not be assigned for post kidney transplant patients who have chronic kidney (CKD) unless a transplant complication such as transplant failure or rejection is documented. If the documentation is unclear as to whether the patient has a complication of the transplant, query the provider.

Conditions that affect the function of the transplanted kidney, other than CKD, should be assigned a code from subcategory T86.1, Complications of transplanted organ, Kidney, and a secondary code that identifies the complication.

For patients with CKD following a kidney transplant, but who do not have a complication such as failure or rejection, see section I.C.14. Chronic kidney disease and kidney transplant status.

4) Complication codes that include the external cause

As with certain other T codes, some of the complications of care codes have the external cause included in the code. The code includes the nature of the complication as well as the type of procedure that caused the complication. No external cause code indicating the type of procedure is necessary for these codes.

5) Complications of care codes within the body system chapters

Intraoperative and postprocedural complication codes are found within the body system chapters with codes specific to the organs and structures of that body system. These codes should be sequenced first, followed by a code(s) for the specific complication, if applicable.

20. Chapter 20: External Causes of Morbidity (VØØ-Y99)

The external causes of morbidity codes should never be sequenced as the first-listed or principal diagnosis.

External cause codes are intended to provide data for injury research and evaluation of injury prevention strategies. These codes capture how the injury or health condition happened (cause), the intent (unintentional or accidental; or intentional, such as suicide or assault), the place where the event occurred the activity of the patient at the time of the event, and the person's status (e.g., civilian, military).

There is no national requirement for mandatory ICD-10-CM external cause code reporting. Unless a provider is subject to a state-based external cause code reporting mandate or these codes are required by a particular payer, reporting of ICD-10-CM codes in Chapter 20, External Causes of Morbidity, is not required. In the absence of a mandatory reporting requirement, providers are encouraged to voluntarily report external cause codes, as they provide valuable data for injury research and evaluation of injury prevention strategies.

a. General External Cause Coding Guidelines

1) Used with any code in the range of AØØ.Ø-T88.9, ZØØ-Z99

An external cause code may be used with any code in the range of A00.0-T88.9, Z00-Z99, classification that is a health condition due to an external cause. Though they are most applicable to injuries, they are also valid for use with such things as infections or diseases due to an external source, and other health conditions, such as a heart attack that occurs during strenuous physical activity.

2) External cause code used for length of treatment

Assign the external cause code, with the appropriate 7th character (initial encounter, subsequent encounter or sequela) for each encounter for which the injury or condition is being treated.

Most categories in chapter 20 have a 7th character requirement for each applicable code. Most categories in this chapter have three 7th character values: A, initial encounter, D, subsequent encounter and S, sequela. While the patient may be seen by a new or different provider over the course of treatment for an injury or condition, assignment of the 7th character for external cause should match the 7th character of the code assigned for the associated injury or condition for the encounter.

3) Use the full range of external cause codes

Use the full range of external cause codes to completely describe the cause, the intent, the place of occurrence, and if applicable, the activity of the patient at the time of the event, and the patient's status, for all injuries, and other health conditions due to an external cause.

4) Assign as many external cause codes as necessary

Assign as many external cause codes as necessary to fully explain each cause. If only one external code can be recorded, assign the code most related to the principal diagnosis.

5) The selection of the appropriate external cause code

The selection of the appropriate external cause code is guided by the Alphabetic Index of External Causes and by Inclusion and Exclusion notes in the Tabular List.

6) External cause code can never be a principal diagnosis

An external cause code can never be a principal (first-listed) diagnosis.

7) Combination external cause codes

Certain of the external cause codes are combination codes that identify sequential events that result in an injury, such as a fall which results in striking against an object. The injury may be due to either event or both.

The combination external cause code used should correspond to the sequence of events regardless of which caused the most serious injury.

8) **No external cause code needed in certain circumstances**
No external cause code from Chapter 20 is needed if the external cause and intent are included in a code from another chapter (e.g. T36.ØX1- Poisoning by penicillins, accidental (unintentional)).

b. Place of Occurrence Guideline
Codes from category Y92, Place of occurrence of the external cause, are secondary codes for use after other external cause codes to identify the location of the patient at the time of injury or other condition.

Generally, a place of occurrence code is assigned only once, at the initial encounter for treatment. However, in the rare instance that a new injury occurs during hospitalization, an additional place of occurrence code may be assigned. No 7th characters are used for Y92.

Do not use place of occurrence code Y92.9 if the place is not stated or is not applicable.

c. Activity Code
Assign a code from category Y93, Activity code, to describe the activity of the patient at the time the injury or other health condition occurred.

An activity code is used only once, at the initial encounter for treatment. Only one code from Y93 should be recorded on a medical record.

The activity codes are not applicable to poisonings, adverse effects, misadventures or sequela.

Do not assign Y93.9, Unspecified activity, if the activity is not stated.

A code from category Y93 is appropriate for use with external cause and intent codes if identifying the activity provides additional information about the event.

d. Place of Occurrence, Activity, and Status Codes Used with other External Cause Code
When applicable, place of occurrence, activity, and external cause status codes are sequenced after the main external cause code(s). Regardless of the number of external cause codes assigned, generally there should be only one place of occurrence code, one activity code, and one external cause status code assigned to an encounter. However, in the rare instance that a new injury occurs during hospitalization, an additional place of occurrence code may be assigned.

e. If the Reporting Format Limits the Number of External Cause Codes
If the reporting format limits the number of external cause codes that can be used in reporting clinical data, report the code for the cause/intent most related to the principal diagnosis. If the format permits capture of additional external cause codes, the cause/intent, including medical misadventures, of the additional events should be reported rather than the codes for place, activity, or external status.

f. Multiple External Cause Coding Guidelines
More than one external cause code is required to fully describe the external cause of an illness or injury. The assignment of external cause codes should be sequenced in the following priority:

If two or more events cause separate injuries, an external cause code should be assigned for each cause. The first-listed external cause code will be selected in the following order:

External codes for child and adult abuse take priority over all other external cause codes.

See Section I.C.19., Child and Adult abuse guidelines.

External cause codes for terrorism events take priority over all other external cause codes except child and adult abuse.

External cause codes for cataclysmic events take priority over all other external cause codes except child and adult abuse and terrorism.

External cause codes for transport accidents take priority over all other external cause codes except cataclysmic events, child and adult abuse and terrorism.

Activity and external cause status codes are assigned following all causal (intent) external cause codes.

The first-listed external cause code should correspond to the cause of the most serious diagnosis due to an assault, accident, or self-harm, following the order of hierarchy listed above.

g. Child and Adult Abuse Guideline

Adult and child abuse, neglect and maltreatment are classified as assault. Any of the assault codes may be used to indicate the external cause of any injury resulting from the confirmed abuse.

For confirmed cases of abuse, neglect and maltreatment, when the perpetrator is known, a code from YØ7, Perpetrator of maltreatment and neglect, should accompany any other assault codes.

See Section I.C.19. Adult and child abuse, neglect and other maltreatment

h. Unknown or Undetermined Intent Guideline

If the intent (accident, self-harm, assault) of the cause of an injury or other condition is unknown or unspecified, code the intent as accidental intent. All transport accident categories assume accidental intent.

1) Use of undetermined intent

External cause codes for events of undetermined intent are only for use if the documentation in the record specifies that the intent cannot be determined.

i. Sequelae (Late Effects) of External Cause Guidelines

1) Sequelae external cause codes

Sequela are reported using the external cause code with the 7th character "S" for sequela. These codes should be used with any report of a late effect or sequela resulting from a previous injury.

See Section I.B.10 Sequela (Late Effects)

2) Sequela external cause code with a related current injury

A sequela external cause code should never be used with a related current nature of injury code.

3) Use of sequela external cause codes for subsequent visits

Use a late effect external cause code for subsequent visits when a late effect of the initial injury is being treated. Do not use a late effect external cause code for subsequent visits for follow-up care (e.g., to assess healing, to receive rehabilitative therapy) of the injury when no late effect of the injury has been documented.

j. Terrorism Guidelines

1) Cause of injury identified by the Federal Government (FBI) as terrorism

When the cause of an injury is identified by the Federal Government (FBI) as terrorism, the first-listed external cause code should be a code from category Y38, Terrorism. The definition of terrorism employed by the FBI is found at the inclusion note at the beginning of category Y38. Use additional code for place of occurrence (Y92.-). More than one Y38 code may be assigned if the injury is the result of more than one mechanism of terrorism.

2) **Cause of an injury is suspected to be the result of terrorism**
When the cause of an injury is suspected to be the result of terrorism a code from category Y38 should not be assigned. Suspected cases should be classified as assault.

3) **Code Y38.9, Terrorism, secondary effects**
Assign code Y38.9, Terrorism, secondary effects, for conditions occurring subsequent to the terrorist event. This code should not be assigned for conditions that are due to the initial terrorist act.

It is acceptable to assign code Y38.9 with another code from Y38 if there is an injury due to the initial terrorist event and an injury that is a subsequent result of the terrorist event.

k. External cause status
A code from category Y99, External cause status, should be assigned whenever any other external cause code is assigned for an encounter, including an Activity code, except for the events noted below. Assign a code from category Y99, External cause status, to indicate the work status of the person at the time the event occurred. The status code indicates whether the event occurred during military activity, whether a non-military person was at work, whether an individual including a student or volunteer was involved in a non-work activity at the time of the causal event.

A code from Y99, External cause status, should be assigned, when applicable, with other external cause codes, such as transport accidents and falls. The external cause status codes are not applicable to poisonings, adverse effects, misadventures or late effects.

Do not assign a code from category Y99 if no other external cause codes (cause, activity) are applicable for the encounter.

An external cause status code is used only once, at the initial encounter for treatment. Only one code from Y99 should be recorded on a medical record.

Do not assign code Y99.9, Unspecified external cause status, if the status is not stated.

21. Chapter 21: Factors influencing health status and contact with health services (ZØØ-Z99)
Note: The chapter specific guidelines provide additional information about the use of Z codes for specified encounters.

a. Use of Z codes in any healthcare setting
Z codes are for use in any healthcare setting. Z codes may be used as either a first-listed (principal diagnosis code in the inpatient setting) or secondary code, depending on the circumstances of the encounter. Certain Z codes may only be used as first-listed or principal diagnosis.

b. Z Codes indicate a reason for an encounter
Z codes are not procedure codes. A corresponding procedure code must accompany a Z code to describe any procedure performed.

c. Categories of Z Codes

1) **Contact/Exposure**
Category Z20 indicates contact with, and suspected exposure to, communicable diseases. These codes are for patients who do not show any sign or symptom of a disease but are suspected to have been exposed to it by close personal contact with an infected individual or are in an area where a disease is epidemic.

Category Z77, Other contact with and (suspected) exposures hazardous to health, indicates contact with and suspected exposures hazardous to health.

Contact/exposure codes may be used as a first-listed code to explain an encounter for testing, or, more commonly, as a secondary code to identify a potential risk.

2) Inoculations and vaccinations

Code Z23 is for encounters for inoculations and vaccinations. It indicates that a patient is being seen to receive a prophylactic inoculation against a disease. Procedure codes are required to identify the actual administration of the injection and the type(s) of immunizations given. Code Z23 may be used as a secondary code if the inoculation is given as a routine part of preventive health care, such as a well-baby visit.

3) Status

Status codes indicate that a patient is either a carrier of a disease or has the sequelae or residual of a past disease or condition. This includes such things as the presence of prosthetic or mechanical devices resulting from past treatment. A status code is informative, because the status may affect the course of treatment and its outcome. A status code is distinct from a history code. The history code indicates that the patient no longer has the condition.

A status code should not be used with a diagnosis code from one of the body system chapters, if the diagnosis code includes the information provided by the status code. For example, code Z94.1, Heart transplant status, should not be used with a code from subcategory T86.2, Complications of heart transplant. The status code does not provide additional information. The complication code indicates that the patient is a heart transplant patient.

For encounters for weaning from a mechanical ventilator, assign a code from subcategory J96.1, Chronic respiratory failure, followed by code Z99.11, Dependence on respirator [ventilator] status.

The status Z codes/categories are:

Z14 Genetic carrier

Genetic carrier status indicates that a person carries a gene, associated with a particular disease, which may be passed to offspring who may develop that disease. The person does not have the disease and is not at risk of developing the disease.

Z15 Genetic susceptibility to disease

Genetic susceptibility indicates that a person has a gene that increases the risk of that person developing the disease.

Codes from category Z15 should not be used as principal or first-listed codes. If the patient has the condition to which he/she is susceptible, and that condition is the reason for the encounter, the code for the current condition should be sequenced first. If the patient is being seen for follow-up after completed treatment for this condition, and the condition no longer exists, a follow-up code should be sequenced first, followed by the appropriate personal history and genetic susceptibility codes. If the purpose of the encounter is genetic counseling associated with procreative management, code Z31.5, Encounter for genetic counseling, should be assigned as the first-listed code, followed by a code from category Z15. Additional codes should be assigned for any applicable family or personal history.

Z16 Resistance to antimicrobial drugs

This code indicates that a patient has a condition that is resistant to antimicrobial drug treatment. Sequence the infection code first.

Z17 Estrogen receptor status

Z18 Retained foreign body fragments

Z19 **Hormone sensitivity malignancy status**

Z21 Asymptomatic HIV infection status

This code indicates that a patient has tested positive for HIV but has manifested no signs or symptoms of the disease.

Z22 Carrier of infectious disease

Carrier status indicates that a person harbors the specific organisms of a disease without manifest symptoms and is capable of transmitting the infection.

Z28.3 Underimmunization status

Z33.1 Pregnant state, incidental

This code is a secondary code only for use when the pregnancy is in no way complicating the reason for visit. Otherwise, a code from the obstetric chapter is required.

Z66 Do not resuscitate

This code may be used when it is documented by the provider that a patient is on do not resuscitate status at any time during the stay.

Z67 Blood type

Z68 Body mass index (BMI)

As with all other secondary diagnosis codes, the BMI codes should only be assigned when they meet the definition of a reportable diagnosis (see Section III, Reporting Additional Diagnoses).

Z74.Ø1 Bed confinement status

Z76.82 Awaiting organ transplant status

Z78 Other specified health status

Code Z78.1, Physical restraint status, may be used when it is documented by the provider that a patient has been put in restraints during the current encounter. Please note that this code should not be reported when it is documented by the provider that a patient is temporarily restrained during a procedure.

Z79 Long-term (current) drug therapy

Codes from this category indicate a patient's continuous use of a prescribed drug (including such things as aspirin therapy) for the long-term treatment of a condition or for prophylactic use. It is not for use for patients who have addictions to drugs. This subcategory is not for use of medications for detoxification or maintenance programs to prevent withdrawal symptoms in patients with drug dependence (e.g., methadone maintenance for opiate dependence). Assign the appropriate code for the drug dependence instead.

Assign a code from Z79 if the patient is receiving a medication for an extended period as a prophylactic measure (such as for the prevention of deep vein thrombosis) or as treatment of a chronic condition (such as arthritis) or a disease requiring a lengthy course of treatment (such as cancer). Do not assign a code from category Z79 for medication being administered for a brief period of time to treat an acute illness or injury (such as a course of antibiotics to treat acute bronchitis).

Z88 Allergy status to drugs, medicaments and biological substances

Except: Z88.9, Allergy status to unspecified drugs, medicaments and biological substances status

Z89 Acquired absence of limb

Z9Ø Acquired absence of organs, not elsewhere classified

Z91.Ø- Allergy status, other than to drugs and biological substances

Z92.82 Status post administration of tPA (rtPA) in a different facility within the last 24 hours prior to admission to a current facility

Assign code Z92.82, Status post administration of tPA (rtPA) in a different facility within the last 24 hours prior to admission to current facility, as a secondary diagnosis when a patient is received by transfer into a facility and documentation indicates they were administered tissue plasminogen activator (tPA) within the last 24 hours prior to admission to the current facility.

This guideline applies even if the patient is still receiving the tPA at the time they are received into the current facility.

The appropriate code for the condition for which the tPA was administered (such as cerebrovascular disease or myocardial infarction) should be assigned first.

Code Z92.82 is only applicable to the receiving facility record and not to the transferring facility record.

Z93 Artificial opening status

Z94 Transplanted organ and tissue status

Z95 Presence of cardiac and vascular implants and grafts

Z96 Presence of other functional implants

Z97 Presence of other devices

Z98 Other postprocedural states

Assign code Z98.85, Transplanted organ removal status, to indicate that a transplanted organ has been previously removed. This code should not be assigned for the encounter in which the transplanted organ is removed. The complication necessitating removal of the transplant organ should be assigned for that encounter.

See section I.C19. for information on the coding of organ transplant complications.

Z99 Dependence on enabling machines and devices, not elsewhere classified

Note: Categories Z89-Z9Ø and Z93-Z99 are for use only if there are no complications or malfunctions of the organ or tissue replaced, the amputation site or the equipment on which the patient is dependent.

4) History (of)

There are two types of history Z codes, personal and family. Personal history codes explain a patient's past medical condition that no longer exists and is not receiving any treatment, but that has the potential for recurrence, and therefore may require continued monitoring.

Family history codes are for use when a patient has a family member(s) who has had a particular disease that causes the patient to be at higher risk of also contracting the disease.

Personal history codes may be used in conjunction with follow-up codes and family history codes may be used in conjunction with screening codes to explain the need for a test or procedure. History codes are also acceptable on any medical record regardless of the reason for visit. A history of an illness, even if no longer present, is important information that may alter the type of treatment ordered.

The history Z code categories are:

Z8Ø Family history of primary malignant neoplasm

Z81 Family history of mental and behavioral disorders

Z82 Family history of certain disabilities and chronic diseases (leading to disablement)

Z83 Family history of other specific disorders

Z84 Family history of other conditions
Z85 Personal history of malignant neoplasm
Z86 Personal history of certain other diseases
Z87 Personal history of other diseases and conditions
Z91.4- Personal history of psychological trauma, not elsewhere classified
Z91.5 Personal history of self-harm
Z91.8- Other specified personal risk factors, not elsewhere classified
Exception:
Z91.83, Wandering in diseases classified elsewhere
Z92 Personal history of medical treatment
Except: Z92.Ø, Personal history of contraception
Except: Z92.82, Status post administration of tPA (rtPA) in a different facility within the last 24 hours prior to admission to a current facility

5) Screening

Screening is the testing for disease or disease precursors in seemingly well individuals so that early detection and treatment can be provided for those who test positive for the disease (e.g., screening mammogram).

The testing of a person to rule out or confirm a suspected diagnosis because the patient has some sign or symptom is a diagnostic examination, not a screening. In these cases, the sign or symptom is used to explain the reason for the test.

A screening code may be a first-listed code if the reason for the visit is specifically the screening exam. It may also be used as an additional code if the screening is done during an office visit for other health problems. A screening code is not necessary if the screening is inherent to a routine examination, such as a pap smear done during a routine pelvic examination.

Should a condition be discovered during the screening then the code for the condition may be assigned as an additional diagnosis.

The Z code indicates that a screening exam is planned. A procedure code is required to confirm that the screening was performed.

The screening Z codes/categories:

Z11 Encounter for screening for infectious and parasitic diseases
Z12 Encounter for screening for malignant neoplasms
Z13 Encounter for screening for other diseases and disorders
Except: Z13.9, Encounter for screening, unspecified
Z36 Encounter for antenatal screening for mother

6) Observation

There are **three** observation Z code categories. They are for use in very limited circumstances when a person is being observed for a suspected condition that is ruled out. The observation codes are not for use if an injury or illness or any signs or symptoms related to the suspected condition are present. In such cases the diagnosis/symptom code is used with the corresponding external cause code.

The observation codes are to be used as principal diagnosis only. **The only exception to this is when the principal diagnosis is required to be a code from category Z38, Liveborn infants according to place of birth and type of delivery. Then a code from category ZØ5, Encounter for observation and evaluation of newborn for suspected diseases and conditions ruled out, is sequenced after the Z38 code.** Additional codes may be used in addition to the observation code, but only if they are unrelated to the suspected condition being observed.

Codes from subcategory Z03.7, Encounter for suspected maternal and fetal conditions ruled out, may either be used as a first-listed or as an additional code assignment depending on the case. They are for use in very limited circumstances on a maternal record when an encounter is for a suspected maternal or fetal condition that is ruled out during that encounter (for example, a maternal or fetal condition may be suspected due to an abnormal test result). These codes should not be used when the condition is confirmed. In those cases, the confirmed condition should be coded. In addition, these codes are not for use if an illness or any signs or symptoms related to the suspected condition or problem are present. In such cases the diagnosis/symptom code is used.

Additional codes may be used in addition to the code from subcategory ZØ3.7, but only if they are unrelated to the suspected condition being evaluated.

Codes from subcategory ZØ3.7 may not be used for encounters for antenatal screening of mother. *See Section I.C.21. Screening.*

For encounters for suspected fetal condition that are inconclusive following testing and evaluation, assign the appropriate code from category O35, O36, O4Ø or O41.

The observation Z code categories:

ZØ3	Encounter for medical observation for suspected diseases and conditions ruled out
ZØ4	Encounter for examination and observation for other reasons Except: ZØ4.9, Encounter for examination and observation for unspecified reason
ZØ5	**Encounter for observation and evaluation of newborn for suspected diseases and conditions ruled out**

7) **Aftercare**

Aftercare visit codes cover situations when the initial treatment of a disease has been performed and the patient requires continued care during the healing or recovery phase, or for the long-term consequences of the disease. The aftercare Z code should not be used if treatment is directed at a current, acute disease. The diagnosis code is to be used in these cases. Exceptions to this rule are codes Z51.Ø, Encounter for antineoplastic radiation therapy, and codes from subcategory Z51.1, Encounter for antineoplastic chemotherapy and immunotherapy. These codes are to be first-listed, followed by the diagnosis code when a patient's encounter is solely to receive radiation therapy, chemotherapy, or immunotherapy for the treatment of a neoplasm. If the reason for the encounter is more than one type of antineoplastic therapy, code Z51.Ø and a code from subcategory Z51.1 may be assigned together, in which case one of these codes would be reported as a secondary diagnosis.

The aftercare Z codes should also not be used for aftercare for injuries. For aftercare of an injury, assign the acute injury code with the appropriate 7th character (for subsequent encounter).

The aftercare codes are generally first-listed to explain the specific reason for the encounter. An aftercare code may be used as an additional code when some type of aftercare is provided in addition to the reason for admission and no diagnosis code is applicable. An example of this would be the closure of a colostomy during an encounter for treatment of another condition.

Aftercare codes should be used in conjunction with other aftercare codes or diagnosis codes to provide better detail on the specifics of an aftercare encounter visit, unless otherwise directed by the classification. Should a patient receive multiple types of antineoplastic therapy during the same encounter, code Z51.Ø, Encounter for antineoplastic radiation therapy, and codes from subcategory Z51.1, Encounter for antineoplastic chemotherapy and immunotherapy, may be used together on a record. The sequencing of multiple aftercare codes depends on the circumstances of the encounter.

Certain aftercare Z code categories need a secondary diagnosis code to describe the resolving condition or sequelae**.** For others, the condition is included in the code title.

Additional Z code aftercare category terms include fitting and adjustment, and attention to artificial openings.

Status Z codes may be used with aftercare Z codes to indicate the nature of the aftercare. For example code Z95.1, Presence of aortocoronary bypass graft, may be used with code Z48.812, Encounter for surgical aftercare following surgery on the circulatory system, to indicate the surgery for which the aftercare is being performed. A status code should not be used when the aftercare code indicates the type of status, such as using Z43.Ø, Encounter for attention to tracheostomy, with Z93.Ø, Tracheostomy status.

The aftercare Z category/codes:

Z42	Encounter for plastic and reconstructive surgery following medical procedure or healed injury
Z43	Encounter for attention to artificial openings
Z44	Encounter for fitting and adjustment of external prosthetic device
Z45	Encounter for adjustment and management of implanted device
Z46	Encounter for fitting and adjustment of other devices
Z47	Orthopedic aftercare
Z48	Encounter for other postprocedural aftercare
Z49	Encounter for care involving renal dialysis
Z51	Encounter for other aftercare **and medical care**

8) Follow-up

The follow-up codes are used to explain continuing surveillance following completed treatment of a disease, condition, or injury. They imply that the condition has been fully treated and no longer exists. They should not be confused with aftercare codes, or injury codes with a 7th character for subsequent encounter, that explain ongoing care of a healing condition or its sequelae. Follow-up codes may be used in conjunction with history codes to provide the full picture of the healed condition and its treatment. The follow-up code is sequenced first, followed by the history code.

A follow-up code may be used to explain multiple visits. Should a condition be found to have recurred on the follow-up visit, then the diagnosis code for the condition should be assigned in place of the follow-up code.

The follow-up Z code categories:

ZØ8	Encounter for follow-up examination after completed treatment for malignant neoplasm
ZØ9	Encounter for follow-up examination after completed treatment for conditions other than malignant neoplasm
Z39	Encounter for maternal postpartum care and examination

9) Donor

Codes in category Z52, Donors of organs and tissues, are used for living individuals who are donating blood or other body tissue. These codes are only for individuals donating for others, not for self-donations. They are not used to identify cadaveric donations.

10) Counseling

Counseling Z codes are used when a patient or family member receives assistance in the aftermath of an illness or injury, or when support is required in coping with family or social problems. They are not used in conjunction with a diagnosis code when the counseling component of care is considered integral to standard treatment.

The counseling Z codes/categories:

Z30.Ø-	Encounter for general counseling and advice on contraception
Z31.5	Encounter for genetic counseling
Z31.6-	Encounter for general counseling and advice on procreation
Z32.2	Encounter for childbirth instruction
Z32.3	Encounter for childcare instruction
Z69	Encounter for mental health services for victim and perpetrator of abuse
Z7Ø	Counseling related to sexual attitude, behavior and orientation
Z71	Persons encountering health services for other counseling and medical advice, not elsewhere classified
Z76.81	Expectant mother prebirth pediatrician visit

11) Encounters for Obstetrical and Reproductive Services

See Section I.C.15. Pregnancy, Childbirth, and the Puerperium, for further instruction on the use of these codes.

Z codes for pregnancy are for use in those circumstances when none of the problems or complications included in the codes from the Obstetrics chapter exist (a routine prenatal visit or postpartum care). Codes in category Z34, Encounter for supervision of normal pregnancy, are always first-listed and are not to be used with any other code from the OB chapter.

Codes in category Z3A, Weeks of gestation, may be assigned to provide additional information about the pregnancy. **Category Z3A codes should not be assigned for pregnancies with abortive outcomes (categories OØØ-OØ8), elective termination of pregnancy (code Z33.32), nor for postpartum conditions, as category Z3A is not applicable to these conditions.** The date of the admission should be used to determine weeks of gestation for inpatient admissions that encompass more than one gestational week.

The outcome of delivery, category Z37, should be included on all maternal delivery records. It is always a secondary code. Codes in category Z37 should not be used on the newborn record.

Z codes for family planning (contraceptive) or procreative management and counseling should be included on an obstetric record either during the pregnancy or the postpartum stage, if applicable.

Z codes/categories for obstetrical and reproductive services:

Z3Ø	Encounter for contraceptive management
Z31	Encounter for procreative management
Z32.2	Encounter for childbirth instruction
Z32.3	Encounter for childcare instruction
Z33	Pregnant state
Z34	Encounter for supervision of normal pregnancy
Z36	Encounter for antenatal screening of mother

Z3A	Weeks of gestation
Z37	Outcome of delivery
Z39	Encounter for maternal postpartum care and examination
Z76.81	Expectant mother prebirth pediatrician visit

12) Newborns and Infants

See Section I.C.16. Newborn (Perinatal) Guidelines, for further instruction on the use of these codes.

Newborn Z codes/categories:

Z76.1	Encounter for health supervision and care of foundling
Z00.1-	Encounter for routine child health examination
Z38	Liveborn infants according to place of birth and type of delivery

13) Routine and administrative examinations

The Z codes allow for the description of encounters for routine examinations, such as, a general check-up, or, examinations for administrative purposes, such as, a pre-employment physical. The codes are not to be used if the examination is for diagnosis of a suspected condition or for treatment purposes. In such cases the diagnosis code is used. During a routine exam, should a diagnosis or condition be discovered, it should be coded as an additional code. Pre-existing and chronic conditions and history codes may also be included as additional codes as long as the examination is for administrative purposes and not focused on any particular condition.

Some of the codes for routine health examinations distinguish between "with" and "without" abnormal findings. Code assignment depends on the information that is known at the time the encounter is being coded. For example, if no abnormal findings were found during the examination, but the encounter is being coded before test results are back, it is acceptable to assign the code for "without abnormal findings." When assigning a code for "with abnormal findings," additional code(s) should be assigned to identify the specific abnormal finding(s).

Pre-operative examination and pre-procedural laboratory examination Z codes are for use only in those situations when a patient is being cleared for a procedure or surgery and no treatment is given.

The Z codes/categories for routine and administrative examinations:

Z00	Encounter for general examination without complaint, suspected or reported diagnosis
Z01	Encounter for other special examination without complaint, suspected or reported diagnosis
Z02	Encounter for administrative examination Except: Z02.9, Encounter for administrative examinations, unspecified
Z32.0-	Encounter for pregnancy test

14) Miscellaneous Z codes

The miscellaneous Z codes capture a number of other health care encounters that do not fall into one of the other categories. Certain of these codes identify the reason for the encounter; others are for use as additional codes that provide useful information on circumstances that may affect a patient's care and treatment.

Prophylactic Organ Removal

For encounters specifically for prophylactic removal of an organ (such as prophylactic removal of breasts due to a genetic susceptibility to cancer or a family history of cancer), the principal or first-listed code should be a code from category Z40, Encounter for prophylactic surgery, followed by the appropriate codes to identify the associated risk factor (such as genetic susceptibility or family history).

If the patient has a malignancy of one site and is having prophylactic removal at another site to prevent either a new primary malignancy or metastatic disease, a code for the malignancy should also be assigned in addition to a code from subcategory Z40.0, Encounter for prophylactic surgery for risk factors related to malignant neoplasms. A Z40.0 code should not be assigned if the patient is having organ removal for treatment of a malignancy, such as the removal of the testes for the treatment of prostate cancer.

Miscellaneous Z codes/categories:

Z28	Immunization not carried out Except: Z28.3, Underimmunization status
Z29	**Encounter for other prophylactic measures**
Z40	Encounter for prophylactic surgery
Z41	Encounter for procedures for purposes other than remedying health state Except: Z41.9, Encounter for procedure for purposes other than remedying health state, unspecified
Z53	Persons encountering health services for specific procedures and treatment, not carried out
Z55	Problems related to education and literacy
Z56	Problems related to employment and unemployment
Z57	Occupational exposure to risk factors
Z58	Problems related to physical environment
Z59	Problems related to housing and economic circumstances
Z60	Problems related to social environment
Z62	Problems related to upbringing
Z63	Other problems related to primary support group, including family circumstances
Z64	Problems related to certain psychosocial circumstances
Z65	Problems related to other psychosocial circumstances
Z72	Problems related to lifestyle **Note: These codes should be assigned only when the documentation specifies that the patient has an associated problem**
Z73	Problems related to life management difficulty
Z74	Problems related to care provider dependency Except: Z74.01, Bed confinement status
Z75	Problems related to medical facilities and other health care
Z76.0	Encounter for issue of repeat prescription
Z76.3	Healthy person accompanying sick person
Z76.4	Other boarder to healthcare facility
Z76.5	Malingerer [conscious simulation]
Z91.1-	Patient's noncompliance with medical treatment and regimen
Z91.83	Wandering in diseases classified elsewhere
Z91.89	Other specified personal risk factors, not elsewhere classified

15) Nonspecific Z codes

Certain Z codes are so non-specific, or potentially redundant with other codes in the classification, that there can be little justification for their use in the inpatient setting. Their use in the outpatient setting should be limited to those instances when there is no further documentation to permit more precise coding. Otherwise, any sign or symptom or any other reason for visit that is captured in another code should be used.

Nonspecific Z codes/categories:

Z02.9	Encounter for administrative examinations, unspecified
Z04.9	Encounter for examination and observation for unspecified reason
Z13.9	Encounter for screening, unspecified
Z41.9	Encounter for procedure for purposes other than remedying health state, unspecified
Z52.9	Donor of unspecified organ or tissue
Z86.59	Personal history of other mental and behavioral disorders
Z88.9	Allergy status to unspecified drugs, medicaments and biological substances status
Z92.0	Personal history of contraception

16) Z Codes That May Only be Principal/First-Listed Diagnosis

The following Z codes/categories may only be reported as the principal/first-listed diagnosis, except when there are multiple encounters on the same day and the medical records for the encounters are combined:

Z00	Encounter for general examination without complaint, suspected or reported diagnosis Except: Z00.6
Z01	Encounter for other special examination without complaint, suspected or reported diagnosis
Z02	Encounter for administrative examination
Z03	Encounter for medical observation for suspected diseases and conditions ruled out
Z04	Encounter for examination and observation for other reasons
Z33.2	Encounter for elective termination of pregnancy
Z31.81	Encounter for male factor infertility in female patient
Z31.83	Encounter for assisted reproductive fertility procedure cycle
Z31.84	Encounter for fertility preservation procedure
Z34	Encounter for supervision of normal pregnancy
Z39	Encounter for maternal postpartum care and examination
Z38	Liveborn infants according to place of birth and type of delivery
Z42	Encounter for plastic and reconstructive surgery following medical procedure or healed injury
Z51.0	Encounter for antineoplastic radiation therapy
Z51.1-	Encounter for antineoplastic chemotherapy and immunotherapy
Z52	Donors of organs and tissues Except: Z52.9, Donor of unspecified organ or tissue
Z76.1	Encounter for health supervision and care of foundling
Z76.2	Encounter for health supervision and care of other healthy infant and child
Z99.12	Encounter for respirator [ventilator] dependence during power failure

Section II. Selection of Principal Diagnosis

The circumstances of inpatient admission always govern the selection of principal diagnosis. The principal diagnosis is defined in the Uniform Hospital Discharge Data Set (UHDDS) as "that condition established after study to be chiefly responsible for occasioning the admission of the patient to the hospital for care."

The UHDDS definitions are used by hospitals to report inpatient data elements in a standardized manner. These data elements and their definitions can be found in the July 31, 1985, Federal Register (Vol. 50, No, 147), pp. 31038-40.

Since that time the application of the UHDDS definitions has been expanded to include all non-outpatient settings (acute care, short term, long term care and psychiatric hospitals; home health agencies; rehab facilities; nursing homes, etc). **The UHDDS definitions also apply to hospice services (all levels of care).**

In determining principal diagnosis**,** coding conventions in the ICD-10-CM, the Tabular List and Alphabetic Index take precedence over these official coding guidelines.

(See Section I.A., Conventions for the ICD-10-CM)

The importance of consistent, complete documentation in the medical record cannot be overemphasized. Without such documentation the application of all coding guidelines is a difficult, if not impossible, task.

A. Codes for symptoms, signs, and ill-defined conditions
Codes for symptoms, signs, and ill-defined conditions from Chapter 18 are not to be used as principal diagnosis when a related definitive diagnosis has been established.

B. Two or more interrelated conditions, each potentially meeting the definition for principal diagnosis.
When there are two or more interrelated conditions (such as diseases in the same ICD-10-CM chapter or manifestations characteristically associated with a certain disease) potentially meeting the definition of principal diagnosis, either condition may be sequenced first, unless the circumstances of the admission, the therapy provided, the Tabular List, or the Alphabetic Index indicate otherwise.

C. Two or more diagnoses that equally meet the definition for principal diagnosis
In the unusual instance when two or more diagnoses equally meet the criteria for principal diagnosis as determined by the circumstances of admission, diagnostic workup and/or therapy provided, and the Alphabetic Index, Tabular List, or another coding guidelines does not provide sequencing direction, any one of the diagnoses may be sequenced first.

D. Two or more comparative or contrasting conditions
In those rare instances when two or more contrasting or comparative diagnoses are documented as "either/or" (or similar terminology), they are coded as if the diagnoses were confirmed and the diagnoses are sequenced according to the circumstances of the admission. If no further determination can be made as to which diagnosis should be principal, either diagnosis may be sequenced first.

E. A symptom(s) followed by contrasting/comparative diagnoses
GUIDELINE HAS BEEN DELETED EFFECTIVE OCTOBER 1, 2014

F. Original treatment plan not carried out
Sequence as the principal diagnosis the condition, which after study occasioned the admission to the hospital, even though treatment may not have been carried out due to unforeseen circumstances.

G. Complications of surgery and other medical care
When the admission is for treatment of a complication resulting from surgery or other medical care, the complication code is sequenced as the principal diagnosis. If the complication is classified to the T8Ø-T88 series and the code lacks the necessary specificity in describing the complication, an additional code for the specific complication should be assigned.

H. Uncertain Diagnosis
If the diagnosis documented at the time of discharge is qualified as "probable", "suspected", "likely", "questionable", "possible", or "still to be ruled out", or other similar terms indicating uncertainty, code the condition as if it existed or was established. The bases for these guidelines are the diagnostic workup, arrangements for further workup or observation, and initial therapeutic approach that correspond most closely with the established diagnosis.

Note: This guideline is applicable only to inpatient admissions to short-term, acute, long-term care and psychiatric hospitals.

I. Admission from Observation Unit

1. Admission Following Medical Observation
When a patient is admitted to an observation unit for a medical condition, which either worsens or does not improve, and is subsequently admitted as an inpatient of the same hospital for this same medical condition, the principal diagnosis would be the medical condition which led to the hospital admission.

2 Admission Following Post-Operative Observation
When a patient is admitted to an observation unit to monitor a condition (or complication) that develops following outpatient surgery, and then is subsequently admitted as an inpatient of the same hospital, hospitals should apply the Uniform Hospital Discharge Data Set (UHDDS) definition of principal diagnosis as "that condition established after study to be chiefly responsible for occasioning the admission of the patient to the hospital for care."

J. Admission from Outpatient Surgery
When a patient receives surgery in the hospital's outpatient surgery department and is subsequently admitted for continuing inpatient care at the same hospital, the following guidelines should be followed in selecting the principal diagnosis for the inpatient admission:

- If the reason for the inpatient admission is a complication, assign the complication as the principal diagnosis.
- If no complication, or other condition, is documented as the reason for the inpatient admission, assign the reason for the outpatient surgery as the principal diagnosis.
- If the reason for the inpatient admission is another condition unrelated to the surgery, assign the unrelated condition as the principal diagnosis.

K. Admissions/Encounters for Rehabilitation
When the purpose for the admission/encounter is rehabilitation, sequence first the code for the condition for which the service is being performed. For example, for an admission/encounter for rehabilitation for right-sided dominant hemiplegia following a cerebrovascular infarction, report code I69.351, Hemiplegia and hemiparesis following cerebral infarction affecting right dominant side, as the first-listed or principal diagnosis. If the condition for which the rehabilitation service is no longer present, report the appropriate aftercare code as the first-listed or principal diagnosis. For example, if a patient with severe degenerative osteoarthritis of the hip, underwent hip replacement and

the current encounter/admission is for rehabilitation, report code Z47.1, Aftercare following joint replacement surgery, as the first-listed or principal diagnosis.

See Section I.C.21.c.7, Factors influencing health states and contact with health services, Aftercare.

Section III. Reporting Additional Diagnoses

GENERAL RULES FOR OTHER (ADDITIONAL) DIAGNOSES

For reporting purposes the definition for "other diagnoses" is interpreted as additional conditions that affect patient care in terms of requiring:

clinical evaluation; or
therapeutic treatment; or
diagnostic procedures; or
extended length of hospital stay; or
increased nursing care and/or monitoring.

The UHDDS item #11-b defines Other Diagnoses as "all conditions that coexist at the time of admission, that develop subsequently, or that affect the treatment received and/or the length of stay. Diagnoses that relate to an earlier episode which have no bearing on the current hospital stay are to be excluded." UHDDS definitions apply to inpatients in acute care, short-term, long term care and psychiatric hospital setting. The UHDDS definitions are used by acute care short-term hospitals to report inpatient data elements in a standardized manner. These data elements and their definitions can be found in the July 31, 1985, Federal Register (Vol. 50, No, 147), pp. 31038-40.

Since that time the application of the UHDDS definitions has been expanded to include all non-outpatient settings (acute care, short term, long term care and psychiatric hospitals; home health agencies; rehab facilities; nursing homes, etc). **The UHDDS definitions also apply to hospice services (all levels of care).**

The following guidelines are to be applied in designating "other diagnoses" when neither the Alphabetic Index nor the Tabular List in ICD-10-CM provide direction. The listing of the diagnoses in the patient record is the responsibility of the attending provider.

A. Previous conditions

If the provider has included a diagnosis in the final diagnostic statement, such as the discharge summary or the face sheet, it should ordinarily be coded. Some providers include in the diagnostic statement resolved conditions or diagnoses and status-post procedures from previous admission that have no bearing on the current stay. Such conditions are not to be reported and are coded only if required by hospital policy.

However, history codes (categories Z8Ø-Z87) may be used as secondary codes if the historical condition or family history has an impact on current care or influences treatment.

B. Abnormal findings

Abnormal findings (laboratory, x-ray, pathologic, and other diagnostic results) are not coded and reported unless the provider indicates their clinical significance. If the findings are outside the normal range and the attending provider has ordered other tests to evaluate the condition or prescribed treatment, it is appropriate to ask the provider whether the abnormal finding should be added.

Please note: This differs from the coding practices in the outpatient setting for coding encounters for diagnostic tests that have been interpreted by a provider.

C. Uncertain Diagnosis

If the diagnosis documented at the time of discharge is qualified as "probable", "suspected", "likely", "questionable", "possible", or "still to be ruled out" or other similar terms indicating uncertainty, code the condition as if it existed or was established. The bases for these guidelines are the diagnostic workup, arrangements for further workup or observation, and initial therapeutic approach that correspond most closely with the established diagnosis.

Note: This guideline is applicable only to inpatient admissions to short-term, acute, long-term care and psychiatric hospitals.

Section IV. Diagnostic Coding and Reporting Guidelines for Outpatient Services

These coding guidelines for outpatient diagnoses have been approved for use by hospitals/ providers in coding and reporting hospital-based outpatient services and provider-based office visits. **Guidelines in Section I, Conventions, general coding guidelines and chapter-specific guidelines, should also be applied for outpatient services and office visits.**

Information about the use of certain abbreviations, punctuation, symbols, and other conventions used in the ICD-10-CM Tabular List (code numbers and titles), can be found in Section IA of these guidelines, under "Conventions Used in the Tabular List." Section I.B. contains general guidelines that apply to the entire classification. Section I.C. contains chapter-specific guidelines that correspond to the chapters as they are arranged in the classification. Information about the correct sequence to use in finding a code is also described in Section I.

The terms encounter and visit are often used interchangeably in describing outpatient service contacts and, therefore, appear together in these guidelines without distinguishing one from the other.

Though the conventions and general guidelines apply to all settings, coding guidelines for outpatient and provider reporting of diagnoses will vary in a number of instances from those for inpatient diagnoses, recognizing that:

The Uniform Hospital Discharge Data Set (UHDDS) definition of principal diagnosis **does not apply to hospital-based outpatient services and provider-based office visits.**

Coding guidelines for inconclusive diagnoses (probable, suspected, rule out, etc.) were developed for inpatient reporting and do not apply to outpatients.

A. Selection of first-listed condition

In the outpatient setting, the term first-listed diagnosis is used in lieu of principal diagnosis.

In determining the first-listed diagnosis the coding conventions of ICD-10-CM, as well as the general and disease specific guidelines take precedence over the outpatient guidelines.

Diagnoses often are not established at the time of the initial encounter/visit. It may take two or more visits before the diagnosis is confirmed.

The most critical rule involves beginning the search for the correct code assignment through the Alphabetic Index. Never begin searching initially in the Tabular List as this will lead to coding errors.

1. **Outpatient Surgery**
   When a patient presents for outpatient surgery (same day surgery), code the reason for the surgery as the first-listed diagnosis (reason for the encounter), even if the surgery is not performed due to a contraindication.

2. **Observation Stay**
   When a patient is admitted for observation for a medical condition, assign a code for the medical condition as the first-listed diagnosis.

   When a patient presents for outpatient surgery and develops complications requiring admission to observation, code the reason for the surgery as the first reported diagnosis (reason for the encounter), followed by codes for the complications as secondary diagnoses.

B. Codes from AØØ.Ø through T88.9, ZØØ-Z99
The appropriate code(s) from AØØ.Ø through T88.9, ZØØ-Z99 must be used to identify diagnoses, symptoms, conditions, problems, complaints, or other reason(s) for the encounter/visit.

C. Accurate reporting of ICD-10-CM diagnosis codes
For accurate reporting of ICD-10-CM diagnosis codes, the documentation should describe the patient's condition, using terminology which includes specific diagnoses as well as symptoms, problems, or reasons for the encounter. There are ICD-10-CM codes to describe all of these.

D. Codes that describe symptoms and signs
Codes that describe symptoms and signs, as opposed to diagnoses, are acceptable for reporting purposes when a diagnosis has not been established (confirmed) by the provider. Chapter 18 of ICD-10-CM, Symptoms, Signs, and Abnormal Clinical and Laboratory Findings Not Elsewhere Classified (codes RØØ-R99) contain many, but not all codes for symptoms.

E. Encounters for circumstances other than a disease or injury
ICD-10-CM provides codes to deal with encounters for circumstances other than a disease or injury. The Factors Influencing Health Status and Contact with Health Services codes (ZØØ-Z99) are provided to deal with occasions when circumstances other than a disease or injury are recorded as diagnosis or problems.

See Section I.C.21. Factors influencing health status and contact with health services.

F. Level of Detail in Coding

1. **ICD-10-CM codes with 3, 4, 5, 6 or 7 characters**
   ICD-10-CM is composed of codes with 3, 4, 5, 6 or 7 characters. Codes with three characters are included in ICD-10-CM as the heading of a category of codes that may be further subdivided by the use of fourth, fifth, sixth or seventh characters to provide greater specificity.

2. **Use of full number of characters required for a code**
   A three-character code is to be used only if it is not further subdivided. A code is invalid if it has not been coded to the full number of characters required for that code, including the 7th character, if applicable.

G. ICD-10-CM code for the diagnosis, condition, problem, or other reason for encounter/visit
List first the ICD-10-CM code for the diagnosis, condition, problem, or other reason for encounter/visit shown in the medical record to be chiefly responsible for the services provided. List additional codes that describe any coexisting conditions. In some cases the first-listed diagnosis may be a symptom when a diagnosis has not been established (confirmed) by the physician.

H. Uncertain diagnosis
Do not code diagnoses documented as "probable", "suspected," "questionable," "rule out," or "working diagnosis" or other similar terms indicating uncertainty. Rather, code the condition(s) to the highest degree of certainty for that encounter/visit, such as symptoms, signs, abnormal test results, or other reason for the visit.

Please note: This differs from the coding practices used by short-term, acute care, long-term care and psychiatric hospitals.

I. Chronic diseases
Chronic diseases treated on an ongoing basis may be coded and reported as many times as the patient receives treatment and care for the condition(s)

J. Code all documented conditions that coexist
Code all documented conditions that coexist at the time of the encounter/visit, and require or affect patient care treatment or management. Do not code conditions that were previously treated and no longer exist. However, history codes (categories Z8Ø-Z87) may be used as secondary codes if the historical condition or family history has an impact on current care or influences treatment.

K. Patients receiving diagnostic services only
For patients receiving diagnostic services only during an encounter/visit, sequence first the diagnosis, condition, problem, or other reason for encounter/visit shown in the medical record to be chiefly responsible for the outpatient services provided during the encounter/visit. Codes for other diagnoses (e.g., chronic conditions) may be sequenced as additional diagnoses.

For encounters for routine laboratory/radiology testing in the absence of any signs, symptoms, or associated diagnosis, assign ZØ1.89, Encounter for other specified special examinations. If routine testing is performed during the same encounter as a test to evaluate a sign, symptom, or diagnosis, it is appropriate to assign both the Z code and the code describing the reason for the non-routine test.

For outpatient encounters for diagnostic tests that have been interpreted by a physician, and the final report is available at the time of coding, code any confirmed or definitive diagnosis(es) documented in the interpretation. Do not code related signs and symptoms as additional diagnoses.

Please note: This differs from the coding practice in the hospital inpatient setting regarding abnormal findings on test results.

L. Patients receiving therapeutic services only
For patients receiving therapeutic services only during an encounter/visit, sequence first the diagnosis, condition, problem, or other reason for encounter/visit shown in the medical record to be chiefly responsible for the outpatient services provided during the encounter/visit. Codes for other diagnoses (e.g., chronic conditions) may be sequenced as additional diagnoses.

The only exception to this rule is that when the primary reason for the admission/encounter is chemotherapy or radiation therapy, the appropriate Z code for the service is listed first, and the diagnosis or problem for which the service is being performed listed second.

M. Patients receiving preoperative evaluations only
For patients receiving preoperative evaluations only, sequence first a code from subcategory ZØ1.81, Encounter for pre-procedural examinations, to describe the pre-op consultations. Assign a code for the condition to describe the reason for the surgery as an additional diagnosis. Code also any findings related to the pre-op evaluation.

N. Ambulatory surgery
For ambulatory surgery, code the diagnosis for which the surgery was performed. If the postoperative diagnosis is known to be different from the

preoperative diagnosis at the time the diagnosis is confirmed, select the postoperative diagnosis for coding, since it is the most definitive.

O. Routine outpatient prenatal visits
See Section I.C.15. Routine outpatient prenatal visits.

P. Encounters for general medical examinations with abnormal findings
The subcategories for encounters for general medical examinations, ZØØ.Ø-, provide codes for with and without abnormal findings. Should a general medical examination result in an abnormal finding, the code for general medical examination with abnormal finding should be assigned as the first-listed diagnosis. **An examination with abnormal findings refers to a condition/diagnosis that is newly identified or a change in severity of a chronic condition (such as uncontrolled hypertension, or an acute exacerbation of chronic obstructive pulmonary disease) during a routine physical examination.** A secondary code for the abnormal finding should also be coded.

Q. Encounters for routine health screenings
See Section I.C.21. Factors influencing health status and contact with health services, Screening

Appendix I. Present on Admission Reporting Guidelines

Introduction

These guidelines are to be used as a supplement to the *ICD-10-CM Official Guidelines for Coding and Reporting* to facilitate the assignment of the Present on Admission (POA) indicator for each diagnosis and external cause of injury code reported on claim forms (UB-04 and 837 Institutional).

These guidelines are not intended to replace any guidelines in the main body of the *ICD-10-CM Official Guidelines for Coding and Reporting*. The POA guidelines are not intended to provide guidance on when a condition should be coded, but rather, how to apply the POA indicator to the final set of diagnosis codes that have been assigned in accordance with Sections I, II, and III of the official coding guidelines. Subsequent to the assignment of the ICD-10-CM codes, the POA indicator should then be assigned to those conditions that have been coded.

As stated in the Introduction to the ICD-10-CM Official Guidelines for Coding and Reporting, a joint effort between the healthcare provider and the coder is essential to achieve complete and accurate documentation, code assignment, and reporting of diagnoses and procedures. The importance of consistent, complete documentation in the medical record cannot be overemphasized. Medical record documentation from any provider involved in the care and treatment of the patient may be used to support the determination of whether a condition was present on admission or not. In the context of the official coding guidelines, the term "provider" means a physician or any qualified healthcare practitioner who is legally accountable for establishing the patient's diagnosis.

These guidelines are not a substitute for the provider's clinical judgment as to the determination of whether a condition was/was not present on admission. The provider should be queried regarding issues related to the linking of signs/symptoms, timing of test results, and the timing of findings.

Please see the CDC website for the detailed list of ICD-10-CM codes that do not require the use of a POA indicator (ftp://ftp.cdc.gov/pub/Health_Statistics/NCHS/Publications/ICD10CM/2017/). The conditions on this exempt list represent categories

and/or codes for circumstances regarding the healthcare encounter or factors influencing health status that do not represent a current disease or injury or are always present on admission.

General Reporting Requirements

All claims involving inpatient admissions to general acute care hospitals or other facilities that are subject to a law or regulation mandating collection of present on admission information.

Present on admission is defined as present at the time the order for inpatient admission occurs -- conditions that develop during an outpatient encounter, including emergency department, observation, or outpatient surgery, are considered as present on admission.

POA indicator is assigned to principal and secondary diagnoses (as defined in Section II of the Official Guidelines for Coding and Reporting) and the external cause of injury codes.

Issues related to inconsistent, missing, conflicting or unclear documentation must still be resolved by the provider.

If a condition would not be coded and reported based on UHDDS definitions and current official coding guidelines, then the POA indicator would not be reported.

Reporting Options

Y - Yes

N - No

U - Unknown

W – Clinically undetermined

Unreported/Not used – (Exempt from POA reporting)

Reporting Definitions

Y = present at the time of inpatient admission

N = not present at the time of inpatient admission

U = documentation is insufficient to determine if condition is present on admission

W = provider is unable to clinically determine whether condition was present on admission or not

Timeframe for POA Identification and Documentation

There is no required timeframe as to when a provider (per the definition of "provider" used in these guidelines) must identify or document a condition to be present on admission. In some clinical situations, it may not be possible for a provider to make a definitive diagnosis (or a condition may not be recognized or reported by the patient) for a period of time after admission. In some cases it may be several days before the provider arrives at a definitive diagnosis. This does not mean that the condition was not present on admission. Determination of whether the condition was present on admission or not will be based on the applicable POA guideline as identified in this document, or on the provider's best clinical judgment.

If at the time of code assignment the documentation is unclear as to whether a condition was present on admission or not, it is appropriate to query the provider for clarification.

Assigning the POA Indicator

Condition is on the "Exempt from Reporting" list

Leave the "present on admission" field blank if the condition is on the list of ICD-10-CM codes for which this field is not applicable. This is the only circumstance in which the field may be left blank.

POA Explicitly Documented

Assign Y for any condition the provider explicitly documents as being present on admission.

Assign N for any condition the provider explicitly documents as not present at the time of admission.

Conditions diagnosed prior to inpatient admission

Assign "Y" for conditions that were diagnosed prior to admission (example: hypertension, diabetes mellitus, asthma)

Conditions diagnosed during the admission but clearly present before admission

Assign "Y" for conditions diagnosed during the admission that were clearly present but not diagnosed until after admission occurred.

Diagnoses subsequently confirmed after admission are considered present on admission if at the time of admission they are documented as suspected, possible, rule out, differential diagnosis, or constitute an underlying cause of a symptom that is present at the time of admission.

Condition develops during outpatient encounter prior to inpatient admission

Assign Y for any condition that develops during an outpatient encounter prior to a written order for inpatient admission.

Documentation does not indicate whether condition was present on admission

Assign "U" when the medical record documentation is unclear as to whether the condition was present on admission. "U" should not be routinely assigned and used only in very limited circumstances. Coders are encouraged to query the providers when the documentation is unclear.

Documentation states that it cannot be determined whether the condition was or was not present on admission

Assign "W" when the medical record documentation indicates that it cannot be clinically determined whether or not the condition was present on admission.

Chronic condition with acute exacerbation during the admission

If a single code identifies both the chronic condition and the acute exacerbation, see POA guidelines pertaining to **codes that contain multiple clinical concepts.**

If a single code only identifies the chronic condition and not the acute exacerbation (e.g., acute exacerbation of chronic leukemia), assign "Y."

Conditions documented as possible, probable, suspected, or rule out at the time of discharge

If the final diagnosis contains a possible, probable, suspected, or rule out diagnosis, and this diagnosis was based on signs, symptoms or clinical findings suspected at the time of inpatient admission, assign "Y."

If the final diagnosis contains a possible, probable, suspected, or rule out diagnosis, and this diagnosis was based on signs, symptoms or clinical findings that were not present on admission, assign "N".

Conditions documented as impending or threatened at the time of discharge

If the final diagnosis contains an impending or threatened diagnosis, and this diagnosis is based on symptoms or clinical findings that were present on admission, assign "Y".

If the final diagnosis contains an impending or threatened diagnosis, and this diagnosis is based on symptoms or clinical findings that were not present on admission, assign "N".

Acute and Chronic Conditions

Assign "Y" for acute conditions that are present at time of admission and N for acute conditions that are not present at time of admission.

Assign "Y" for chronic conditions, even though the condition may not be diagnosed until after admission.

If a single code identifies both an acute and chronic condition, see the POA guidelines for codes **that contain multiple clinical concepts**.

Codes **That Contain Multiple Clinical Concepts**

Assign "N" if **at least** one **of the clinical concepts included in the** code was not present on admission (e.g., COPD with acute exacerbation and the exacerbation was not present on admission; gastric ulcer that does not start bleeding until after admission; asthma patient develops status asthmaticus after admission).

Assign "Y" if all of the **clinical concepts included in the code** were present on admission (e.g., **duodenal ulcer that perforates prior to admission**).

For infection codes that include the causal organism, assign "Y" if the infection (or signs of the infection) **were** present on admission, even though the culture results may not be known until after admission (e.g., patient is admitted with pneumonia and the provider documents Pseudomonas as the causal organism a few days later).

Same Diagnosis Code for Two or More Conditions

When the same ICD-10-CM diagnosis code applies to two or more conditions during the same encounter (e.g. two separate conditions classified to the same ICD-10-CM diagnosis code):

Assign "Y" if all conditions represented by the single ICD-10-CM code were present on admission (e.g. bilateral unspecified age-related cataracts).

Assign "N" if any of the conditions represented by the single ICD-10-CM code was not present on admission (e.g. traumatic secondary and recurrent hemorrhage and seroma is assigned to a single code T79.2, but only one of the conditions was present on admission).

Obstetrical conditions

Whether or not the patient delivers during the current hospitalization does not affect assignment of the POA indicator. The determining factor for POA assignment is whether the pregnancy complication or obstetrical condition described by the code was present at the time of admission or not.

If the pregnancy complication or obstetrical condition was present on admission (e.g., patient admitted in preterm labor), assign "Y".

If the pregnancy complication or obstetrical condition was not present on admission (e.g., 2nd degree laceration during delivery, postpartum hemorrhage that occurred during current hospitalization, fetal distress develops after admission), assign "N".

If the obstetrical code includes more than one diagnosis and any of the diagnoses identified by the code were not present on admission assign "N".

(e.g., Category O11, Pre-existing hypertension with pre-eclampsia)

Perinatal conditions

Newborns are not considered to be admitted until after birth. Therefore, any condition present at birth or that developed in utero is considered present at admission and should be assigned "Y". This includes conditions that occur during delivery (e.g., injury during delivery, meconium aspiration, exposure to streptococcus B in the vaginal canal).

Congenital conditions and anomalies

Assign "Y" for congenital conditions and anomalies except for categories QØØ-Q99, Congenital anomalies, which are on the exempt list. Congenital conditions are always considered present on admission.

External cause of injury codes

Assign "Y" for any external cause code representing an external cause of morbidity that occurred prior to inpatient admission (e.g., patient fell out of bed at home, patient fell out of bed in emergency room prior to admission)

Assign "N" for any external cause code representing an external cause of morbidity that occurred during inpatient hospitalization (e.g., patient fell out of hospital bed during hospital stay, patient experienced an adverse reaction to a medication administered after inpatient admission)

Appendix 3: Mapping Tables

Chapter 1: Infectious and Parasitic Diseases

Sepsis (Systemic, Generalized, Complication)

ICD-9-CM Terminology	Category	ICD-10-CM Terminology	Category
Enterobacter Septicemia	**Ø38**	(Other) Gram-negative Sepsis (Enterobacter)	**A41**
Escherichia coli Septicemia	**Ø38**	Escherichia coli Sepsis	**A41**
Friedlander's Sepsis (gram-negative)	**Ø38**	(Other) Gram-negative organism (Klebsiella) (Friedlander's) Sepsis	**A41**
Gram-negative Septicemia (unspecified)	**Ø38**	Gram-negative Sepsis (unspecified)	**A41**
Proteus Septicemia	**Ø38**	(Other) Gram-negative Sepsis	**A41**
Pseudomonas Septicemia	**Ø38**	(Other) Gram-negative Sepsis	**A41**
Staphylococcal Septicemia	**Ø38**	Staphylococcus Sepsis	**A41**
Streptococcal (Group B) Septicemia	**Ø38**	Streptococcus, group B Sepsis	**A4Ø**
Neonatal Streptococcus group B Septicemia	**771, Ø38**	Streptococcus, neonatal, group B	**P36**
Pneumococcal Septicemia (streptococcus pneumoniae)	**Ø38**	Pneumococcal Sepsis (streptococcus pneumoniae)	**A4Ø**
Septicemia	**Ø38**	Sepsis	**A4Ø, A41**
Viral Septicemia	**Ø79**	Viral agent as cause of diseases classified elsewhere	**A41 B97**
Disseminated Candidiasis	**112**	Candidal Sepsis	**B37**
Sepsis	**995**	Sepsis	**A41**
Severe Sepsis	**995**	Severe Sepsis	**R65**
Newborn Sepsis	**771**	Newborn Sepsis	**P36**
Complication due to surgery	**998**	Complication due to surgery	**T81**
Complication tracheostomy/stoma	**519**	Complication tracheostomy stoma	**J95**
Resulting from infusion, injection, transfusion, vaccination	**999**	Resulting from infusion, injection, transfusion, vaccination	**T8Ø, T88**
Resulting from insemination	**999**	Resulting from insemination	**T8Ø**
Complication due to any device, implant and graft	**996**	Complication due to any device, implant and graft	**T82, T83, T84, T85, T86**
Complication of pregnancy, labor, postpartum, postabortal	**639, 659, 67Ø**	Complication of following pregnancy, labor, postpartum, postabortal	**OØ3, OØ4, OØ7, OØ8, O75, O85**

Gastroenteritis (Viral, Bacterial, Protozoan)

ICD-9-CM Terminology	Category	ICD-10-CM Terminology	Category
Adenovirus Enteritis	**ØØ8**	Adenovirus Enteritis	**AØ8**
Astrovirus Enteritis	**ØØ8**	Astrovirus Enteritis	**AØ8**
Campylobacter Enteritis	**ØØ8**	Enteritis, infectious due to Campylobacter	**AØ4**
Clostridium difficile Enteritis	**ØØ8**	Clostridium difficile Enteritis	**AØ4**
Cryptosporidiosis	**ØØ7**	Gastroenteritis due to Cryptosporidium	**AØ7**
Enteritis, Escherichia coli	**ØØ8**	Enteritis, infectious due to Escherichia coli	**AØ4**
Giardial Enteritis	**ØØ7**	Giardial Enteritis	**AØ7**
Infectious Gastroenteritis (presumed)	**ØØ9**	Infectious Enteritis NOS	**AØ9**
Enteritis due to Norovirus	**ØØ8**	Norovirus Enteritis	**AØ8**
Enteritis Norwalk-like agent	**ØØ8**	Gastroenteropathy, acute, due to Norwalk agent	**AØ8**
Enteritis, due to rotavirus	**ØØ8**	Rotaviral Gastroenteritis	**AØ8**
Salmonella Gastroenteritis	**ØØ3**	Salmonella Gastroenteritis	**AØ2**
Shigella Enteritis	**ØØ4**	Shigella Infection	**AØ3**
Staphylococcal Enteritis	**ØØ8**	Staphylococcal Enteritis	**AØ4**
Viral Gastroenteritis, unspecified	**ØØ8**	Viral Gastroenteritis, NEC	**AØ8**

Foodborne Intoxication (and Infection)

ICD-9-CM Terminology	Category	ICD-10-CM Terminology	Category
Food Poisoning (unspecified)	**ØØ5**	Foodborne Intoxication (unspecified)	**AØ5**
Botulism (Clostridium) Food Poisoning	**ØØ5**	Foodborne Intoxication, due to Clostridium botulism (classical)	**AØ5**
Intestinal infection due to Campylobacter	**ØØ8**	Campylobacter enteritis	**AØ4**
Clostridium difficile Food Poisoning	**ØØ5**	Enteritis, Clostridium difficile (foodborne intoxication)	**AØ4**
E. coli enteritis	**ØØ8**	Enteritis, infectious, due to Escherichia coli	**AØ4**
Enteritis due to Norovirus	**ØØ8**	Norovirus Enteritis	**AØ8**
Salmonella Food Poisoning	**ØØ3**	Foodborne Intoxication, due to Salmonella with gastroenteritis	**AØ2**
Staphylococcal Food Poisoning	**ØØ5**	Staphylococcal Foodborne Intoxication	**AØ5**
Listeriosis infection	**Ø27, ØØ8**	Listeria, other forms	**A32**

Human Immunodeficiency Virus (HIV) Disease (AIDS)

ICD-9-CM Terminology	Category	ICD-10-CM Terminology	Category
Human Immunodeficiency virus (symptomatic)	**Ø42**	Human Immunodeficiency virus disease	**B2Ø**

Chapter 2: Neoplasms

Malignant Neoplasm of Liver and Intrahepatic Bile Ducts

ICD-9-CM Terminology	Category	ICD-10-CM Terminology	Category
Malignant neoplasm of liver primary	**155**	[Diagnoses specify type:] Liver cell carcinoma Hepatoblastoma Angiosarcoma of liver Other sarcoma of liver Other specified carcinomas of liver Malignant neoplasm of liver, primary, unspecified as to type	**C22**

Malignant Neoplasm of Breast

ICD-9-CM Terminology	Category	ICD-10-CM Terminology	Category
Malignant neoplasm of (female) breast (anatomic site/quadrant)	**174**	Malignant neoplasm of (female) breast (anatomic site/quadrant): Laterality included: Right Left Unspecified	**C5Ø**
Malignant neoplasm of (male) breast: Nipple and areola Other & unspecified sites	**175**	Malignant neoplasm of male breast (aligned with female anatomic site classifications and laterality: Central portion Quadrant Axillary tail Overlapping sites Right/Left/Unspecified	**C5Ø**
Carcinoma in situ of breast	**233**	Carcinoma in situ of breast	**DØ5**

Malignant Neoplasm of Unspecified Site

ICD-9-CM Terminology	Category	ICD-10-CM Terminology	Category
Malignant neoplasm, primary, secondary, disseminated	**199**	Malignant neoplasm, primary, secondary, disseminated	**C79, C8Ø**
Carcinoma in situ, unspecified	**234**	Carcinoma in situ, unspecified	**DØ9**
Other malignant neoplasm of unspecified site	**199**	Malignant (primary) neoplasm, unspecified	**C8Ø**

Chapter 3: Diseases of the Blood & Blood-Forming Organs and Certain Disorders Involving the Immune Mechanism

Iron Deficiency Anemia

ICD-9-CM Terminology	Category	ICD-10-CM Terminology	Category
Iron deficiency anemia	**280**	Iron deficiency anemia	**D50**

Acquired Hemolytic Anemia

ICD-9-CM Terminology	Category	ICD-10-CM Terminology	Category
Autoimmune/ non-autoimmune hemolytic anemias	**283**	Drug-induced autoimmune hemolytic anemia Other autoimmune/nonautoimmune hemolytic anemia	**D59**
Hemoglobinuria due to hemolysis from external causes	**283**	Paroxysmal nocturnal hemoglobinuria Other acquired hemolytic anemias	**D59**

Postoperative Anemia

ICD-9-CM Terminology	Category	ICD-10-CM Terminology	Category
Postoperative, due to (acute) blood loss anemia	**285**	Postoperative, due to (acute) blood loss anemia	**D62**
Postoperative, due to chronic blood loss anemia	**280**	Postoperative, due to chronic blood loss anemia	**D50**

Chapter 4: Endocrine, Nutritional and Metabolic Diseases

Diabetes Type 2

ICD-9-CM Terminology	Category	ICD-10-CM Terminology	Category
Diabetes (by type) with complications/ manifestations:	**Example Type II:**	[Combination codes eliminate or reduce multiple coding, such as:]	**Example Type II:**
Renal	**25Ø.4X**	Type 2 DM w/ nephropathy	**E11**
ophthalmic	**25Ø.5X**	Type 2 DM w/ retinopathy/macular edema	**E11**
Neurological	**25Ø.6X**	Type 2 DM w/ diabetic polyneuropathy	**E11**
Peripheral circulatory	**25Ø.7X**	Type 2 DM w/ angiopathy/gangrene	**E11**
Other	**25Ø.8X**	Type 2 DM w/diabetic dermatitis	**E11**
(Use additional code to specify manifestation)		(assign appropriate 4th–6th characters)	
		Instructional notes prompt necessity of additional codes	

Diabetes Secondary, Other Specified or Due to Underlying Condition

ICD-9-CM Terminology	Category	ICD-10-CM Terminology	Category
Secondary DM w/o complication controlled or unspecified	**249**	Diabetes due to underlying condition w/o complications	**EØ8**
		Drug or chemical induced diabetes mellitus without complications	**EØ9**
		Other specified diabetes mellitus without complications	**E13**
Secondary diabetes w/o complication uncontrolled	**249**	Diabetes due to underlying condition w/ hyperglycemia	**EØ8**
		Drug or chemical induced diabetes w/ hyperglycemia	**EØ9**

Diabetes Type 1

ICD-9-CM Terminology	Category	ICD-10-CM Terminology	Category
Diabetes w/o complication type I (juvenile) controlled	**25Ø**	Type 1 diabetes mellitus without complications	**E1Ø**
Diabetes w/o complication type I (juvenile) uncontrolled	**25Ø**	Type 1 diabetes with hyperglycemia	**E1Ø**

Chapter 5: Mental, Behavioral and Neurodevelopmental Disorders

Alcohol, Drug, Nicotine and Substance Abuse, Dependence, or Use

ICD-9-CM Terminology	Category	ICD-10-CM Terminology	Category
Alcoholism, dependent	**303**	Dependence, alcohol	**F10**
Abuse, alcohol, non-dependent	**305**	Abuse, alcohol (non-dependent)	**F10**
Use of nonprescribed drugs (alcohol)	**305**	Use, alcohol	**F10**
Dependence, drug (specified drug or category)	**304**	Dependence, drug (specified drug or category)	**F11, F12, F13, F14, F15, F16, F18, F19**
Abuse, drugs, nondependent	**305**	Abuse, drug (nondependent)	**F11, F12, F13, F14, F15, F16, F18, F19**
Use (of), (specified drug or category)	**305**	Use of (specified drug or category)	**F11, F12, F13, F14, F15, F16, F18, F19**
Dependence, nicotine	**305**	Dependence, drug, nicotine	**F17**
Abuse, tobacco	**305**	Dependence, drug, nicotine	**F17**
Use of, nonprescribed drugs (nicotine)	**305**	Use (of), tobacco, with dependence (nicotine)	**F17**
Dependence, caffeine	**304**	Dependence, drug, stimulant NEC (caffeine)	**F15**
Abuse, drugs, caffeine	**305**	Abuse, drug, stimulant NEC	**F15**
Use of, nonprescribed drugs (caffeine)	**305**	Use, stimulant NEC(caffeine)	**F15**
Dependence, inhalant	**304**	Dependence, drug, inhalant	**F18**
Abuse, drugs, inhalant	**305**	Abuse, drug, inhalant	**F18**
Use, substance	**305**	Use of, inhalants	**F18**

Major Depression

ICD-9-CM Terminology	Category	ICD-10-CM Terminology	Category
Depression, major, recurrent episode	**296**	Disorder, depressive, recurrent	**F33**
Depression, major, single episode	**296**	Depression, major, single episode	**F32**
Depression, major, severe, specified as with psychotic behavior	**296**	Depression, major, with psychotic symptoms	**F32**

Chapter 6: Diseases of the Nervous System

Encephalopathy

ICD-9-CM Terminology	Category	ICD-10-CM Terminology	Category
Anoxic encephalopathy	**348**	Anoxic encephalopathy	**G93**
Metabolic encephalopathy	**348**	Metabolic encephalopathy	**G93**
Septic encephalopathy		Septic encephalopathy	
Toxic encephalitis and encephalomyelitis, myelitis	**323**	Toxic encephalitis, myelitis	**G92**
Toxic encephalopathy	**349**	Toxic encephalopathy	**G92**
Toxic metabolic encephalopathy	**349**	Toxic metabolic encephalopathy	**G92**
Other encephalopathy	**348**	Other encephalopathy	**G93**
Encephalopathy, unspecified	**348**	Encephalopathy, unspecified	**G93**

Epilepsy and Seizure (Disorder, Recurrent)

ICD-9-CM Terminology	Category	ICD-10-CM Terminology	Category
Convulsions: (as) Specified as: Epileptic	 **345**	Convulsions (as): Specified as: Epileptic	 **G40**
Seizure disorder Seizure, recurrent	**345** **345**	Seizure disorder Seizure, recurrent	**G40** **G40**
Epilepsy (type): w/ or w/o intractable epilepsy	**345**	Epilepsy (type): w/ or w/o intractable epilepsy ALSO: w/ or w/o status epilepticus	**G40**
Generalized epilepsy: w/ or w/o intractable epilepsy Nonconvulsive Convulsive Petit mal Grand mal	**345**	Generalized idiopathic epilepsy: Intractable/not intractable w/ or w/o status epilepticus	**G40**
Localization-related (focal) (partial) epilepsy and epileptic syndromes with simple partial seizures: w/ intractable epilepsy w/o intractable epilepsy	**345**	Localization-related (focal) (partial) *idiopathic* epilepsy and epileptic syndromes with seizures of localized onset Localization-related (focal) (partial) *symptomatic* epilepsy and epileptic syndromes with simple partial seizures	**G40** **G40**
Localization-related (focal) (partial) epilepsy and epileptic syndromes with complex partial seizures w/ intractable epilepsy w/o intractable epilepsy	**345**	Localization-related (focal) (partial) symptomatic epilepsy and epilepsy syndromes with complex partial seizures: Not intractable w/ or w/o status epilepticus Intractable w/ or w/o status epilepticus	**G40**

Migraine

ICD-9-CM Terminology	Category	ICD-10-CM Terminology	Category
Migraine (type): Intractable Not intractable w/ status migrainosus w/o status migrainosus	**346**	Migraine (type): Intractable Not intractable w/ status migrainosus w/o status migrainosus	**G43**
Variants of migraine, not elsewhere classified Intractable Not intractable w/ status migrainosus w/o status migrainosus	**346**	[Diagnoses specify type as:] Other Cyclical Ophthalmoplegic Periodic headache syndromes (adult/child) Abdominal [Also status and severity:] Intractable Not intractable w/ status migrainosus w/o status migrainosus	**G43**

Transient Cerebral Ischemia

ICD-9-CM Terminology	Category	ICD-10-CM Terminology	Category
Other/unspecified transient cerebral ischemia	**435**	[Specify affected anatomic site:] Carotid artery syndrome Multiple/bilateral precerebral artery syndrome Middle cerebral artery syndrome Anterior cerebral artery syndrome Posterior cerebral artery syndrome	 **G45** **G45** **G46** **G46** **G46**
Other Ill/defined cerebrovascular disease	**437**	Brain stem stroke syndrome Cerebellar stroke syndrome Pure motor lacunar syndrome Pure sensory lacunar syndrome	**G46** **G46** **G46** **G46**

Chapter 7: Diseases of the Eye and Adnexa

ICD-9-CM Terminology	Category	ICD-10-CM Terminology	Category
Senile	**Terminology**	Age-related	**Terminology**
Glaucoma: Use additional code for stage	**365**	Glaucoma: [Diagnoses specify type/laterality] Stage included in 7th character	**H4Ø** **H42**
Nuclear sclerosis	**366**	Age-related cataract	**H25**
Nuclear cataract, nonsenile	**366**	Infantile and juvenile nuclear cataract	**H26**
Toxic cataract	**366**	Drug-induced cataract	**H26**
After-cataract	**366**	Other secondary cataract	**H26**

Chapter 8: Diseases of the Ear and Mastoid Process

ICD-9-CM Terminology	Category	ICD-10-CM Terminology	Category
Noise-induced hearing loss	**388**	Noise effects on (specify laterality) inner ear	**H83**
Unspecified sudden hearing loss	**388**	Sudden idiopathic hearing loss	**H91**
Tinnitus: Subjective Objective	**388**	Tinnitus (specify laterality)	**H93**
Conductive hearing loss: (unilateral/bilateral) External ear Tympanic membrane Middle ear Inner ear Combined	**389**	Conductive hearing loss: Bilateral Right Left with unrestricted hearing contralateral side	**H9Ø**
Sensorineural hearing loss: Unilateral Bilateral Asymmetrical	**389**	Sensorineural hearing loss: Bilateral Unilateral With unrestricted hearing contralateral side	**H9Ø**
Disorders of acoustic nerve	**388**	Disorders of acoustic nerve: (specify laterality) Right/left/bilateral/unspecified	**H93**

Chapter 9: Diseases of the Circulatory System

ICD-9-CM Terminology	Category	ICD-10-CM Terminology	Category
Subsequent (refers to episode of care)	**41Ø**	Subsequent (refers to consecutive AMIs)	**I22**
Postmyocardial infarction syndrome	**411**	Dressler's syndrome	**I24**
Intermediate coronary syndrome	**411**	Unstable angina	**I2Ø** **I25**
Other second degree AV block (Mobitz I)	**426**	AV block, second degree (both Mobitz I & II)	**I44**
Left bundle branch hemiblock	**426**	Left anterior fascicular block Left posterior fascicular block Other/unspecified fascicular block	**I44**
Right bundle branch block	**426**	Right fascicular block Other/unspecified right bundle branch block	**I45**
Right bundle branch block and (right) (left) (anterior) (posterior) fascicular block	**426**	Bifascicular block	**I45**

ICD-9-CM Terminology	Category	ICD-10-CM Terminology	Category
Lown-Ganong-Levine syndrome	**426**	Pre-excitation syndrome	**I45**
Paroxysmal supraventricular tachycardia	**427**	Supraventricular tachycardia Junctional premature depolarization	**I47** **I49**
Paroxysmal ventricular tachycardia	**427**	Re-entry ventricular arrhythmia Ventricular tachycardia	**I47**
Atrial flutter	**427**	Persistent/Atypical/Typical atrial flutter	**I48**
Supraventricular premature beats	**427**	Atrial premature depolarization	**I49**
Sinoatrial node dysfunction	**427**	Sick sinus syndrome	**I49**
Congestive heart failure, unspecified	**428**	Heart failure, unspecified	**I5Ø**
Left heart failure	**428**	Left ventricular failure	**I5Ø**
Secondary renovascular hypertension, unspecified	**4Ø5**	Secondary renovascular hypertension	**I15**
Acute myocardial infarction (site) (episode of care)	**41Ø**	STEMI involving (site) Non-ST elevation (NSTEMI) myocardial infarction	**I21**
Acute coronary occlusion without MI	**411**	Acute coronary thrombosis not resulting in MI	**I24**
Angina decubitus	**413**	Other forms of angina pectoris	**I2Ø**
Prinzmetal Angina	**413**	Angina pectoris with documented spasm	**I2Ø**
Coronary atherosclerosis of (native) (bypass) (transplant) vessel	**414**	Atherosclerotic heart disease of (native) (bypass) (transplant) with or w/o angina (type)	**I25**
Other specified forms of chronic ischemic heart disease	**414**	Ischemic cardiomyopathy Silent myocardial ischemia Chronic ischemic heart disease	**I25**
Acute cor pulmonale	**415**	[Combination codes with underlying etiology:] Septic pulmonary embolism with acute cor pulmonale Saddle embolus of pulmonary artery with acute cor pulmonale Other pulmonary embolism with acute cor pulmonale	**I26**
Iatrogenic embolism and infarction	**415**	[As complication of procedure:] Air embolism following infusion, transf..., init Complication of artery following a procedure Embolism of cardiac prosth device/graft Embolism of vascular prosth dev/graft [As complication of infection or specific iatrogenic cause (code also):] Pulmonary embolism	 **T8Ø** **T81** **T82** **T82** **I26**
Unspecified chronic pulmonary heart disease	**416**	Cor pulmonale (chronic)	**I27**
Idiopathic myocarditis	**422**	Isolated myocarditis	**I4Ø**
Septic myocarditis	**422**	Infective myocarditis	**I4Ø**

ICD-9-CM Terminology	Category	ICD-10-CM Terminology	Category
Other certain sequelae MI	**429**	[Diagnoses specify MI sequelae condition:] Hemopericardium as complication MI Rupture of cardiac wall as complication MI Thrombosis (site) as current complication MI	**I23**
Occlusion & stenosis (cerebral/precerebral artery) w/Infarction	**433**	Cerebral infarction due to (thrombosis, embolism, occlusion)	**I63**
Cerebral embolism (with/without infarction)	**434**	Cerebral infarction due to embolism (specify site) Occlusion and stenosis of (specify site)	**I63** **I66**
Other Ill/defined cerebrovascular disease	**437**	Cerebral amyloid angiopathy	**I68**
Postoperative hypertension	**997.91**	Postoperative hypertension	**I97.3**

Chapter 10: Diseases of the Respiratory System

ICD-9-CM Terminology	Category	ICD-10-CM Terminology	Category
Mechanical complication (e.g., tracheostomy stoma)	**519**	Malfunction (e.g., tracheostomy stoma)	**J95**
Chronic airway obstruction, NEC	**496**	Chronic obstructive pulmonary disease	**J44.9**
Other pulmonary insufficiency, NEC	**518**	Acute respiratory distress syndrome	**J8Ø**
Acute respiratory failure following trauma and surgery	**518**	Postprocedural respiratory failure	**J95**
Influenza with pneumonia	**487**	[Diagnoses specify influenza type (with pneumonia):] Flu due to identified influenza virus Flu due to other identified influenza virus Flue due to unidentified influenza virus	**J1Ø** **J11**
Avian Influenza virus (pneumonia, other resp infection)	**488**	Identified novel influenza A virus (with manifestation: pneumonia, other respiratory)	**JØ9**
Influenza due to 2009 H1N1 virus	**488**	Influenza due to identified novel influenza A virus	**JØ9**
Other emphysema	**498**	Unilateral pulmonary emphysema Panlobular emphysema Centrilobar emphysema	**J43**
Extrinsic asthma/ Intrinsic asthma	**493**	[Diagnoses specify severity:] Mild intermittent asthma Mild persistent asthma Moderate persistent asthma Severe persistent asthma	**J45**

ICD-9-CM Terminology	Category	ICD-10-CM Terminology	Category
Pulmonary collapse	**518**	Atelectasis Other pulmonary collapse	**J98**
Acute/chronic respiratory failure	**518**	[Acute or chronic RF with the following:] Respiratory failure with hypoxia Respiratory failure with hypercapnia Respiratory failure with hypoxia or hypercapnia	**J96**

Chapter 11: Diseases of the Digestive System

ICD-9-CM Terminology	Category	ICD-10-CM Terminology	Category
Pseudopolyposis	**556**	Inflammatory polyps [Combination diagnoses specify assoc. complications:] Inflammatory polyps with rectal bleeding Inflammatory polyps with intestinal obstruction Inflammatory polyps of colon with fistula Inflammatory polyps with abscess	**K51**
Ulcerative colitis	**556**	[Combination diagnoses specify assoc. complications:] Inflammatory polyps with rectal bleeding Inflammatory polyps with intestinal obstruction Inflammatory polyps of colon with fistula Inflammatory polyps with abscess	**K51**
Universal ulcerative colitis	**556**	Ulcerative pancolitis	**K51**
Abscess of anal and rectal regions	**566**	[Combination diagnoses specify underlying cause:] Crohn's disease with (site-specific) abscess [Diagnoses specify anatomic site:] Anal abscess Rectal abscess Ischiorectal abscess Intrasphincteric abscess	 **K5Ø** **K61**
Abscess of intestine	**569**	[Combination diagnoses specify underlying cause:] Crohn's disease with (site-specific) abscess Ulcerative colitis (site-specific) with abscess Diverticulitis (site-specific) with abscess	 **K5Ø** **K51** **K57**

ICD-9-CM Terminology	Category	ICD-10-CM Terminology	Category
Fistula of intestine	**569**	[Combination diagnoses specify underlying cause:] Crohn's disease with (site-specific) fistula Ulcerative colitis (site-specific) with fistula Inflammatory polyps with fistula	 **K5Ø** **K51** **K51**
Hemorrhoids	**455**	Hemorrhoids and perianal venous thrombosis	**K64**

Chapter 12: Diseases of the Skin and Subcutaneous Tissue

ICD-9-CM Terminology	Category	ICD-10-CM Terminology	Category
Cellulitis & abscess	**682**	[Diagnoses specify site/laterality:] Cutaneous abscess Cellulitis Acute lymphangitis	 **LØ2** **LØ3**
Pressure ulcer (site) (Use additional code to specify stage)	**7Ø7**	Pressure ulcer: [Diagnoses specify site/laterality/stage] Example: Pressure ulcer of left hip stage 2	**L89** **L89.222**
Chronic ulcer of other specified site	**7Ø7**	Non-pressure ulcer of (site): [Diagnoses specify severity:] Limited to breakdown of skin With fat layer exposed With necrosis of muscle With necrosis of bone With unspecified severity	**L98**

Debridement (Excisional)

ICD-9-CM Terminology	Category	ICD-10-PCS Terminology	Category
Debridement, excisional (skin or subcutaneous tissue)	**86**	Excision (skin) (subcutaneous tissue and fascia)	**ØHB, ØJB**

Chapter 13: Diseases of the Musculoskeletal System and Connective Tissue

ICD-9-CM Terminology	Category	ICD-10-CM Terminology	Category
Spondylosis (site): w/ or w/o myelopathy	**721**	Spondylosis (type) (site): w/ radiculopathy w/o myelopathy	**M46–M48**
Cervical spondylosis with myelopathy	**721**	Anterior spinal artery compression syndromes Vertebral artery compression syndromes	**M47**
Spinal stenosis (site)	**723**	Spinal stenosis (site) [Diagnoses specify causal pathology:] Subluxation stenosis Osseous stenosis Connective tissue stenosis Intervertebral disc stenosis	**M48**
Partial tear of rotator cuff	**726**	Incomplete rotator cuff tear/rupture of shoulder, nontraumatic (specify laterality)	**M75**
Other affections of shoulder region NEC	**726**	(of shoulder): Osteophyte Calcific tendonitis Impingement syndrome Other/unspecified shoulder lesion	 **M25** **M75** **M75** **M75**
Enthesopathy (of site)	**726**	[Diagnosis specify pathology according to site:] Example (hip) Gluteal tendonitis Ilial crest spur Iliotibial band syndrome	 **M76** **M76** **M76**
Acute osteomyelitis (specify site)	**730**	Acute osteomyelitis (of site): [Specify as:] Acute hematogenous osteomyelitis Subacute osteomyelitis Other acute osteomyelitis	**M86**
Chronic osteomyelitis (specify site)	**730**	Chronic osteomyelitis (of site): [Specify assoc complication:] Chronic multifocal osteomyelitis Chronic osteomyelitis with draining sinus Other chronic hematogenous Other chronic osteomyelitis	**M86**
Senile osteoporosis	**733**	Age-related osteoporosis w/o current pathological fracture	**M81**
Osteoporosis: Idiopathic Disuse	**733**	Other osteoporosis without current pathological fracture	**M81**

ICD-9-CM Terminology	Category	ICD-10-CM Terminology	Category
Pathological fracture (specify site)	**733**	[Diagnoses specify anatomic site and underlying disease if applicable:] Age-related osteoporosis with current pathological fracture Other osteoporosis w/current pathological fracture Pathological fracture in neoplastic disease Pathological fracture in other disease	 **M8Ø** **M8Ø** **M84** **M84**
Stress fracture (specify site)	**733**	Stress fracture (of site) Fatigue fracture (of vertebra; specify site)	**M84** **M48**
Scoliosis, idiopathic	**737**	Idiopathic scoliosis (as): Juvenile (site) Adolescent (site) Other (site)	**M41**
Infantile scoliosis: Resolving Infantile	**737**	Infantile idiopathic scoliosis (specify spinal site)	**M41**

Chapter 14: Diseases of the Genitourinary System

ICD-9-CM Terminology	Category	ICD-10-CM Terminology	Category
Acute kidney failure with lesion: (specify as) Tubular necrosis Renal cortical necrosis Medullary necrosis	**584**	Acute kidney failure (specify as with): Tubular necrosis Renal cortical necrosis Medullary necrosis	**N17**
Acute pyelonephritis w/ or w/o lesion of medullary necrosis	**59Ø**	Acute tubulo-interstitial nephritis	**N1Ø**
Chronic pyelonephritis w/ or w/o lesion of medullary necrosis	**59Ø**	Nonobstructive reflux-associated chronic pyelonephritis Chronic obstructive pyelonephritis Other chronic tubulo-interstitial nephritis	**N11**
Unspecified pyelonephritis	**59Ø**	Chronic tubulo-interstitial nephritis, unspecified Tubulo-interstitial nephritis, not spec as acute or chronic Pyelonephritis	**N11** **N12** **N13**
Hematuria: Benign Essential Idiopathic	**599**	Hematuria: Persistent/recurrent *see* Hematuria, idiopathic w/ glomerular lesion (specify)	 **NØ2** **NØ2**
Hypertrophy of prostate	**6ØØ**	Enlarged prostate	**N4Ø**

ICD-9-CM Terminology	Category	ICD-10-CM Terminology	Category
Impotence of organic origin	**6Ø7**	[Diagnoses classify underlying pathology or cause:] Examples: Erectile dysfunction due to arterial insufficiency Drug-induced erectile dysfunction Erectile dysfunction (following specific surgery)	**N52**

Chapter 15: Pregnancy, Childbirth, and the Puerperium

Hypertension Complicating Pregnancy, Childbirth, and the Puerperium

ICD-9-CM Terminology	Category	ICD-10-CM Terminology	Category
Hypertension complicating pregnancy, childbirth, or the puerperium	**642**	Hypertension complicating, childbirth, pregnancy, and the puerperium	**O1Ø, O11, O13, O16**

Chapter 16: Certain Conditions Originating in the Perinatal Period

Respiratory Distress of Newborn

ICD-9-CM Terminology	Category	ICD-10-CM Terminology	Category
Respiratory distress syndrome in newborn	**769**	Respiratory distress syndrome of newborn	**P22**
Cardiorespiratory distress syndrome of newborn	**769**	Cardiorespiratory distress syndrome of newborn	**P22**
Hyaline membrane disease (pulmonary)	**769**	Hyaline membrane disease	**P22**
Idiopathic respiratory distress syndrome [IRDS or RDS] of newborn	**769**	Idiopathic respiratory distress syndrome [IRDS or RDS] of newborn	**P22**
Pulmonary hypoperfusion syndrome	**769**	Pulmonary hypoperfusion syndrome	**P22**
Type I respiratory distress of the newborn	**769**	Respiratory distress syndrome, type I	**P22**
Transitory tachypnea of newborn	**77Ø**	Transient tachypnea of newborn	**P22**
Idiopathic tachypnea of newborn	**77Ø**	Idiopathic tachypnea of newborn	**P22**
Wet lung syndrome	**77Ø**	Wet lung syndrome	**P22**

ICD-9-CM Terminology	Category	ICD-10-CM Terminology	Category
Type II respiratory distress of the newborn	**770**	Respiratory distress syndrome, type II	**P22**
Other respiratory problems after birth	**770**	Other respiratory distress of newborn	**P22**
Other respiratory problems after birth	**770**	Respiratory distress of newborn, unspecified	**P22**

Chapter 17: Congenital Malformations, Deformation, and Chromosomal Abnormalities

ICD-9-CM Terminology	Category	ICD-10-CM Terminology	Category
Other congenital anomalies of the circulatory system	**747**	Congenital malformation of great arteries	**Q25**

Chapter 18: Symptoms, Signs and Abnormal Clinical and Laboratory Findings, Not Elsewhere Classified

ICD-9-CM Terminology	Category	ICD-10-CM Terminology	Category
Respiratory arrest	**799**	Respiratory arrest	**R09**
Coma	**780**	Coma, unspecified [Individual and total coma scores √ 6th & add required 7th character]: Coma scale, eyes open Coma scale, best verbal response Coma scale best motor response Glasgow coma scale, total score	**R40**
Altered mental status	**780**	Disorientation, unspecified Altered mental status, unspecified	**R41**
Amnesia Memory loss	**790**	Anterograde amnesia Retrograde amnesia Other amnesia	**R41**
Senility without mention of psychosis	**797**	Age-related cognitive decline	**R41**

Chapter 19: Injury, Poisoning and Certain Other Consequences of External Causes

ICD-9-CM Terminology	Category	ICD-10-CM Terminology	Category
Injury: Type of injury: [Fracture, open wound] Injury subclassification: [Open, closed, complicated] Anatomic site [Skull, vertebrae] Site subclassification [Frontal bone, cervical vertebrae] Associated injury: [Intracranial injury][Spinal cord injury]		Injury: Anatomic site of injury [Head, neck, thorax, abdomen] Site subclassification: [Scalp, eyelid, cervical esophagus] Type of injury: [Superficial, open wound, fracture, internal injury] Injury subclassification: [Open, closed, partial, complete] Seventh characters report nature of encounter: [Initial treatment, subsequent tx, sequelae]	
Closed fracture of shaft of femur	**82Ø**	Fracture of femur: [Diagnoses specify site, type of fracture, laterality, nature of encounter, complications] Example: *Nondisplaced* spiral fracture of shaft of right femur, displaced, initial encounter for *closed* fracture	**S72**
Open fracture subtrochanteric section femur	**82Ø**	Fracture of femur: [Diagnoses specify site, type of fracture, laterality, nature of encounter, complications] Example: *Displaced* subtrochanteric fracture right femur, initial encounter for *open* fracture type 1 or 2	**S72**
Poisoning, overdose: Drug or substance classification [Anticoagulant, anti-infective] Substance subclassification [Coumadin, sulfonamides] (Use additional external cause code to report intent] Example: Coumadin overdose, accidental	**964** **E858**	Poisoning, overdose, underdosing: Drug or substance classification [Systemic hematologic, systemic antibiotics] Substance subclassification [Anticoagulant, anti-infective] Drug subclassification: [Coumadin, sulfonamides] Nature of poisoning/intent: [Unintentional, intentional self-harm, underdosing] Example: Coumadin overdose, accidental	**T45**
Adverse effect of drug: Nature of adverse effect Substance/intent Example: Petechiae due to Adverse effects of Coumadin therapy	**782** **E934**	Adverse effect of drug: Nature of adverse effect Substance/intent Example: Petechiae due to Adverse effects of Coumadin therapy	**R23** **T45**
Complications of surgical and medical care, not elsewhere classified	**996–999**	Complications of surgical and medical care, not elsewhere classified	**T8Ø–T88**

ICD-9-CM Terminology	Category	ICD-10-CM Terminology	Category
Complications of surgical and medical care, not elsewhere classified	**996–999**	Certain intraoperative and postprocedural complications and disorders of (body system), not elsewhere classified: Examples: Endocrine system Nervous system Eye and adnexa Ear and mastoid	**[Included in body system chapter]** **E89** **G97** **H59** **H95**
Mechanical complication CABG	**996**	Breakdown (mechanical) of coronary artery bypass graft, initial Displacement of CABG, initial Leakage of CABG, initial Mechanical complication of CABG, initial	**T82**

Chapter 20: External Causes of Morbidity

ICD-9-CM Terminology	Category	ICD-10-CM Terminology	Category
Unspecified procedure as the cause of abnormal reaction of patient, or of later complication, without mention of misadventure at time of procedure	**E879.8**	Prosthetic and other implants, materials and accessory cardiovascular devices associated with adverse incidents	**Y71**

Chapter 21: Factors Influencing Health Status and Contact with Health Services

ICD-9-CM Terminology	Category	ICD-10-CM Terminology	Category
Routine general medical examination at health care facility	**V7Ø**	Encounter for general adult medical examination	**ZØØ**